TICS AND RELATED DISORDERS

CLINICAL NEUROLOGY AND NEUROSURGERY MONOGRAPHS
Volume 7

Titles already published

Benson: *Aphasia, Alexia and Agraphia*
Fenichel: *Neonatal Neurology*
Halliday: *Evoked Potentials in Clinical Testing*
Rudge: *Clinical Neuro-otology*
Oosterhuis: *Myasthenia Gravis*
Harding: *The Hereditary Ataxias and Related Disorders*

TICS AND RELATED DISORDERS

A. J. Lees MD, MRCP
Consultant Neurologist, National Hospitals for Nervous Diseases, University College Hospital and Whittington Hospital, London, UK

Foreword by
MACDONALD CRITCHLEY CBE, MD, MBChB, FRCP

CHURCHILL LIVINGSTONE
EDINBURGH LONDON MELBOURNE AND NEW YORK 1985

CHURCHILL LIVINGSTONE
Medical Division of Longman Group Limited

Distributed in the United States of America by Churchill Livingstone Inc., 1560 Broadway, New York, N.Y. 10036, and by associated companies, branches and representatives throughout the world.

First published 1985

ISBN 0 443 02677 7

British Library Cataloguing in Publication Data

Lees, A. J.
  Tics and related disorders. — (Clinical neurology
  and neurosurgery monographs; v. 7)
  1. Tic
  I. Title   II. Series
  616.8'49   RC552.T5

Printed and bound by
Clark Constable, Edinburgh, London, Melbourne

Foreword

Early in my neurological apprenticeship I chanced upon a copy of the treatise on *Tics* by Meige and Feindel. I read and re-read the volume and my interest was all the greater because it had been translated into English by one of my chiefs. These miscellaneous movement-disorders have continued to intrigue me.

From my student days and from my residency at Great Ormond Street I was, of course, all too familiar with the diverse habit-spasms of the nervous child. But this was only the tip of an iceberg. I now became increasingly aware of the manifold mannerisms that most of my seniors seemed to show, ranging from a slow and solemn closure of one eye to a veritable saraband of sniffs, snorts and grimacing. A visiting professor of great eminence startled us all by his Jack-in-the-box display. No one among my elders seemed to be immune — academics, actors, barristers, politicians, clerics — and a subtle correlation with showmanship could be detected. Medical students were quick to seize upon the quirks, oddities and twists of their teachers and to utilize them mercilessly during the Christmas theatricals.

Then there were those instances of spasmodic torticollis that baffled us so often and so much. Did they represent symbolic gestures of aversion and abhorrence, psychologically determined? Many psychiatric colleagues were of that opinion, but none would ever embark upon their treatment. Could it be that torticollis was organic in nature and perhaps capable of alleviation by such mechanical measures as sectioning of either the muscles involved or their nerve-supply? A growing minority shared this suspicion but could not suggest any pathology other than 'deep-seated mischief'; that is, until the advent of epidemic encephalitis lethargica. The sequelae of that disorder were grave and protean, and many were in the nature of tics including torticollis. As to their intractability, James Collier used to proclaim that all muscle-attachments in the neck might be destroyed and every cervical nerve-root be severed, but the jerkings would continue, presumably through the musculature of the oesophagus.

In my experience, the only surgeon to have had any hint of success with torticollic sufferers has been Irving Cooper with his repeated and punctilious stereotactic approaches.

Craft palsies were another allied problem that worried us in those days. Their aetiology was obscure and their management perplexing. Here again the whole subject was fraught with debates as to psychogenesis versus organicity.

Nowadays, and in some regions, it seems to be the practice to assemble all these clinical bits and pieces as though they were components of a neurological jigsaw, to be spoken of as the Tourette syndrome. Is this line of thinking justified?

Dr Lees has had the courage to grasp the nettle. He has embarked upon the exciting but hazardous task of studying in depth each representative of non-volitional movement and to discuss whether a common denominator exists, permeating the clinical aberrations: a formidable, but rewarding, assignment.

Here then is a monograph of distinction which takes up the story where the pens of Meige and of Feindel were laid down. Dr Lees has given us a survey of contemporary ideas in the context of *Bewegungserkentniss*. The contributions of science — chemical, pharmacological, electrophysiological — have added much to our stockpile of information about these enigmatical disorders. Whether a corresponding advance in our understanding of their fundamental nature has resulted is another thing.

Throughout his writing, Dr Lees has been scrupulous in defining each particular movement-disorder before proceeding to a most detailed clinical description.

May I wish this volume not only an appreciative reception, but even acclaim? Its future, I am confident, is assured.

1985   M.C.

Preface

Kinnier Wilson's translation of Meige and Feindel's monograph *Les Tics et leur Traitement* in 1907 proved to have a profound and lasting influence on the Anglo-Saxon concept of tic. In his subsequent lectures and writings Wilson reaffirmed the French School's view that tics were volitional cortical events occurring in emotionally immature and neurotic individuals. The growth of psychoanalytical theory in the early part of this century strengthened this view and, as a consequence, a whole score of fanciful theories based on case studies appeared in the literature. This alienated many psychiatrists and neurologists, and tics were discounted as unworthy of serious attention, being explained away to patients and their relatives as 'bad habits'.

The pioneering work of the Shapiros in New York in the 1960s and the resounding success of the American Tourette Association have drawn the medical profession's attention to the plight of patients with Gilles de la Tourette syndrome and have stimulated a resurgence of interest in tic disorders in the United States emulating that which occurred in Paris at the turn of the century. A new generation of neuropsychiatrists has adopted tic as its *cause célèbre*, perceiving it as the ideal paradigm for studying the interrelationship between emotions and motor behaviour. The occurrence of iatrogenic dyskinesias and tics occurring in association with structural neurological diseases has also stimulated the interest of neurologists.

The rapidly expanding literature is now widely dispersed within psychiatric, psychoanalytical and neurological journals and although there are two comprehensive multi-author textbooks devoted solely to Gilles de la Tourette syndrome, no up-to-date reference work covers the whole subject of tics and the other heterogeneous complex movements with which they are so frequently confused. In this book, I have attempted to draw together the most important strands of what remains a largely phenomenological literature in the hope of providing a modern successor to Meige and Feindel's monograph. My approach has been eclectic as befits a topic with so few established facts and I have attempted to integrate my own work on the subject impartially into the text.

I have encompassed most of the abnormal movements which currently possess no distinctive neurochemical or histological pathology. The abnormal movements seen in the psychotic, mentally retarded and the blind are covered as they are so frequently misdiagnosed as tics, and the adult onset focal dystonias and hyperekplexias are included on historical grounds. I have arbitrarily excluded the myoclonic syndromes, generalised idiopathic torsion dystonia, paroxysmal dyskinesias, neuroleptic-induced rabbit syndrome, hereditary chin quivering and hemifacial spasm. Although drug-induced tics are rare, I have reviewed them in some detail and also covered the constellation of other iatrogenic abnormal involuntary movements. A greater understanding of these unwanted side-effects may well provide further insight into the pathogenesis of spontaneously occurring dyskinesias and tic.

Meige and Feindel hoped that their book would allot to the word tic a definite position in medical terminology. My own aspirations are equally modest and if, as a result of this book, progress can be made in the precise classification and definition of these bewildering disorders I will rest content. However, I also hope that the book may serve as a primer and reference source for those who might be tempted to work on this neglected and challenging group of movement disorders.

1985   A.J.L.

Acknowledgements

I am grateful to Mrs Joan Wolfe, President of the Gilles de la Tourette Syndrome Association of the United Kingdom, and to my collaborators Dr Mary Robertson and Dr Michael Trimble without whose help the data for the United Kingdom study on Gilles de la Tourette syndrome could not have been obtained. Dr Gerald Stern, my colleague and mentor at University College Hospital, has provided inspiration and well-timed nudges of encouragement. Dr Lieh Mak of Hong Kong and Dr Nomura of Japan were good enough to amplify their published studies for inclusion and Dr John Rothwell generously supplied the neurophysiological material depicted in Figures 1.1 to 1.3. I am especially indebted to Miss Elaine Edwards for painstakingly typing endless false starts and final drafts and to my father for proof-reading. The emotional support and forbearance provided by Juana my wife, and George and Nathalie my children, have been crucial in seeing the book through to completion.

Contents

1

Definition and Classification of Tic Disorders

The implausible nature of many of the abnormal movement disorders, their intimate connection with emotional upset, and the dearth of associated structural pathology have hampered rational classification. Semantic controversies persist despite a spate of well-meaning workshops and the recent publication by the Research Group on Extrapyramidal Disorders of an internationally agreed nomenclature (Lakke, 1981). In some respects understanding has advanced little since Charcot, exactly one hundred years ago, expressed the inherent difficulties as follows:

> Epilepsy, chorea, hysteria . . . come to us like so many sphinxes . . . symptomatic combinations deprived of anatomical substratum do not present themselves to the mind of the physician with that appearance of solidity, of objectivity, of affections connected with an appreciable organic lesion.
>
> There are even some who see in some of these affections only an assemblage of odd incoherent phenomena inaccessible to analysis, and which had better perhaps be banished to the category of the unknown.

Early 19th-century attempts at devising a working terminology depended on careful bedside observations and led to a steady proliferation of colourful eponyms such as Dubini's electric chorea, paramyoclonus multiplex of Friedreich and the variable chorea of Brissaud. Very few of these have stood the test of time as distinct nosological entities and most remain now only as monuments to the shortcomings of written descriptions in the field of abnormal movement disorders. Predictably this era of over-enthusiastic 'splitting' was followed by a sceptical volte-face in which all rapid involuntary jerks were lumped once more under a single rubric; this time myoclonus instead of chorea.

The last 20 years have witnessed modest progress in certain areas. Detection of specific enzyme defects, the discovery of physiological and neurotransmitter abnormalities and a greater understanding of underlying modes of inheritance have led to improved classifications of the choreas, dystonias and myoclonic syndromes. The capture of ephemeral dyskinesias on video-film and the greater use of audio-visual aids at medical meetings have also helped to iron out some of the prevailing dialectical arguments.

Tics, on the other hand, remain as *terra incognita*, sitting uneasily within the uncharted borderlands of neurology and psychiatry, the term being often

Table 1.1. CLASSIFICATION OF TICS AND RELATED CONDITIONS

I Idiopathic tics
    (a) Acute transient
    (b) Persistent simple or multiple
    (c) Chronic simple or multiple

II Gilles de la Tourette syndrome

III Tics occurring in association with structural brain damage
    (a) Post-encephalitic
    (b) Carbon monoxide poisoning
    (c) Head injury
    (d) Post-stroke
    (e) Post-rheumatic chorea

IV Drug-induced
    (a) Psychomotor stimulants
    (b) L-dopa
    (c) Neuroleptics

Related disorders
1. The hyperekplexias
2. Habitual manipulations of the body
3. Stereotypies
4. Mannerisms
5. Hyperkinetic syndrome
6. Adult onset focal dystonias
7. Clonic spasms

---

employed as a receptacle for all miscellaneous dyskinesias. They remain no more than a phenomenological concept and any attempt at tentative categorisation must insist on rigid definition and unvarying terminology. The system used in this book (see Table 1.1) aims to avoid questionable distinctions between functional and organic tics. However, its subdivisions are arbitrary and inevitably artificial. Gilles de la Tourette syndrome, for example, is distinguished merely by virtue of its severity. The tonic tics of Meige and Feindel are reclassified in the light of current thinking as focal dystonias, and tic douloureux and hemifacial spasm are considered as clonic spasms. Habitual manipulations of the body, such as thumb sucking and nail biting, are delineated from tics as are the legion of mannerisms and stereotypies so commonly encountered in mental asylums.

Definitions *A tic* is an abrupt, jerky, repetitive movement which involves discrete muscle groups. It mimics a normal co-ordinated movement, varies in intensity and lacks rhythmicity. It may be temporarily suppressed by will power and is relatively easy to imitate. It consists of a brief contraction of the prime

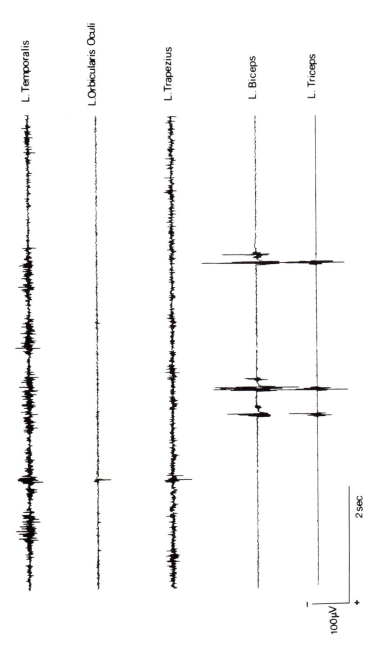

Figure 1.1 *Surface electromyographic record of a 22-year-old man with simple tics in the left arm. (By kind permission of Dr John Rothwell.)*

mover or simultaneous co-activation of agonist and antagonist lasting 50–500 ms (Fig. 1.1).

A *mannerism* is a bizarre mode of carrying out a purposeful act which usually occurs as a result of the incorporation of a stereotyped action into goal-directed behaviour.

A *gesture* is a culturally determined expressive movement calculated to indicate a particular state of mind and which may also be used as a means of adding emphasis to oratory.

Habitual manipulations of the body. These are self-gratifying socially offensive co-ordinated movements which occur particularly at times of anxiety, boredom, tiredness or self-consciousness.

Stereotypies are purposeless voluntary movements carried out in a uniform repetitive fashion often for long periods of time and at the expense of all other activities. In contradistinction to tics, whole areas of the body are involved.

Hyperactivity syndrome is characterised by an abnormal degree of aimless motor restlessness sufficiently severe to disturb attention and concentration and impede the ability to perform structured tasks.

Hyperekplexia is a pathologically exaggerated startle reflex.

Clonic spasms are rapid involuntary movements which follow strict anatomical localisation and can be accurately imitated only by electrical stimulation of the nerve supplying the affected muscle group. These movements may occur during sleep.

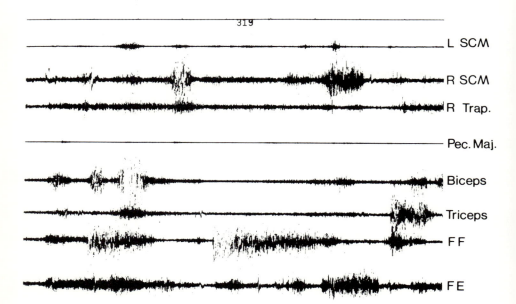

Figure 1.2 *Surface electromyographic record of an 8-year-old boy with benign hereditary chorea showing the random pattern of muscle activity. Time marker 1 s. (By kind permission of Dr John Rothwell.)*

Chorea is a forcible, rapid, irregular, involuntary and unpatterned jerk which is never integrated into a co-ordinated act but may match it in complexity. It is fleeting, unpredictable and presents a comical, playful appearance. It also tends to be aggravated by voluntary movement. Electrophysiologically it is characterised by its unpredictability. The burst of muscle activity may be brief, sustained or interrupted lasting 200 ms–1 s or more (Fig. 1.2).

Myoclonus is an irregular or rhythmical muscle jerk which originates in the central nervous system. The muscle contraction is brief resembling electric shocks and cannot be controlled by will power. The burst of muscle activity closely resembles that seen in tics.

Dystonia is a sustained involuntary torsion which may affect muscle groups of all sizes. The movements are usually slow and may be present continually or only appear during specific motor acts. When severe a relatively fixed abnormal posture may occur and secondary contractures develop. Co-contraction of agonist and antagonist occurs with a long duration of muscle activity lasting 1 s or more (Fig. 1.3). Dystonic spasm is a term applied to more rapid, repetitive, tic-like movements which lack the flowing character of chorea.

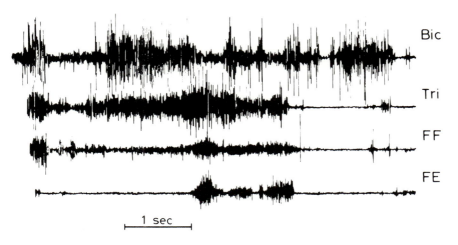

Figure 1.3. Surface electromyographic record of a 40-year-old man with dystonia of the right arm showing long co-contracting bursts of muscle activity in antagonist muscles. (By kind permission of Dr John Rothwell.)

2

Idiopathic Tic

Synonyms Habit spasm, habit chorea, variable chorea, pseudo-chorea.

Definition *A tic* is an abrupt, jerky repetitive movement which involves discrete muscle groups. It mimics a normal co-ordinated movement, varies in intensity and lacks rhythmicity. It may be temporarily suppressed by will power and because of its patterned appearance is relatively easy to imitate.

Sub-varieties *Acute transient tic* appears in childhood, usually involves a single muscle group and remits spontaneously within a year.

Persistent simple or multiple tic is one or more tics occurring in childhood which persist for several years before disappearing in adolescence or early adult life.

Chronic simple or multiple tic is one or occasionally more tics which persist throughout life and vary little in frequency or intensity.

Descriptions of tic probably go back as far as Hippocrates, although there is little justification in regarding the rictus caninus and tortura oris of the ancients as tics. Thomas Willis observed:

> . . . that in the cases of children who have not yet become accustomed to affections of the heart and torments of the external parts, spasmodic matter very often flows into the closest nerves, those of the third, fifth and sixth pairs. As a result, the area of the face and mouth is particularly distorted in these cases.

The word *ticque* was in current use in France as early as the 17th century to describe the behavioural vices of horses and in 18th century literature it was used in the sense of a 'recurrent distasteful act' particularly common in eccentric individuals. The derivation of the word is probably onomatopoeic, communicating the idea of sudden repetition as in tick-tack. *Tucken, ticken* and *tick* in German, *ticque* in French, tug or tick in English, *ticchio* in Italian and *tico* in Spanish are all probably derived from the same etymological root. André was the first to allude to tic douloureux of the face in 1756 but until the end of the 19th century dyskinesias were generally referred to as motor incoordinations and diagnosed as chorea. The first major medical work was that of

Bouteille (1810) who, in his *Traité de chorée*, distinguished a group of move-ment disorders he termed pseudo-chorea and which he defined as follows:

> I use the name pseudo-chorea or false chorea to distinguish those different, nervous, spasmodic, convulsive or hysterical afflictions which fail to show the characteristic features of true chorea, the only resemblance between them and chorea being facial grimacing and involuntary movements.

Sir Charles Bell used the term spasmodic twitching to describe tics in 1830, and in 1852 Marshall Hall clearly described the clonic nature of muscular tics giving examples such as violent frowning, facial distortion and shaking of the head. Trousseau (1873), however, provided the first clear description of tics although at that time he considered them a sort of incomplete chorea related to the occupational neuroses:

> Non-dolorous tic consists of abrupt momentary muscular contractions more or less limited as a general rule, involving preferably the face, but affecting also neck, trunk and limbs. Their exhibition is a matter of everyday experience. In one case it may be a blinking of the eyelids, a spasmodic twitch of cheek, nose or lip; in another it is a toss of the head, a sudden transient, yet ever recurring contortion of the neck, in a third it is a shrug of the shoulder, a convulsive movement of diaphragm or abdominal muscles — in fact the term embodies an infinite variety of bizarre actions that defy analysis.
>
> These tics are not infrequently associated with a highly characteristic cry or ejaculation — a sort of laryngeal or diaphragmatic chorea which may of itself constitute the condition; or there may be a more elaborate symptom in the form of a curious impulse to repeat the same word or the same exclamation. Sometimes the patient is driven to utter aloud what he would fain conceal.

Friedreich (1881) regarded tics as remembrance spasms suggesting that at the time of an intense fright in childhood the ticqueur had reacted with a series of muscle movements and that when external events replicated this experience spontaneous reproduction of the original movement occurred, and sustained excitability finally led to the occurrence of co-ordinated spasms without an external stimulus. Charcot was the first to appreciate that impulsive involuntary ideas or psychical tics commonly occurred together with bodily tics. Railton (1886) considered that occasional discharges from irritable nerve cells near the motor and speech areas in the cerebral cortex might underlie tics and Hammond (1892) developed this idea, postulating an irritative lesion of the motor cortex and subcortical structures as the cause of tics. Despite these early attempts to implicate a structural cause for tics the prevailing view was that they were psychologically determined and difficult to distinguish from hysterical convulsions. The monograph by Meige and Feindel published in 1902 consoli-dated the view that tics were a psychiatric illness. Their definition of tic runs as follows:

> A coordinated purposive act, provoked in the first instance by some external cause or by an idea; repetition leads to it becoming habitual, and finally to its involuntary reproduction without cause and for no purpose; at the same time as its form, inten-sity and frequency are exaggerated; it thus assumes the characters of a convulsive

movement, inopportune and excessive; its execution is often preceded by an irresistible impulse, its suppression associated with malaise. The effect of distraction or of volitional effort is to diminish its activity; in sleep it disappears. It occurs in predisposed individuals who usually show other indications of mental instability

The psychological nature of tics was subscribed to by eminent neurologists such as Brain and Kinnier Wilson and was taken a stage further by Ferenczi (1921) who attempted to determine the underlying psychical traumas by psycho-analysis. Influenced by Freudian concepts he believed that masturbatory conflicts were at the root of tic production whereas others subsequently blamed narcissism or sublimated aggression. A wide range of incompatible doctrinaire theories appeared over the next 40 years, most extrapolated from observations on single patients.

In the last 20 years greater attention has been paid to the epidemiology of tics and there has been a swing towards a more eclectic view on their nature and how they should best be managed. The recent revelation that dopamine may modulate mood and behaviour in subcortical structures has provided further fuel for those who have always believed tics to be organically determined, and has led to the hypothesis that tics might result from a dopaminergic preponderance in an as yet undetermined region of the brain.

EPIDEMIOLOGY

Tics are primarily a disorder of childhood, the majority appearing between the ages of 6 and 8 years. They are common, occurring in at least one in 20 children but are a relatively rare reason for psychiatric referral (Zausmer, 1954; Debray-Ritzen and Dubois, 1980). Chronic simple tics may develop for the first time in adult life although an antecedent history of acute transient tics is often unearthed.

The first epidemiological survey was conducted by Boncour (1910) on 1759 French children aged between 2 and 13 years. An overall prevalence of 24% was found with an unexplained peak frequency in the 54 12-year-old boys of 50%. Tics occurred approximately equally in boys and girls and rudimentary tic-like movements were noted in children below the age of 6 years. Contrary to the accepted view at the time, Boncour found no appreciable difference between ticqueurs and normal children in scholastic achievements or conduct. Unfortunately, this study is marred by the failure of the author to define his diagnostic criteria and there is no information as to whether the tics were transient or persistent.

In the National Child Development Study, examination of 7970 healthy 7-year-olds revealed tics in 4% with an equal sex incidence (Kellmer Pringle et al, 1967). An overall frequency of 4% was also found in a large American study with a peak incidence of 10% in 6- and 7-year-olds (MacFarlane et al, 1954). 12% of a randomly selected group of 482 children living in Buffalo, aged between 6 and 12 years, were found to have tics. Again an equal sex incidence occurred and a slightly higher frequency of 18% was found in the 63 black children (Lapouse and Monk, 1964).

Several other studies, however, have reported a marked male preponderance. Mahler et al (1945) noted a ratio of 3.5 boys to 1 female in 33 children referred for psychiatric treatment and Zausmer (1954) reported a 2:1 male preponderance in 96 children seen in a child psychiatry department. In two recent French studies even higher male: female ratios of 3:1 and 4.5:1 were observed (Dugas et al, 1975; Debray-Ritzen and Dubois, 1980) and an excess of male sufferers has also been reported in the German literature (Boenheim, 1930; Albrecht, 1949).

Abe and Oda (1980) carried out a five year follow-up study of children whose parents had been ticqueurs and found that 20% in the index group compared with 10% in the controls developed tics, a statistically significant difference. No evidence for a higher incidence of psychoneurosis in the index group was found and it was concluded that genetic factors were important in the pathogenesis of tic.

The most careful recent epidemiological investigations are those by Torup in Denmark, Corbett and his colleagues in London, and Debray-Ritzen and Dubois in France. Torup (1962) assessed the disabilities and course of 237 ticqueurs treated in the Paediatric and Child Psychiatry Departments, in a large hospital in Copenhagen, between 1946 and 1957. A male preponderance of 3:1 was found and 80–95% of the children had developed tics by their 10th birthday, the peak incidence occurring between 5 and 8 years. A disproportionately large number were referred between 1947 and 1948 which the author attributes to the insecurity engendered by the Second World War. Serious domestic conflicts and poor home conditions were the commonest identifiable precipitating cause but in at least one-third of cases no obvious explanation could be found. 30–40% of immediate family members had suffered from, or were still experiencing, tics. As a generalisation the children tended to be oversensitive (78%), restless (49%), lack confidence (37%) be anxious (27%) and exhibit obsessional traits (27%).

In their retrospective follow-up study on patients who had attended the Children's and Adolescent Department of the Maudsley Psychiatric Hospital and the Brixton Child Guidance Clinic between 1948 and 1965, Corbett et al (1969) identified 180 children with tics and subsequently conducted careful follow-up interviews and home visits. In the 122 instances where it was accurately recorded, the mean age of onset of tics was found to be 7.3 years (s.d. 2.8 years) and the mean age at first attendance was 10.2 years (s.d. 2.9 years). There was a male: female ratio of 3.6:1 and a family history of tics in 10%. Tics of the eyes, nose and face were commonest but isolated vocal tics were found in 11.6%. No difference was found between the mean intelligence quotients of the patients and age-matched controls, although the ticqueurs were superior on motor speed tests. Virtually all the children with tics had symptoms of emotional disturbance but comparison of neurotic traits with those occurring in a group of age-matched disturbed non-psychotic children revealed that only obsessional traits (12.5% compared with 7.5%) and to a lesser degree speech disorders, encopresis and hypochondriasis occurred more frequently. 30% of both groups had sleep disorders, tension habits, tempers and aggression, disturbed relationships with parents, peers and school, were rebellious and manifested symptoms of anxiety. 31% of the ticqueurs had one or both parents who had suffered a psychiatric illness compared with 19.3% in the general Maudsley Hospital population and only 6.2% from a dental clinic.

Debray-Ritzen and Dubois (1980) examined 4258 children attending 15 schools in the Paris suburbs and found a prevalence of tics as low as 8.7 per 1000. The mean age at onset was 7 years 11 months and 90% had developed them before the age of 12. In the large majority of their 93 cases with tics, no precipitating cause could be found. In one-third of the children motor instability was evident, 17% had reading difficulties and 7% stammered. A high incidence of insomnia, enuresis and other neurotic traits was also reported. Soft neurological abnormalities with features suggestive of the hyperactivity syndrome were present in about one-fifth but the mean intelligence quotient did not differ from that found in age-matched controls.

A high incidence of associated stammering has also been reported by Dugas et al (1975) who found an incidence of 16% in 98 ticqueurs compared with 4% in age-matched controls. They also observed a tendency to immaturity and ambivalence in some patients and obsessional traits in others. The percentage of sinistrals and the mean IQ did not differ significantly from the figures found in the general population.

ANIMAL DATA

Behavioural motor disorders in domesticated and zoo animals have been recognised for centuries. Rudler and Chomel, almost a century ago, drew analogies between the stereotyped licking and masticatory spasms of bad-tempered horses and human tics. They suggested that these motor disorders in the horse were initiated by gluttony, dental problems and trauma to the mouth, and then became automatic and stereotyped (Rudler and Chomel; 1903, 1904).

Glossal tics and torticollis-like spasms occur in cattle and jumping attacks may be seen in captive antelopes. Behavioural vices of this sort also occur in farmyard animals and include tail biting in pigs, wool biting in sheep, crib biting in horses and licking disease in cows. Many of these disturbances more closely resemble stereotypies than tics and have been attributed to lack of environmental stimuli and in some instances to dietary deficiencies.

Sharman (1978) has recently shown that dopaminergic systems may be abnormal in pigs that exhibit stereotyped snout rubbing, a behaviour which can be induced by preventing early weaned piglets from suckling. In controlled studies a small but significant reduction in homovanillic acid in the nucleus accumbens and putamen was found. Sharman also suggested that the animals might carry out these repetitive motor acts in order to restore their dopamine levels which had been decreased by reduced sensory input. Alternatively, dopaminergic neurones which innervate cells concerned with repetitive behaviour may also supply neurones concerned with other functions such as reward systems. As long ago as 1875, Feser reported the effects of apomorphine on domesticated animals and observed that stereotyped tongue movements indistinguishable from those seen in licking sickness in cattle could be provoked by its administration. In the pig, apomorphine, a dopamine receptor agonist, causes intense snout rubbing, chewing and salivation, closely resembling normal rooting. Sharman has also noted snout rubbing in pigs following critical doses of metoclopramide, a dopamine receptor antagonist. A series of further studies using guinea pigs has led him to suggest that different receptor subtypes may explain these disparities, as low doses of both metoclopramide and halo-peridol block apomorphine-induced gnawing and nose rubbing, but no drug could be found to block metoclopramide-induced dyskinesias.

Another potentially useful model which enables cortical/subcortical inter-actions to be studied is the acoustic/tactile startle response. In this, rats show a reflex behavioural response to sudden auditory or tactile stimuli which is mediated through a series of brain-stem circuits and is markedly attenuated by clonidine or neuroleptics (Davis, 1980). Tics, however, are not generally stimulated by startle and this paradigm may well be more relevant to the hyperekplexias.

Tail-pinching in rats may induce stereotyped gnawing, licking and biting which is dependent on dopamine release from nigro-striatal pathways (Antelman et al, 1975). Neuroleptics and drugs which enhance 5 hydroxytryptamine trans-mission have been shown to block this response. Tic-like movements, which then persist throughout the animal's life, can also be induced in rats after a seven-day course of beta-iminodipropionitrile. These movements were poten-tiated by amphetamine and blocked by low doses of apomorphine and halo-peridol (Diamond et al, 1982).

What data exist, therefore, suggest that behavioural vices attributed to boredom and restriction of movement in animals may be mediated through dopaminergic mechanisms. Whether any of these can serve as models for tics is, of course, highly debatable.

AETIOLOGY

The cause of tics is unknown and the available evidence is sufficiently equivocal to permit interpretation according to personal dogma. The French school considered mental infantilism an essential prerequisite for the occur-rence of tics. Meige and Feindel, for instance, believed most adult ticqueurs to have the weak and capricious minds of children with difficulties attending to the completion of a task, and to exhibit lack of will power, sociopathic pro-clivities and egocentricity. Ballet believed that, although some ticqueurs might be exceptionally gifted in one limited sphere of life, development of other mental faculties remained embryonic. An association with obsessions such as *folie de pourquoi*, arithromania and onomatomania was also recognised and Charcot regarded a tic as a psychical disorder masquerading in a physical form. Kinnier

Wilson (1927) also believed that the common association of tics with mental retardation, psychoses and affective illness favoured a psychical predisposition. He considered tics to be the outward expression of a desire half-concealed from consciousness and arising out of a constant quest for pleasurable sensations.

Psycho-analysts have explained tics as symbolic expressions of internal conflict. Fenichel (1945) believed they constituted the involuntary motor equivalents of emotional activity allowing previously repressed sexual and aggressive impulses to appear in disguised form. In other words, the body musculature is used for the immediate discharge of carnal infantile wishes or, in Ferenczi's words (1921), tics may be looked on as stereotyped masturbatory equivalents. Other equally fanciful interpretations include the suggestion that they represent an atavistic identification with the behaviour of animals, a manifestation of mental loneliness or an intense aggression towards a particular person or thing. MacDonald (1963) has suggested that tics occur at a time when the child is struggling for ego control and may be having difficulties with the controlled expression of affect. Morphew and Sim (1969) were struck by the symbolic sexuality, inhibited hostility and obsessional traits present in both ticqueurs and stammerers. Zausmer (1954) found that as a group the parents of his patients were anxious, restrictive and rigid and the children were wiry, asthenic, restless, sensitive, irritable and stubborn. Piatrowski (1945) administered the Rorschach test to 12 children with tics and felt that typically they had had many undesirable experiences which they found difficult to integrate, that they had a high level of neurotic anxiety and showed poor initiative. Most of the recent studies of children with tics have reported a very high incidence of coexisting neurotic traits and emotional upset (Corbett et al, 1969). Occasionally acute stresses such as sexual assault or seeing a pet dog run over have been incriminated retrospectively as aetiological factors, but a history of chronic emotional trauma such as parental illness may be more significant.

The learning theorists such as Yates (1958) have considered tics to occur as a result of a conditioned avoidance response evoked by a particular stress which is then reinforced by an associated reduction in anxiety. A generalisation of the initial stimulus then leads to the occurrence of anxiety in other situations and the tic becomes an increasingly strong habit.

Crown (1953) found that ticqueurs had superior reaction times for skilled movements compared with controls. Corbett et al (1969) also noted a superiority in children with tics on the coding subtest of the WISC and suggested that an exaggerated motor response to stress may be a characteristic feature of ticqueurs. Recent studies, however, have found the opposite result in children with Gilles de la Tourette syndrome (Incagnoli and Kane, 1982; Sutherland et al, 1982). A striking similarity between the nature and distribution of tics and the movements seen in the physiological startle response has been pointed out. Tics most frequently involve the eyelids, the face, the head and neck and then the limbs in that order. This closely parallels the distribution of motor activity in startle. Furthermore, high-speed photography and videotape recordings show that, as in the case of multiple tics, the average latent period between eye blink and upper limb movements in the startle reflex is of the order of

100 m.sec the whole movement being complete in half a second. The occasional occurrence of vocalisations in the startle response and its ability to be conditioned to neutral stimuli are other points in favour of this notion. Neurophysiological accompaniments of the startle reaction such as the galvanic skin response may also occur in tics. Corbett (1971, 1976) believes that these similarities may serve to explain the original nature of tics and that the learning theory hypothesis may then account for their perpetuation.

A developmental defect independent of any psychogenic factors has also been suggested as an aetiological possibility. Normal control of motor activity may in some way remain immature in children with tics rendering them susceptible to faulty conditioning processes. If intolerable emotional stress then supervenes the child's neurosis may take the form of a tic. The restricted age of onset, the predisposition of tics for boys and the high remission rate are all in keeping with this view; many ticqueurs also have other developmental disorders such as bed-wetting and encopresis.

Finally, there is a view that tics should be regarded as symptoms of basal ganglia disease in much the same way as chorea. According to Ferenczi, Freud was of the opinion that organic factors would ultimately be found responsible for tics and this approach to aetiology has always been favoured in the German literature. It leans heavily on the occasional occurrence of tics in association with organic diseases such as epidemic encephalitis lethargica and following drugs known to modify basal ganglia function. There is also some supportive evidence from electroencephalographic studies. Ungher et al (1962) have reported frequent maturational abnormalities, disturbed background activity with discharges of spikes and waves in some children with tics, suggesting that cerebral damage from birth trauma or encephalitis might have occurred. Pasamanick and Kawi (1956) investigated the antenatal and postnatal histories of 83 children with tics but other than a higher incidence of maternal complications during pregnancy (21 compared with 10 in controls) no differences could be found. In particular the incidence of prematurity and neonatal problems was the same in patients and controls. Upper respiratory tract infections have been invoked as an important aetiological factor (Selling, 1929) but there is little confirmatory statistical support for this (Corbett et al, 1969).

PATHOPHYSIOLOGY

Tics have been regarded as pathological habits of cortical origin believed by some to germinate in response to an unwanted sensation. The inapposite motor reaction has been considered to be caused by constitutionally defective inhibitory responses within the brain leading to an exaggerated sensitivity to emotional stimuli. Kinnier Wilson (1929) believed that tics should be considered as voluntary movements low in the ladder of volition but reinforced the view that they were mediated through cortical mechanisms:

Any purposive coordinated act passes by dint of repetition into a habit, an acquired automatism, nor does its character of necessity change if its raison d'être disappears. Should the now purposeless habit assume an exaggerated form and haphazard incidence it has degenerated into a tic, cortical intervention determines its continuance when removal or disappearance of the cause could otherwise cause its death from inanition. Once this state in its turn is passed, the motor phenomena persist independently of volition. In many commonplace tics no more recondite origin than this can be traced; no conscious pleasurable element accompanies them still less any suggestion of a hidden sexual conflict between the ego and repression. Not a few of the simple and limited tics of youthful subjects arise in this fashion making faces across the nursery table in a wet-day competition, experimentation with the phonatory capacities of the larynx, visual or auditory mimicry of the habits of others are examples of the initiatory mechanisms for habit-tic formation. In a sense, these habits constitute a kind of reflex cortical activity and illustrate the escape of function of cortical areas.

Support for an important role of subcortical structures comes from the apparent alleviation of multiple tics by stereotactic thalamic surgery and the occurrence of tic-like movements in a woman with focal epilepsy two weeks after the insertion of electrodes 5 mm lateral to the caudate nucleus. Stimulation at 3 Hz produced hyperkinesias of the limbs and a curious catatonic state in which speech was restricted to monosyllabic utterances. These phenomena disappeared immediately on discontinuing the stimulation and the patient was not known to have any predisposition to tic (Bickford, 1957).

Recent work by Obeso et al (1981) suggests that tics differ from cortically-triggered, self-paced willed movements. In a series of elegant studies they were able to show that tics occur as a result of synchronous contraction of agonist and antagonist muscles lasting about 100 ms. More importantly, by means of back-averaging techniques triggered by the electromyographic discharge, they showed that no time-locked cortical potential was evident preceding the tics but large evoked potentials occurred with the movement. The six adult patients were then asked to simulate their tics as accurately as possible by willed movement. In every case, a typical Bereitschafts readiness potential (negative bilateral wave of 500 ms and 7 μV amplitude) was seen prior to the EMG burst. This study, whilst providing no concrete evidence that tics originate in the basal ganglia, certainly strengthens the view that they are not totally under voluntary control in the sense that purposive co-ordinated movements are (Fig. 2.1 and 2.2). It is possible, however, that if a voluntary movement is repeated often enough the cortical Bereitschafts potential might disappear.

The virtual total lack of any hard data makes a Cartesian insistence that tics are psychogenic or organic unhelpful. One of the characteristic features of tics is the emotional relief engendered by their enactment. This is reminiscent of the familiar release from tension achieved by doing something one feels impelled to do. A disturbance of motivational mechanisms or a derangement of the neural transmission between motivation and motor circuits might be incriminated. The limbic system is believed to be of importance in modulating motivation and, furthermore, in the squirrel monkey the anterior cingulate cortex is involved in vocalisation. Recent demonstrations of the extensive limbic

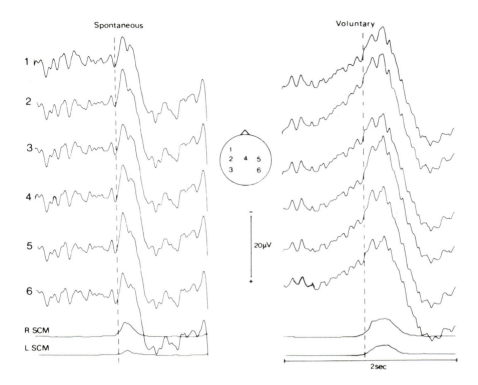

Figure 2.1. *Averaged electroencephalographic response time-locked to muscle jerks in the right sternocleidomastoid muscle. Records on the left (60 trials) are from spontaneous tic, those on the right from voluntarily mimicked tics. The top six electroencephalographic traces are recordings referred to a linked mastoid reference; the bottom two traces are the rectified electromyograph. The vertical dotted line indicates the start of the muscle jerk in sternocleidomastoid. (By kind permission of Dr Obeso and colleagues, 1983. In: Advances in Neurology, vol. 35. Raven Press, New York.)*

inputs into the striatum suggest that close examination of the interplay between these systems might provide a way forward.

CLINICAL DESCRIPTION

Tics are rapid, co-ordinated caricatures of normal motor acts. One hallmark is their irresistibility; as one of Kinnier Wilson's patients remarked: 'You can't help it any more than you can help sneezing.' Any voluntary attempt at suppression inevitably leads to rising tension and disquiet and a compulsive execution of the desired motor reaction will then always culminate in momentary relief. In a few instances, tics appear to begin as a physiological response

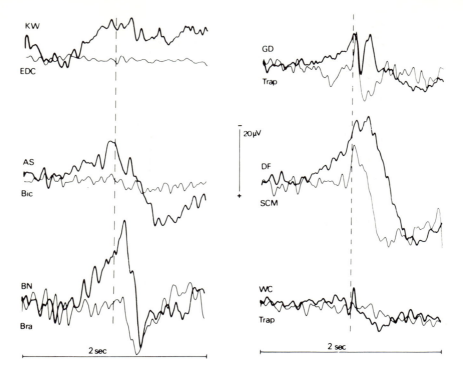

Figure 2.2. EEG *recording from the electrode at C3 point contralateral to the muscle involved in the tic in six patients during spontaneous (light traces) and voluntarily mimicked (heavy traces) jerks. The vertical dotted lines indicate the start of the jerk in the selected muscle labelled under each pair of recordings (average 30–128 sweeps). (By kind permission of Dr Obeso and colleagues, 1984. In: Advances in Neurology, vol. 35. Raven Press, New York.)*

to some source of physical irritation but practice outlives the stimulus and they remain as inapposite, incongruous, embarrassing and occasionally harmful parasite functions. They are attenuated by intense concentration, pleasurable pastimes, sexual arousal and alcohol, they disappear in sleep and can be prevented for a time by will power. Pyrexial illnesses also seem temporarily to reduce their severity in some patients. Tics are profoundly affected by affective stimuli and tend to be worse at times of anxiety, anger or self-consciousness. They are more evident in public places and social gatherings than, for example, in the doctor's consulting rooms and in a number of individuals they are most severe when alone at home. Polymorphism is a characteristic feature and sometimes the movements closely resemble myoclonus or chorea. In general, however, they disturb the normal movements of the affected part of the body to a lesser degree.

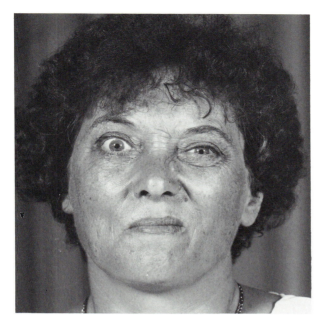

Figure 2.3. *A left eye blink tic.*

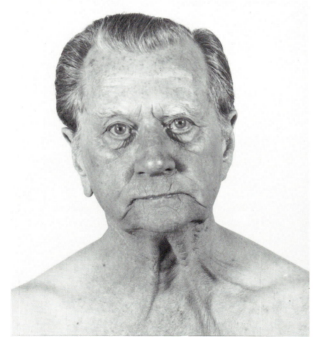

Figure 2.4. *A left platysmal tic.*

LOCALISATION AND VARIETIES

The varieties of tic are limited only by the number of voluntary movements they imitate (Figs 2.3 and 2.4). Most wax and wane and periodically migrate and, in Gilles de la Tourette syndrome there is a virtually inexhaustible repertoire of different motor acts and antics. Some individuals, however, keep a single monosymptomatic tic for years. Individuals with a propensity to tic frequently acquire new habits from observing other ticqueurs and complain that tics are infectious. Wilder and Silbermann (1927) analysed the frequency of tics involving different muscle groups in 170 ticqueurs and found a descending order of frequency from the upper part of the face to the feet so that eye blinks were commonest, followed by tics fo the lower face, neck and shoulders, the least frequent being those in the trunk and legs. The diverse function of the facial muscles may explain the preponderance of tics in this part of the body, the face being responsible for all the mimic expressions which portray our sentiments and emotions. A list of commonly occurring tics is shown in Table 2.1. This is far from exhaustive but includes those tics most frequently encountered in my own practice. The eye wink is the commonest of all tics and consists of ·contraction of the upper lid at irregular intervals. It may be unilateral or bilateral and differs only from a blink in its frequency and abruptness. The orbicularis oculi and nasal muscles are affected and there may be associated eyeball rolling. The everyday use of this motor act as an inviting overture can result in highly embarrassing situations when it occurs involuntarily in public.

Table 2.1. A LIST OF BODY TICS

1. Facial	Eye wink. Eye rolling. Curling in of eyelids. Staring. Eyebrow raising. Scalp movements. Frowning. Nose wrinkling. Nostril twitching. Nasal flaring. Mouth opening. Grimacing. Snarling. Pouting. Lip pursing. Lip twitching. Spitting. Tongue Flicking. Nibbling. Licking. Gnawing. Teeth gnashing. Biting inside of mouth. Jaw protrusions. Platysma contractions. Sucking. Chin rubbing.
2. Head, neck and shoulders	Head tossing. Head nodding. Head jerking. Head drooping. Head rolling. Head swivelling. Shoulder shrugging. Shoulder hunching. Neck stretching.
3. Arms	Arm jerks. Fist clenching. Finger stretching. Arm flicks. Piano playing movements. Arm straightening. Arm bends. Shoulder abductions.
4. Body	Pelvic thrusts. Salutation tics. Abdomen jerks. Pectoral twitches. Abdominal protrusion. Buttock tightening. Chest expansion. Sphincter tightening. Shudders. Tightening of rectus abdominis.
5. Legs	Foot and toe shaking. Hip flexion. Hip abductions. Kicking. Toe curls. Foot dorsiflexion. Genuflexion. Knee extensions.

COURSE

The large majority of childhood ticqueurs remit spontaneously in adolescence but the possibility of a subsequent relapse always remains. In Torup's study 50% of patients were tic-free at follow-up on average nine years after diagnosis. A further 46% were improved and only 6% were unchanged, none of whom were incapacitated. The average age of the patients at follow-up was 18 years (6–26 years) and the average age at cessation of the tics was 12–13 years with a mean duration of symptoms of four to six years. Prognosis for recovery was worse in those who had relatives with tics in adult life (Torup, 1962). In the Maudsley study half the patients had tics as their primary symptom and data were obtained on 73 of these (82%) with a follow-up range of 1–18 years and a mean duration of follow-up of 5.4 years. The patients had a mean age at the time of follow-up of 15 years (range 6–29 years). None of the 73 cases was worse and 30 (40%) had completely recovered, 39 (53%) were improved and four (6%) were unchanged. No significant association was found between the age at follow-up and the outcome, although there was a marked increase in the proportion found to be completely recovered from their tics in those followed for eight years or longer. There was also a greater proportion of complete recoveries in the group whose tics started between 6 and 8 years. Vocal tics tended to have a worse prognosis, and anxiety and depression were the commonest psychiatric symptoms at the time of reassessment. In a study by Mahler et al (1945) only one of 10 ticqueurs who reached military service age was rejected because of tics although three others were refused on other medical grounds and one defaulted. In a 10-year follow-up by postal questionnaire and routine assessment only two of 35 patients still had tics after five years (Dugas et al, 1975). Boenheim also found a high remission rate with 65% of 31 ticqueurs free from symptoms two to three years after treatment with the remainder improved.

Zausmer (1954) treated his patients by simple reassurance and explanation, was able to re-examine 39 of his 96 childhood ticqueurs and obtained data on 41 a mean four and a half years after their initial referral. Overall there had been a marked improvement but only 10 (24%) had been tic-free for one year. In the recovered cases the duration of tics ranged from three to eight and a half years (mean four and a half years). Thirty-one patients had improved at the time of follow up but 10 had not and it was apparent that severe tics could persist in some cases for several years. The prognosis was significantly better in girls and all the 10 unimproved cases were boys.

TREATMENT

Simple tics in children should always be treated seriously even though the majority are short-lived and little more than a mild inconvenience. Many children with tics have behavioural problems and tactful enquiry about underlying stresses and worries occasionally reaps therapeutic dividends. A full psychiatric assessment of the child is a mandatory prelude to any form of treatment; a physical examination must also be carried out to exclude local sources of irritation such as conjunctivitis and sinusitis, and to note any neurological abnormalities. Tics can be explained as a manifestation of anxiety and it should be stressed to parents at the outset that they may be perpetuated unnecessarily by over-concern, unrealistic demands or repeated punishment. The family should also be advised to disregard the movements as much as possible and similar guidance should be communicated to the child's teachers. It is a fairly common experience to find an over-exacting parent making excessive demands on a child and adequate time must be allotted for tactful discussion. In most cases a careful reassuring explanation repeated on at least two occasions is all that is required, the child then being asked to return periodically to see how he or she is progressing.

Suggested therapies for tic are legion ranging from hypnosis and abreaction to stereotactic thalamic surgery, but very few have been properly evaluated. Psychotherapeutic approaches founded on psycho-analytical doctrines are still popular but most of the enthusiastic claims for this line of management stem from isolated anecdotal wonder cures. Behavioural techniques and drugs are widely used for the management of persistent multiple tics and will be discussed ·in some detail.

BEHAVIOURAL TECHNIQUES

Many of these techniques are based on the notion that regular repetition of orderly willed movement may ultimately inhibit the abnormal conditioned reflex underlying tics. Meige and Feindel employed mirror drill with reputedly excellent results. This required the simultaneous repetition of prescribed motor acts by homologous muscle groups on the two sides. Tasks of increasing complexity were set for fixed periods each day leading eventually to instructions to write or draw simultaneously with both hands. This method was felt to be particularly valuable for tics affecting the left hand.

Brissaud's muscular drill (Brissaud, 1895; Brissaud and Feindel, 1899) consisted of a series of graduated exercises designed to teach the patient to remain motionless. After this had been achieved in positions where tics rarely occurred the patient then moved on to postures where adventitious movements commonly arose. Again attempts were made not to move for as long as possible and finally the patient was asked to mantain immobility in affected parts of his body even when completing complicated activities like walking or speaking. For success this simple technique depended on cooperation of the patient and enthusiasm and encouragement from the therapist. Other early methods included breathing exercises to re-create self-control and the regular execution of voluntary movements in affected muscle groups performed to the rhythmical accompaniment of a metronome.

Contemporary modification of these techniques falls broadly into three categories. Probably the most popular is massed practice founded on Dunlap's hypothesis (1945) that undesirable habits could be broken by making the subject repeat them over and over again until boredom sets in. The reported results using this approach are conflicting (Rafi, 1962; Sand and Carlson, 1973). One problem that arises is that tics are frequently multiple and therefore often impossible to imitate. Corbett, however, has suggested that eye blink may act as a trigger to tics in other parts of the body and treatment of this by massed practice may alleviate multiple tics. This view is based on his analogy of tics to the startle response. Vocal tics and cursing may be particularly amenable to massed practice but to be successful it must be carried out regularly without fail for five-minute periods several times each day for many weeks. Habit reversal is another form of therapy which may be helpful occasionally (Azrin and Nunn, 1973). In this the sequence of events involved in tic production is analysed and the patients is then asked to reproduce it over and over again in a different or incompatible order. For example, if the normal sequence is a twitch of the eye followed by a grunt, this order must be reversed by the patient during therapy. Finally there is response prevention which demands the forcible interruption of the abnormal sequence of motor acts at an early stage of their instigation. This is most useful in patients with associated obsessional rituals and often the mere continuous presence of a therapist may effectively inhibit tics. Aversion stimuli may be incorporated into this technique, ranging from pricking the patient with a pin every time he tics to playing pleasant music when a child is tic-free and substituting white noise each time tics occur. The impossibility of organising controlled studies and the high incidence of spontaneous cure make the value of these behavioural methods hard to evaluate. Certainly improvement rates of up to 30% should not be taken to indicate a meaningful therapeutic response.

DRUG TREATMENT

This is rarely indicated in children with simple tics. However, in occasional situations where the child's scholastic potential is threatened and bullying at school is leading to secondary neurotic traits, medication may be indicated. The older the patient with tics the more inveterate the symptoms are likely to be, and certainly in adults with chronic simple tics a trial of drug therapy may be appropriate. Ticqueurs who do not want to be treated, however, should never be persuaded to take medicine as this may do considerably more harm than good.

A general rule when prescribing medication of any sort is to attempt a cure with the most innocuous preparation first. In adults, diazepam or clonazepam are useful starting drugs but, if these fail, neuroleptics such as sulpiride or pimozide should be tried.

3

Gilles de la Tourette Syndrome

Synonyms Tourette syndrome, Brissaud's variable chorea, myospasia impulsiva, maladie des tics convulsifs, tic impulsifs, mimische krampfneurose, koordinierte erinnerungskraempfe.

Definition Multiple body and vocal tics beginning in childhood or adolescence which wax and wane in severity, repeatedly change their form and are present for a minimum period of one year. Coprolalia, copropraxia, echophenomena and complex antics and mannerisms are commonly associated.

INTRODUCTION

Possible early examples of Gilles de la Tourette syndrome may be found in medieval texts. Sprengler (1489) described a priest who, whenever he genuflected before the Virgin Mary, was compelled to thrust out his tongue and cry out. Mary Hall of Gadsden in Hertford, described by William Drage in 1663, may have suffered with the condition and Thomas Willis and John Friend reported a remarkable family of barking girls from the small village of Blackthorn in Oxfordshire (Friend, 1701):

> The awful sight of the yelping girls confronted me directly, each of them replying to the other in absolutely strict alternation with a violent shaking of her head, as if encouraging the others by her nod — like a common country piper — to sing their unpleasant tune together. They were not affected by any spasms in the face except for movements which frequently made their mouths go to and fro; and their pulse was like that of the healthy except that it was slightly weak just before the end. The sound, as it seemed to me, resembled not so much the barking of dogs as their howling, except that it was more rapidly repeated. Often, between these howlings, they enjoyed the power of speech and full possession of their senses.

Exorcism was usually used in treating these unfortunate individuals, often with some success, and it is conceivable that all of them were in fact suffering from possession states or conversion hysteria. In fact confusion in the lay mind between Gilles de la Tourette syndrome and possession states persists and it is rumoured that the theme of the recent box-office success *The Exorcist* was based on an American child admitted to hospital with Gilles de la Tourette syndrome. Stevens (1971) reported the case of Prince Condé who was compelled to stuff his mouth with any nearby object including a curtain to suppress an involuntary bark when in the presence of Louis XIV. The strongest case of all, however, can be made for the English literary figure Samuel Johnson who was noted by his friends to have almost constant tics and gesticulations and to make whistling sounds when bored or ill at ease. Itard (1825), better known for his work on feral children and the education of deaf mutes, provided the first clear description of the disorder in the medical literature. The Marquise de Dampierre, a French noblewoman, began to tic at the age of 7 years. She improved temporarily following a cure in Switzerland but subsequently began to make cries and meaningless utterances. Following her marriage her symptoms became worse and an uncontrollable desire to curse in public forced her to live as a recluse, dying at the age of 85, still swearing. Itard considered this unfortunate case not to be a new disorder but 'as one of the most extraordinary forms clonic convulsions can assume'. Roth (1850) and Sandras (1851) both subsequently described this remarkable patient as did Trousseau (1873) who termed the inapposite vocalisations, diaphragmatic chorea. Many years after Itard's original description Charcot demonstrated her in one of his celebrated Tuesday lectures, concluding that the disorder was psychogenically determined (Charcot, 1885). In 1881 Friedreich reported an undoubted case of the syndrome (Freidreich, 1881) and, three years later, before joining Charcot's staff, Georges Gilles de la Tourette translated Beard's paper on the 'Jumping Frenchmen of Maine'. On his return to the Salpetrière as *chef de clinique* Gilles de la Tourette was delegated the task of reclassifying the 'chaos of the choreas', whereupon he immediately set off in search of jumping Frenchmen arguing that if this disorder existed it was more likely to occur in Paris than in the United States of America. He failed to find any but, instead, meticulously described nine patients, six of whom he had observed personally, suffering from what he believed to be a related disorder characterised by uncoordinated jerks, strange cries, echolalia and coprolalia (Gilles de la Tourette, 1885). In his two-part paper Gilles de la Tourette recognised that the condition which was to earn him eponymous fame was a life-long disorder which began in childhood or adolescence, affected males more frequently and fluctuated in severity. He did not consider intellectual deterioration or psychosis to be late sequelae and he noted that some patients were above average intelligence. He did, however, draw attention to the learning difficulties experienced by many and the positive family history of mental instability. Coprolalia he believed to be pathognomonic, although it was present in only five of his original cases. He also considered that vocal tics always occurred simultaneously with a muscular tic elsewhere in the body and that fever had a markedly beneficial effect upon the frequency of tics. In his later papers when already ill (Gilles de la Tourette, 1899), his views changed, to some degree influenced by those of his contemporary Guinon who considered mental instability to be present in all cases and psychosis to be a common final outcome. In a footnote to his seminal paper of 1885 Gilles de la Tourette commented that, during a recent visit to London, Hughlings Jackson had told him that he had never seen or read of such cases. However, perhaps as a result of their conversation, Jackson reported an example in 1884:

I have a patient, the subject of chorea, who for several years has been in the habit of saying, quite involuntarily, the word bloody. A few years ago, he was frightened by a man shouting the word after him, the fright produced chorea and if I may use such a term chorea of his mind too; as for three days he said the word bloody and little else; now he ejaculates it occasionally. The mental process for saying that word, is as little under his control as a few of the muscles of his face are, for the twitching of which he is now attending the London Hospital.

Guinon (1886, 1887), like his teacher Charcot, regarded tic disorders as a clinical continuum, the movements to be identical with the gestures and mannerisms of everyday life, and he believed an underlying psycho-neurosis to be responsible. Five cases were described in his first paper, the first of which would not now fulfil the diagnostic criteria as it more closely resembles startle. Four of Guinon's cases developed a psychosis or severe personality disorder which led to his belief that mental deterioration was almost inevitable. He also drew up criteria for distinguishing Gilles de la Tourette's syndrome, which he believed to be incurable, from hysterical tics which responded to hypnosis. Catrou (1890) in his doctoral thesis believed the disorder to be commoner in males, to occur in often intelligent but unbalanced personalities and to have a relatively poor prognosis because of learning difficulties and laziness. Indeed in virtually all the 23 papers published between 1825 and 1900, Gilles de la Tourette's syndrome was considered to be due to 'neuropathic antecedents' and the patients considered as higher degenerates. Koester (1899) discovered two cases amongst 2500 patients at the Leipzig University Polyclinic and was able to find a total of 50 cases in the literature.

Meige and Feindel believed Gilles de la Tourette syndrome to be a distinct nosological entity characterised by multiple vocal and body tics, coprolalia, and echolalia, often culminating in insanity. Prince (1906) described a man with facial grimacing, purposive head and shoulder jerks and what he termed automatic speech. He believed fear and apprehension to be crucial in the pathogenesis and that many of the movements occurred as a result of mimicry and autosuggestion.

After this flurry of initial reports, interest in the condition receded and no further cases were mentioned in the literature for 30 years. Creak and Guttman (1935) then reported six patients from the Maudsley Hospital explaining the dearth of recent reports on the basis of misdiagnosis and a lack of recognition. Kinnier Wilson (1941) described a 19-year-old girl who developed head, face and arm tics at the age of 8 and then began to repeat swear words in a low monotonous voice or, alternatively, would suddenly interlard her ordinary conversational speech with obscenities. The patient also had marked echolalia and délire de toucher and was eventually certified insane. This report consolidated the misapprehension that psychosis invariably occurred once the patient reached adult life.

Between 1920 and 1960 there followed a series of single case reports mainly from psycho-analysts, most of whom considered the tics to stem from underlying dynamic conflicts usually of a sexual or aggressive nature. The family dynamics and particularly the child's relationship to his parents were thought by many to be crucial aetiological factors. Hammer (1965), for example, considered that his patient and the patient's mother were mutually involved in a sado-masochistic relationship, while others have postulated that tics reflect unconscious muscular eroticism towards the father. Some considered an obsessional compulsive neurosis to be a crucial underlying trigger, whereas feelings of guilt and hostility were favoured by others (Mahler et al, 1945). Oberndorf (1916) believed tics to be a defence against pleasurable thumb sucking. The most striking aspect of all these papers is the general lack of agreement and the singular lack of success of psycho-analysis in managing the disorder.

In 1961 Seignot, and Caprini and Melotti independently reported the beneficial effects of haloperidol in patients with Gilles de la Tourette syndrome. This observation led to a subtle change in the prevailing views regarding the pathogenesis of the condition. Chapel (1966) considered the disorder to be due to an organic brain abnormality activated by psychic stress such as anger towards parents. Furthermore, the availability for the first time of a therapy which held out hope of improvement without necessarily any attached psychiatric implications led to an increasing number of sufferers referring themselves for medical attention. Fernando (1967), on reviewing the English-speaking literature, accepted 65 cases and added four of his own. He emphasised that spontaneous remissions could occur for several years, that as a group they were neurotic and often of high intelligence and that the disorder seldom led to schizophrenia. By 1976, probably as a result of increasing awareness, he was able to collect 102 more cases from the literature (Fernando, 1976). Abuzzahab and Anderson (1976) set up an International Registry for patients with Gilles de la Tourette syndrome obtaining details of 430 cases from all over the world. The comprehensive clinical studies by the Shapiros and their colleagues in New York between 1965 and 1974 have provided a detailed picture of the clinical features and their insistence that the disorder is caused by structural brain damage has stimulated research into the pathogenesis of the condition.

EPIDEMIOLOGY

Although Gilles de la Tourette syndrome is a rare disorder the originally quoted prevalence figure of five per million may be a considerable underestimate. Misdiagnosis, the need to survey large populations to obtain accurate statistics and the reluctance of many ticqueurs and their families to cooperate fully with research have hampered data collection. Study of death certificates is also valueless as the disorder does not cause death and is often considered irrelevant in a moribund patient. On the basis of their membership figures from hundreds of regional chapters throughout the United States, the American Tourette Syndrome Association has estimated that there may be as many as 100 000 Americans with the disorder. Although there may be an element of propagandist over-exaggeration in this figure in fact it does not differ greatly from the rough 0.03% life-time prevalence calculated by Shapiro et al (1978) on the basis of four studies published before 1966. What is clear from both the American experience and my own as medical adviser to the United Kingdom Tourette Syndrome Association is that every radio or television broadcast, magazine or newspaper article or lecture to lay audiences, turns up several new cases, most of whom have never been correctly diagnosed. Probably the best available study is that carried out in Rochester, Minnesota, over a 12-year period in which a total of three new cases were detected giving an incidence of 4.6 per million per year (Lucas et al, 1982).

In a large number of patients studied by Shapiro and colleagues in the New York Metropolitan area, almost half were of Eastern European background (Shapiro et al, 1978). In a further sample of 132 cases Shapiro found the parents were East European Jews in 25% compared with 4% of East European non-Jews, raising the possibility of a higher frequency of the disorder in Ashkenazims. Eldridge et al (1977) also found that 57% of 81 patients surveyed in New York were East European Jews. The high indigenous Jewish population in New York City, however, may have been partly responsible for these findings. More intriguing was the report of an unusually large number of Jewish families in a non-selective epidemiological study on Gilles de la Tourette syndrome in the Minneapolis area where the population is predominantly Northern European (Wassman et al, 1977). However, a number of other studies failed to confirm these findings (Golden, 1977; Nee et al, 1980; Lees et al, 1984) and, although it is possible that Ashkenazi Jews may have a greater genetic predisposition to Gilles de la Tourette's syndrome, it seems likely that referral bias and cultural factors affecting the expression and tolerance of the symptoms are more important.

Gilles de la Tourette syndrome in fact occurs in all races and is distributed equally among different social classes. Large representative series have been published from the United States, Western Europe, Japan, China and Hong Kong. It also occurs on the Indian subcontinent and is known to occur in the black populations of South Africa and the United States. Generally there is a striking cross-cultural uniformity in the clinical picture except for a comparatively low incidence of coprolalia in Japanese patients. All the larger series report a male: female incidence of at least 3:1 with a mean age of onset of 7 years, nearly all cases beginning before the age of 12 (Table 3.1)

GENETICS

There is general agreement that Gilles de la Tourette syndrome shows a familial concentration, especially if one considers idiopathic tic as a minor manifestation. One of Gilles de la Tourette's original cases had a sister with the same disorder and Oppenheim (1887) recorded the remarkable family history of a patient with Gilles de la Tourette syndrome whose four daughters and three grandchildren had the same disease. Another family has been

Table 3.1.

Series	CAUCASIAN		CHINESE	JAPANESE
	United States (Shapiro et al, 1978)	United Kingdom (Lees et al, 1984)	(Lieh Mak et al, 1982) (Chen Han Bai and Lu Fei Han Quin, 1983) (Singer, 1976)	(Nomura and Segawa, 1982)
Number of patients	145	53	37	100
Male: female ratio	3:1	3:1	4:1	5:1
Mean age at onset (years)	7	7	9	6.5
Presenting tic	Eye blink (42%) Head tic (20%) Vocal tic (19%)	Eye blink (35%) Head tic (19%) Vocal tic (15%)	Grimace (30%) Eye blink (30%) Vocal tic (15%)	Eye blink (35%) Head tic (24%) Vocal tic (10%)
Mean age at onset of vocal tics (y)	9	11	9	8
% cases with coprolalia	60%	39%	40%	True — 4% Quasi — 19%
% cases with copropraxia	20%	21%	Not reported	Not reported
% cases with echolalia	35%	46%	30%	Not reported
% cases with echopraxia	10%	21%	Not reported	Not reported

reported in which no fewer than 17 of 43 members were affected (Guggenheim, 1979).

Wilson et al (1978) reviewed the available literature concluding that 30% of close relatives of the proband have tics or Gilles de la Tourette syndrome. Shapiro et al (1978) reported that 36% of their patients had at least one family member with tics and that 7.4% had a family member with Gilles de la Tourette syndrome. Comparable figures from the United Kingdom study were 46% and 4% respectively (Lees et al, 1984). The New York group also noted a higher frequency of a positive family history in females than male patients. Kidd et al (1980) reported a 14.4% incidence of tics in first-degree relatives of patients randomly selected from the American Tourette Syndrome Association membership register, and Pauls et al (1981) obtained a figure of 23.7% in patients attending a Child Study Centre Clinic at Yale University. In a selected group of patients referred to the National Institute of Mental Health in the United States, Nee et al (1980) deduced by exhaustive enquiry the fact that 16 of their 50 cases had a family member with Gilles de la Tourette syndrome, and another 16 a family history of tics; 24 of the families had more than one affected member.

Despite this suggestive data a specific genetic mechanism has not as yet been identified. Wilson et al (1978), taking an iconoclastic line, rightly point out that assuming 10% as a reasonable estimate for the prevalence of tics, family aggregation findings as reported do not provide support for an important genetic factor in Gilles de la Tourette syndrome. Abuzzahab and Anderson (1976) went even further and considered genetic factors to be unimportant in the pathogenesis of the disorder. Preliminary HLA studies of 12 patients and their families have not revealed a particular HLA A or B type to be associated with the disease (Cummings et al, 1982).

Equally the findings from these studies in which families of clinic patients have been examined do not refute a genetic factor and in a further epidemiological survey Kidd et al (1980) provide some evidence for transmission in Gilles de la Tourette syndrome. In this study based on data obtained from the families of 75 patients they concluded that the frequency of Gilles de la Tourette syndrome or tics among relatives was significantly heterogeneous. The data suggested that idiopathic tics were indeed a forme fruste of Gilles de la Tourette syndrome, that there was a real sex difference in prevalence as it was found in the relatives of both male and female probands and that finally the sex difference may be related to a threshold effect. The authors considered it possible that hereditary and non-hereditary subgroups might exist.

Some support for a genetic factor also comes from the limited data on twins. The four reasonably well-documented monozygous twin sets were all concordant, although in two the disorder varied in its time of onset and severity (Shapiro et al, 1978; Wassman et al, 1978; Jenkins and Ashby, 1983; Wasserman et al, 1983). In none was there a family history of tics or Gilles de la Tourette syndrome in the parents. In the four fraternal twins in the literature all were discordant for Gilles de la Tourette syndrome. Merskey (1974) also reported a single patient with the XYY chromosome karyotype and suggested this abnormality might predispose to both tics and essential tremors.

In common with a number of other neuro-behavioural disorders most of the common genetic models have been proposed. An autosomal dominant inheritance with reduced penetrance and variable expressivity has been suggested to explain families with affected parents and offspring (Eldridge et al, 1977), whereas Shapiro et al (1978) considered a polygenic inheritance with a relatively high frequency of responsible genes to be more likely. Other suggested possibilities include the existence of hereditary and non-hereditary forms or the importance of an environmental factor in initiating the process in genetically predisposed individuals. What seems clear, however, is that sex-related thresholds must be in operation to explain the undoubted male preponderance. Baron et al (1980) have recently reanalysed Shapiro's Mount Sinai Hospital data and suggested that the mode of transmission could be explained by a single major locus model but not by a multifactorial-polygenic model. Kidd and Pauls (1982), however, were able to fit their data to two and three allele single major locus models and multifactorial-polygenic models. They point out that discrimination among quite distinct models is extremely difficult if only the trait phenotype is available.

On the basis of the available evidence it would seem reasonable to advise patients that there is no familial incidence in the majority of cases, that the illness is extremely rare and that the chances are overwhelmingly in favour of having an unaffected child. The risks, however, may be somewhat increased if there are several members of the family with tics or Gilles de la Tourette syndrome.

AETIOLOGY

The vagaries of medical fashion have had a most unhelpful influence on understanding the cause of Gilles de la Tourette syndrome. Its recognition around the turn of the century coincided with the rapid growth of psychological theory and it soon became an ideal target for psycho-analytical speculation. The pandemic of von Economo's disease after the First World War left in its wake numerous cases of post-encephalitic tics, raising the alternative idea of a structural or viral cause, and the recent advances in neurochemistry have led to fashionable theories of monoamine dysfunction. The cause is unknown and will probably remain so until mechanisms underlying tics are better understood.

Gilles de la Tourette syndrome's position on the borderlands of neurology and psychiatry has led to familiar historical aetiological conflicts. The lack of convincing histological abnormalities, the occurrence of coprolalia and the capacity of patients to suppress voluntarily the movements have all been marshalled in support of a primary underlying psychogenic cause. At the other pole there are those who consider it to be a degenerative neurological disorder of the central nervous system and point to the occurrence of similar symptoms following structural brain damage or the use of dopaminergic drugs, the presence of subtle neurological abnormalities, and the beneficial response in some instances to dopamine receptor blocking drugs. Others take a middle line and postulate a developmental weakness caused by subtle structural brain damage or biochemical dysfunction of the motor mind which leads to a predisposed vulnerability to psychological factors. Finally, there are those who see within the blanket of Gilles de la Tourette syndrome several discrete disorders some better classified as myoclonus or chorea and others clearly psychogenic.

Shapiro has been a strong advocate of an organic aetiology and considers subcortical lesions to be responsible. 50% of his patients compared with 20% of control normal children had mild motor asymmetries including impairment of rapid alternating movements, drift of the outstretched hand and alterations in muscle tone. Dystonic and choreiform movements were also occasionally noted. 47% had non-specific electroencephalographic abnormalities and 20% were left-handed or ambidextrous. Although IQ tests were in the average range, 50% of his patients compared to 14% of controls had a marked verbal/performance WAIS IQ discrepancy of 15 points and the Bender-Gestalt test was rated as organic in 42% of patients compared with 16% of controls. 57.9% of his patients also exhibited signs and symptoms of the hyperactivity syndrome (Sweet et al, 1973; Shapiro et al, 1978). Other studies have confirmed this high frequency of neuro-developmental 'soft signs' (Golden, 1977a; Nomura and Segawa, 1982). No abnormalities in birth history with respect to birth weight, delivery complications, mother's age or birth order have been found (Shapiro et al, 1978). In the United Kingdom study, neurological examination proved normal except for the associated presence of chorea and focal dystonia in a small percentage of untreated patients (Lees et al, 1984).

The German school has long emphasised the coupling of normal motor activity with emotional and intellectual stimuli within the corpus striatum and thalamus (Hess, 1949; Hassler, 1953). Immaturity of striatal neurones leading to disinhibition with release of tics under emotional stress has been considered a possibility. Bing (1936) in fact suggested that psychological factors in early life might actually be involved in causing structural immaturity. The presence of chorea and focal dystonia in a small minority of untreated patients also raises the possibility of a subgroup with basal ganglia dysfunction. Devinsky (1983) has also speculated that subcortical structures may be deranged in Gilles de la Tourette syndrome and, on the basis of analogies with encephalitis lethargica, circumstantial neurochemical and neuropharmacological evidence and animal studies on vocalisation, he suggested that attention should be centred on the peri-aqueductal grey matter and the midbrain tegmentum. Others, however, following careful neuropsychological testing, have implicated the association cortex (Sutherland et al, 1982).

The link between Gilles de la Tourette syndrome and hyperactivity syndrome is intriguing. Similar aetiological theories have been proposed for both conditions and many of the behavioural and minor neurological abnormalities reported to occur in some patients with Gilles de la Tourette syndrome also occur in hyperkinetic children. It has been suggested that those cases with associated attention deficits might differ from other patients with Gilles de la Tourette syndrome in that a family history is usually lacking (Rapoport et al, 1982). Further possible support for heterogeneity comes from the observation that patients with a family history of tics or Gilles de la Tourette syndrome respond more consistently to haloperidol and tend to have a higher incidence of obsessive compulsive behavioural traits (Moldofsky et al, 1974; Caine et al, 1982). An exaggerated startle response has also been reported in some patients (Lees et al, 1984) suggesting that the distinction between Gilles de la Tourette syndrome, startle neurosis and related culturally conditioned disorders such as latah may not be as clear cut as has recently been suggested.

Evidence that the disorder is caused by a psycho-neurosis is unconvincing. Overactive behaviour preceding the appearance of tics has been reported frequently (Mahler et al, 1945; Rapoport, 1959) raising the possibility of a preceding temperamental susceptibility and, very occasionally, acute emotional distress appears to have precipitated the onset of tics. In a controlled study using the Minnesota Multiphasic Personality Inventory no difference could be found between patients and age-matched psychiatric out-patients with respect to the incidence of overt and underlying psychosis, hysteria, obsessional compulsive traits and inhibition of hostility. Both groups had a high incidence of adjustment problems (Shapiro et al, 1978) and it would seem reasonable to conclude that there is a higher prevalence of psychiatric symptoms in patients with Gilles de la Tourette syndrome. Subgroups of patients may show obsessional compulsive traits (Ascher, 1948; Nee et al, 1980), inappropriate sexual activity (Moldofsky et al, 1974; Nee et al, 1980) and sleep disorders (Zarcone et al, 1972). Morphew and Sim (1969) reviewed 43 case reports concluding that the disorder was psychogenic because of the good response to psychotherapy and the frequency of precipitating emotional stresses. Mahler and Rangell (1943) believed that the disorder sprang from a failure to gratify instinctual urges and coined the term emotional incontinence to explain the preoccupation of many patients with sexual and aggressive impulses (Moldofsky et al, 1974; Eldridge et al, 1977). Indeed, inhibition of hostility is a theme running through much of the psychiatric literature. Gilles de la Tourette syndrome has also been considered in terms of a disordered expression of affect; a notion which has some support from the study of Corbett et al (1969) which revealed that ticqueurs manifested less aggression and depression compared with age-matched psychiatric out-patients. The heterogeneity of the psychiatric symptomatology and the undoubted presence of a substantial number of psychiatrically normal patients are difficult to reconcile with a primary psychogenic hypothesis.

PATHOPHYSIOLOGY

Tics are less automatic than many of the other dyskinesias considered to arise as a result of basal ganglia dysfunction. Nevertheless, they are of great rapidity and become virtually uncontrollable after certain powerful emotional stimuli. Attempts at suppression will result in mounting apprehension and release of the tic produces temporary emotional fulfilment. The characteristic, somewhat truncated, movements strike one not so much as foreign and inhuman but as excessive inopportune caricatures which in certain normal affective states would not appear incongruous. They particularly call to mind the shouts and syncopations of extempore jazz musicians and the rapturous gyrations of those locked in ecstatic possession states. Bliss (1980) in his autobiographical account argues that tics are in a sense voluntary occurring in response to a subjective itch to tic. This echoes Hassler's notion of a 'second will' which lies just beyond an individual's volitional powers but is nevertheless consciously experienced.

The abnormal vocalisations are a central symptom of Gilles de la Tourette syndrome. Usually these are non-verbal consisting of lingual laryngeal, labial and nasal tics, which occur at phrase junctures in speech where in normal conversation a pause might occur. At the beginning and end of clauses, normal speakers produce occasional extraneous movements of the larynx, lips and mouth. Furthermore, vocal tics are usually synchronous with overall speech rhythm suggesting that their origin must be closely linked with the complexities of normal speech planning. What in fact distinguishes them mainly is their excessive force and repetitiveness rather than any disruption of speech flow or content. Verbal tics also occur commonly in Gilles de la Tourette syndrome and Ludlow et al (1982) have raised the possibility that dysfunction in the dominant supplementary motor area may be important. This hypothesis is based on the loss of 'vocal gestures' such as hissing and sniffing following lesions in the third frontal convolution, and the presence in some patients with Gilles de la Tourette syndrome of additional language disorders reminiscent of those found in transcortical motor dysphasia. In this disturbance there is intact speech with normal repetition but a paucity of verbal output. It is now known, however, that lesions within subcortical structures may also produce subtle disorders of word fluency.

It has been proposed that there are two separate speech mechanisms which, in man, may function in parallel producing a dual control over normal social discourse. The first and more primitive is probably important in emotionally charged language and tends to be emptier in content and less open to modification by feedback mechanisms. The cingulate cortex and central grey matter are considered to be important in the mediation of this function. It has been suggested that the existence of this system might explain why Pithecanthropus, despite his small brain, is believed to have spoken. The second, more sophisticated system, includes the pulvinar, Wernickes speech area and the dominant supplementary motor area. It controls speech production and purposive behavioural planning. The system is believed to dominate the older limbic system and is capable of suppressing emotional behaviour during language formulation.

However, the forms of non-verbal vocalisation which characterise Gilles de la Tourette syndrome have not been produced by stimulation of the neo cortex (Penfield and Jasper, 1954) or the anterior cingulate cortex in man (Lewin and Whitty, 1960). Selective lesions of the anterior cingulate cortex also failed to produce vocalisations (Whitty et al, 1952) although there are a few reports of akinetic mutism occurring following damage to both anterior cingulate cortices. In the lower apes the mesencephalic grey matter appears to play a crucial role in initiating vocalisation (Jurgens and Ploog, 1970) and Magoun and colleagues in 1937 demonstrated in several different mammals that species-specific calls, independent of the emotional state, could be induced by stimulating the peri-aqueductal grey matter and tegmentum. In monkeys, specific socially relevant sounds indistinguishable, from those which occur naturally, have been evoked and it has been shown that these are not due to stimulation of contiguous pain fibres. It seems clear, therefore, that in animals at least vocalisations can occur as a result of direct arousal of rostral brain-stem areas without primary stimulation of speech centres.

The mesencephalic grey matter is the final output pathway for fibres passing to the cranial nerve nuclei involved in articulation. Excitation of this area occurs at the highest level from the anterior cingulate cortex and from afferents arriving from the amygdala, septal area and hypothalamus. In one study, stimulation of the anterior cingulate cortex in humans led to a number of different co-ordinated movements which were difficult for the patient to inhibit and at times were executed in a gauche manner. Activities included licking, rubbing of the fingers and thumb together, glancing eye movements, to and fro hand movements and touching the lips (Talairach et al, 1973). These movements bear some similarity to the complicated stereotypies often seen in Gilles de la Tourette syndrome. It is also of interest that bilateral anterior cingulotomies have been claimed to alleviate obsessional compulsive psychoses (Whitty et al, 1952). The anterior cingulate cortex has a rich dopamine innervation from the ventrotegmental area of the midbrain and the unmasking of tics by dopaminergic agonists in post-encephalitic Parkinson's syndrome and their attenuation by neuroleptics has led to the idea that central dopamine receptor supersensitivity might be important in the pathophysiology of tics. Iverson and Alpert (1982) have suggested that attention should be directed to neuronal circuits functionally related to dopaminergic neurones when considering the pathophysiology of Gilles de la Tourette syndrome. Critchley (1982) has also suggested that disorders of chemical messenger regulation within subcortical and limbic structures may be relevant.

The symptom of coprolalia has been difficult for most neurologists to reconcile with an organic condition. It consists of the irresistible urge to utter socially unacceptable words usually of a scatological nature without any apparent provocation and often in the most inappropriate of settings, thus differing clearly from normal cursing. The obscenities are often uttered loudly with an unusual cadence or pitch and sometimes with imprecise pronounciation of phonemes. Like other vocal tics they tend to occur at the beginning or end of phrases interrupting the flow but not the rhythm of conversation. Swearing is a familiar occurrence in most societies and is particularly likely to occur when the speaker is surprised, frightened, disappointed or stressed. It is most commonly heard in adolescent males where it may be used to reinforce masculinity amongst peer groups and relieve inner emotional tensions. Coprolalia has been regarded as a hostile reaction towards authority and, anal-libidinal in nature, it is said by some to be particularly likely to occur in inflexible individuals who are afraid of punishment and have strict over-exigeant parents. As with other psychogenic theories relating to Gilles de la Tourette syndrome no consensus can be obtained from the literature and these quasi-scientific explanations make for unsatisfying reading. Coprolalia can occur in association with organic disorders such as encephalitis lethargica and has been reported together with tics after the administration of drugs known to modify central dopaminergic activity. Aphasics in their efforts to communicate occasionally erupt with a stream of involuntary profanities which are not always obviously linked with frustration. Habitual stutterers may fluently admonish themselves with a series of oaths after struggling for minutes to produce even a single word.

In the Anglo-Saxon culture, obscenities fall into two broad groups; those words related to basic physical acts such as copulation, defecation and urination, and religious profanities. In current parlance these are approximately equally distributed although generally the religious profanities shock less and are more socially acceptable. In patients with coprolalia there is a preponderance of four-letter physical obscenities, words such as God and hell being relatively uncommon.

Using a series of computer programmes which generates letters or spoken phonemes by a Markov process in a random fashion, Nuwer (1982) has shown that in second and third order texts which appear increasingly more like English there is an unexpected repeated occurrence of physical obscenities which, by the fourth order of processing, have virtually disappeared. This study has also been reproduced in second order German. When, rather than the letters being typed, sequences of phonemes are spoken by a computer with a loudspeaker the effect is even more apparent. From this work Nuwer concluded that coprolalia in Gilles de la Tourette syndrome might result from a short circuiting in brain function leading to the production of a series of high probability strings of phonemes.

PATHOLOGICAL DATA

In 1925 Bing reported the case of a patient who committed suicide after psychotherapy had failed to improve his multiple tics. At autopsy, meningitic thickening around the facial nerve was seen but no microscopic study of the basal ganglia was carried out. Two other more detailed neuropathological descriptions are available in the literature. The first case is that of a man who developed involuntary vocalisations and jerks at the age of 18 after an unremarkable childhood. Jerks of the head, facial grimaces, abdominal wall twitches and limb jerks appeared, frequently accompanied by guttural cries and the inapposite use of the word *cochon* and other mild oaths. He was also noted to have right hemifacial spasm and ptosis. Despite his incapacities he remained well balanced and after a non-specific deterioration in his health he died from a convulsion at the age of 30. A careful histological examination of the brain was conducted four hours after death with particular attention to the motor pathways. No evidence of any disease process was found (De Wulf and van Bogaert, 1941). The second case was reported by Clauss and Balthasar in two articles. At the age of 3 a male infant developed facial twitches which got steadily worse over the next two to three years. After scarlet fever the movements subsided for a few years but when aged 10 the child again developed head shaking, limb jerks and foot stamping. By the age of 12 he was uttering inarticulate sounds and involuntary obscenities. Over the next few years he remained restless with body jerks and his speech was interrupted by inappropriate vocal tics. Tongue and lip biting and striking himself in the face to prevent expletives occurred commonly. His last years were spent in institutional care and he died aged 42 from a pulmonary embolus. The autopsy was performed 24 hours after death when the brain was normal to the naked eye examination. Non-specific findings included scattered collections of lymphocytes in the subarachnoid and some perivascular spaces and an area of neuronal loss in one thalamus.

However, what Balthasar believed to be of considerable significance was an increase in the packing density of neurones within the corpus striatum and an increase in the relative number of small neurones per unit volume compared with those found in the normal adult.

These findings were carefully checked by comparative cell counts with normal controls and he concluded that hypoplasia of the corpus striatum was characteristic of Gilles de la Tourette syndrome.

At the First International Gilles de la Tourette Syndrome Symposium in New York in 1981, Richardson (1982) reviewed these two cases, coming down firmly in favour of de Wolf and van Bogaert's conclusion that no distinctive histological abnormality can as yet be attributed to Gilles de la Tourette syndrome. At the end of his presentation Hassler rose to the microphone and informed the audience that he had seen the relevant slides and had discussed them with Oscar Vogt who had himself reviewed them with Balthasar. All three were of the opinion that dwarfism of spiny neurones without gliosis was present in the caudate and putamen.

CLINICAL DESCRIPTION

A solitary eye blink or head toss is the usual presenting feature at around the age of 7 years. Subsequently the child's normal motor behaviour becomes swamped by innumerable constantly changing muscle jerks which ebb and flow in their intensity. Some patients actually present with a whole host of simultaneously occurring tics including vocalisations, but it is more usual for vocal tics to appear one or two years later. As in idiopathic tic there is a strong predilection for the head and neck area, and the relative frequency of tics in various parts of the body bears a rough correlation with the area of the motor cortex which represents that region (Fig. 3.1). The jerking movements are at times so frequent and severe that secondary complications occur including

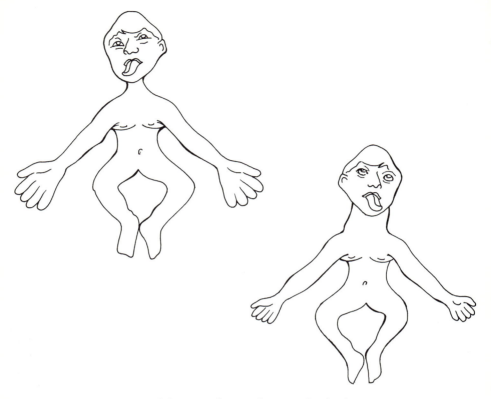

Figure 3.1 *A comparison of the cortical motor homunculus (top) with a similar schematic picture of the relative incidence of tics in different body areas.*

cervical   radiculopathies,   peripheral   nerve   compression   and   chronic conjunctivitis.

Vocal tics Vocal tics are a diagnostic prerequisite of Gilles de la Tourette syndrome and consist of a wide range of inarticulate noises and sounds which vary in intensity and type over time (Table 3.2). They most commonly appear around the age of 10 years, but occur as the presenting feature of the illness in about one-sixth of patients. The noise is often loud and distressing and emitted with an altered pitch and volume. Laryngeal tics are commonest and include barks, grunts, coughs and throat clearing. Lingual tics include hisses and clicks, nasal tics, snorts and sniffs, and labial tics, lip smacking, spitting and raspberry noises. Many of these sounds resemble the cries of animals or collo-quial, emotionally-charged exclamations. Gilles de la Tourette believed that each vocalisation was associated with a muscular movement such as a jump or a tic, but this is not now considered to be an invariable accompaniment. They usually occur during speech rather than in periods of silence and particularly at times when a normal speaker would produce hesitation phenomena such as

Table 3.2. VOCAL TICS

Grunt	Deep breathing
Throat clearing	Belch
Bark	Hoot
Sniff	Ooh
Snort	Hum
Ugh	Hiss
Ah	Sucking noise
Gulp	Growl
Squeak	Yahoo
Shriek	Pant
Spitting	Sh, sh, sh
Hiccough	Wa wa
Click	Quack
Raspberry noises	T, T, T, T
Gasp	Ha, ha, ha

filled pauses, word repetitions and interjections. Frank (1978) reported that vocal tics most commonly occur at the end of sentences or clauses, thus occurring in synchrony with the overall speech rhythm and not impeding normal communication. Martindale (1977) noted that the average length of sentence containing a vocal tic was 23 words compared with 12 words in those without a tic. Vocal tics occurred most commonly at syntactical breaking points between phrases and sentences and tended to occur most before words of low information or uncertainty and after words of high information or certainty. Sentences containing a tic also tended to have more words with connotations of passivity, goodness and weakness. Vocal tics also tended to occur before words conveying the meaning of strength and badness and after words implying goodness and weakness.

About one-third of patients utter emotionally charged words in inappropriate settings which are of great personal significance to the individual. These words are often spoken oddly with unusual emphasis on particular syllables as a result of contraction of the diaphragm or abdominal muscles. Normal prosody can be severely disrupted as a result of staccato, harsh intonations or sudden inaudible whispers. One of the patients at the National Hospital would occasionally shout out the word 'cat' and another repeated the word 'Elvis'. Some patients also have mild language difficulties with poor speech output and excessive false starts, repetitions and hesitations. A few patients stammer as well and I have also seen a boy with associated spasmodic dysphonia.

Coprolalia Coprolalia occurs in up to 60% of Northern European, American and Chinese patients, but is relatively rare in the Japanese (Table 3.3). It usually appears in early adolescence (Table 3.3) and remissions are common. Shapiro et al (1978) reported the exceptional case of an 11-year-old

Table 3.3.

	United States (Shapiro et al, 1978)	United Kingdom (Lees et al, 1984)	COPROLALIA Hong Kong (Lieh Mak et al, 1982)	Japan (Nomura and Segawa, 1982)
Mean age at onset	12	14	14	9.5
Frequency % total population	60%	39%	58%	Quasi — 19% True — 4%
Commonest words	Fuck Shit Cunt Motherfucker	Fuck Cunt Shit Bastard	Tiu (fuck) Shui (useless person) Tiu ma (motherfucker) Tiu so (aunt fucker)	Kusobaba (shit grandma) Chikusho (son of a bitch) Female genitalia and breasts

boy, the son of middle class parents, who, at the age of 4 when being cradled lovingly by his mother, responded by uttering the word 'fuck'. This sequence of events then occurred regularly and the mother became so upset that she stopped holding the child altogether. By the age of 5 he was rushing to the bathroom uttering strings of foul obscenities and by the age of 11 his swearing was so frequent he had become socially handicapped. In Shapiro's series, coprolalia was the presenting feature of the disorder in 6% but in the United Kingdom study none of the cases presented in this particular way.

Coprolalia must be clearly distinguished from voluntary cursing in response to provocation. It occurs without any appropriate stimulus, and the obscenity is usually emitted in a loud abrupt fashion sometimes with imprecise pronunciation of phonemes. In common with vocal tics it usually breaks through in the pauses between sentences but there are some patients who repeatedly utter the same swear word over and over again. Many patients experience the repetitive thought of an obscene word without actually uttering it — so-called mental coprolalia. Others attempt to conceal or attenuate the curse by verbalising only the first syllable such as 'cu cu' for 'cunt', or altering a letter such as 'cuck' as a substitute for 'fuck'. Other patients use thinly disguised euphemisms. All these seem to be ploys to damp down the social embarrassment while still affording maximal relief from inner tension. Some patients use long strings of obscenities such as 'huckleberry, fuckleberry, fuck, fuck'. Another patient of mine repeated the work 'fuck' over and over again almost like a mantra. Interestingly this young man also experienced frequent neuroleptic-induced oculogyric crises at which time the obscenities would temporarily cease.

Coprolalia is the most distressing and socially disruptive symptom of Gilles de la Tourette syndrome. Children have their mouths washed out with soap and adults are ridiculed or ostracised by workmates and strangers. Social events like going to the cinema or church are precluded and many of the more severely affected patients lead curious subterranean existences hidden away from the mainstream of society. Attempts to suppress the obscenities for any prolonged period of time leads to unbearable mental stress and patients may be forced to excuse themselves to seek a public lavatory where they then release a stream of foul language. In the doctor's surgery or when hard at work symptoms may be mild, but as soon as the individual returns to the haven of his own home swearing increases, occasionally to such a degree that modification to the home has to be made to insulate neighbours from the babble of foul language.

Copropraxia This is less common than coprolalia but occurs in up to one-quarter of patients (see Table 3.4). Most of these have additional coprolalia and in some an obscene gesture occurs as a substitute for a concealed curse. The gestures are culturally determined but in Anglo-Saxon orientated societies the palm-back V sign, simulated masturbation movements, forearm jerks with the fist clenched, and clenched fist with extended index finger are commonest.

Echophenomena Echolalia occurs at some time in about 50% of cases and echopraxia in about 25%. A number also develop palilalia with recurrent

Table 3.4. COMPLEX MOVEMENTS

Touching (objects, others, self)
Hitting (self, objects, others)
Squatting
Jumping
Stamping
Turning in circles
Rocking
Kneeling
Throwing objects
Smelling
Kicking
Walking backwards
Rubbing movements
Making fist
Bending trunk
Cracking fingers
Shooting hand out
Twiddling fingers
Lifting knee to chin
Exaggerated startle
Face covering
Kicking one heel with the other foot
Pulling down pants
Drooping of head
Body hunching
Skipping

perseveration of the last word or two of a sentence. Like coprolalia, echolalia tends to be welded on to the clinical picture in adolescence or early adult life and spontaneous remissions are common. In conversation some patients echo whole sentences whereas others restrict themselves to a few key words. Some will jerk and echo their own name on being called. Many imitate the noises of animals or celebrities' voices on television. I have heard of one patient who was able to channel his compulsion and become a competent impersonator. Another of my own patients repeated words back during a consultation in ventriloquist fashion. A further patient recorded speech on a tape-recorder and then played it back immediately. The comments of Gilles de la Tourette's fourth patient are illuminating:

> In listening to a discussion I was seized by an almost irrepressible urge to repeat a word or the end of a sentence. I needed all my strength and sense of decency to hold back from repeating this word out loud; as I could only restrain myself part way.

The patient would say out loud particular words when reading and when left to his own devices would repeat words incessantly:

> Furthermore, every intellectual faculty for the moment is absorbed by the word or sentence that is being repeated so that my train of thought is usually lost. The word heard or read rises to one's lips to be repeated at varying intervals, but always coincident with or at the end of the tormenting muscle jerks.

Imitation of other people's body language and mannerisms is the commonest form of echopraxia. Some patients also perform senseless non-obscene gestures over and over again such as saluting, thumbs up or victory V signs. Motor perseveration with the repetition of a spontaneously occurring movement or gesture is also common.

Complex movements Strange antics and mannerisms occur very frequently and add to the bizarre appearance of these patients (Table 3.4). Compulsive touching of objects or people is most frequent. Popular items to touch include fires, irons, hot plates, lighted cigarettes, door handles, railings, floors and fabrics with an erotic texture such as fur, velvet, satin and silk. Touching of breasts, bottoms and hair also occurs and other objects which had a particular fascination for individual patients in the United Kingdom study included heads, noses, lips, rounded stones and sharp knives.

Striking, usually directed towards the patient's own body, occurs in about a third of patients and tends to be commoner in females. Punching or hitting the head and head banging are the most frequent manifestations. Less commonly self-inflicted lacerations and bites or walking deliberately into things are seen. Several cases of detached retinae as a result of constant head trauma have now been reported and one patient in the United Kingdom study gouged his eye badly by picking and scratching, and another died from a subdural haematoma caused by repetitive punching of his own head. Lip chewing and finger mutilation do not occur.

BEHAVIOURAL DISORDERS

Emotional disturbances and difficulties in social adaptation are common in children with Gilles de la Tourette syndrome. Many parents report that their affected child behaves differently from their other siblings from an early age, being fretful, restless and over-sensitive. A number of children develop a reactive depression with irritability, withdrawal and temper tantrums or may compensate with vivacious, energetic and often humorous behaviour. Severely affected children experience educational difficulties stemming from restless-ness, poor attention, difficult interpersonal relationships and learning problems. In the United Kingdom study (Lees et al, 1984), 10 of the 18 children were easily distractable, emotionally immature and 'behind at school'. Four of these had selective visual memory defects and three specific reading and writing difficulties. Shapiro et al (1978) considered 58% of their patients to have atten-tion deficit syndrome and Lucas et al (1967) noted similar learning deficits with poor motor control, directional confusion and poor space utilisation and planning in 10 of their 15 patients. Self-destructive behaviour, uncontrollable aggressive outbursts, inappropriate sexual activity and antisocial and delinquent behaviour are all also commonly reported (Nee et al, 1980). Bizarre fantasies including a fascination for knives, sadistic thoughts about hurting children or loved ones and perverse Oedipal fantasies also occasionally occur. Some patients develop obsessional rituals or recurrent short-lived phobias. Wilson et al (1982) found a higher degree of behaviour disturbance in 21 children with Gilles de la Tourette syndrome than in normal age-matched controls, comparing the difficulties in magnitude to those seen in problem children in special classes. They commented that the behaviour disturbance was variable and that those children with higher intelligence quotients and relatively fewer tics were better balanced than the rest. They believed the behaviour disorder to be an integral component of the illness but stressed that reduction in tic severity was not always associated with an improvement in behaviour. Golden (1977a) considered only three of his 15 children with the disorder to have major personality problems, but eight had learning difficulties and three were hyperactive. Shapiro and Shapiro (1981) have reported that up to 85% of their patients continued to show mild to moderate behavioural difficulties into adult life and considered this to be a reactive response to the social handicaps caused by the movement disorder. Asam (1979, 1982) has suggested, however, that the severity of the personality disturbance may decrease to some degree with increasing age. Only 50% of Shapiro's male patients married compared with 72% of females although divorce tended to be higher in the female group (44% compared with 12.5% of the males).

PSYCHOPATHOLOGY

Although there is unquestionably a high psychiatric morbidity in Gilles de la Tourette syndrome it is often remarkable how intact affected individuals remain in the face of the most appalling social and physical handicaps. There is no evidence to support the earlier view that most patients become psychotic during the later stages of the disorder. In the United Kingdom study of 44 adult patients only two exhibited ideas of reference and none were psychotic as defined by the presence of hallucinations or delusions. Fernando (1967) in his review of 69 cases found only two who had become long-stay inmates of a psychiatric hospital as a result of psychotic illness. Shapiro et al (1972) found three schizophrenics and five unspecified psychotics out of a group of 34 patients with Gilles de la Tourette syndrome but concluded that schizophrenia and other psychoses were not major factors in the aetiology nor a concomitant of the condition.

Depression on the other hand seems to be common. Twenty-five of the 44 patients in the United Kingdom study rated themselves as mild to severely depressed on the Beck Depression Rating Scale. The mean scores for neuroticism, borderline personality ratings and obsessional traits were also higher than normal but could possible be explained by the associated presence of depression. High scores also occurred on hostility rating scales and anxiety trait scales when compared with normals and these seemed to be relatively independent of depression.

A number of studies have suggested a high incidence of obsessional compulsive illness (Morphew and Sim, 1969; Nee et al, 1980; Montgomery et al, 1982). Mental fixations are a striking feature in a number of patients who become plagued by the pressure of their own bizarre internal fantasies. The original thought is often seeded during ordinary conversation, but then continues to reverberate in the patient's mind over and over again, often to the exclusion of all other mental activity. A number of patients, including one described originally by Charcot, suffer with arithomania, the repetition of sequences of figures over and over to themselves in their head or the eccentric counting of numbers. One of my patients for example always counted in threes, however large the figures involved, whereas another filled pages of notebooks with arithmetical hieroglyphics. Other patients experience *folie du doute*, some taking elaborate detours to avoid passing certain houses or streets on their way to and from work. It has been pointed out that other features of obsessional compulsive illness may be lacking in these patients such as rigidity, lack of affect, perfectionism, isolation and rationalisation.

It is clear from the available data that there is no single psychiatric illness causing the motor manifestations of Gilles de la Tourette syndrome. Whether neurotic illness could act as a trigger for the development of the disorder or is merely a reactive response to the physical disabilities is unclear. It is known, however, that minor brain damage can increase the incidence of behavioural disorders and that basal ganglia damage such as occurs in Parkinson's disease may lead to a higher incidence of psychopathology than occurs in matched controls with comparable physical disability.

NEUROPSYCHOLOGICAL ABNORMALITIES

Early reports which suggested that patients with multiple tics were above average intelligence (Mahler et al, 1945) have not been confirmed. In fact there appears to be a normal range of intelligence on WAIS or WISC testing in large series of patients (Shapiro et al, 1978; Lees et al, 1984). Gilles de la Tourette syndrome may also occur in the mentally retarded (Ismeuth, 1979). Two studies, however, have reported a significant superiority of verbal over performance abilities (Shapiro et al, 1978; Incagnoli and Kane, 1982). In Shapiro's study this was most marked in the adult patients who appeared to have particular difficulties with the block design test. The performance WISC test of digit symbol and object assembly presented difficulties for the children and 40% of both adults and children were considered organically impaired on the Bender-Gestalt test. These results could not be explained by the patients' medication. Most of these findings were not confirmed in the United Kingdom study in which only three of 50 patients had a verbal IQ greater than the performance IQ by 15 points or more and two had a performance IQ greater than the verbal IQ by a similar margin. Different patient populations might explain the differences.

Specific deficits in non-constructional visuopractic abilities — impaired coding, written arithmetic and copying tasks — (Incagnoli and Kane, 1983) and in spatial memory, verbal fluency and auditory discrimination have also been reported (Sutherland et al, 1982). Dysfunction of the right cerebral hemisphere has been proposed as the cause for all these abnormalities (Sutherland et al, 1982). On the contrary, Bonnet (1982) administered the Luria-Nebraska neuropsychological test battery to four patients who were not receiving medication and concluded that there appeared to be a relatively greater dysfunction in the left parieto-occipital region. In general, however, he concluded that the abnormalities were subtle and the patients appeared functionally intact when compared with controls. Joschko and Rourke (1982) also failed to find any major neuropsychological abnormalities, although they did note some perseveration on tests in which no feedback regarding performance was given to the child.

BIOCHEMICAL DATA

The measurement of monoamines and neuropeptides and receptor binding studies have not as yet been carried out on post-mortem brain tissue. Biochemical abnormalities have been reported in urine, blood and cerebrospinal fluid although the small number of samples, methodological differences between studies, medication effects and the usual drawbacks of these indirect methods preclude any definite conclusions.

A number of investigators have determined baseline lumbar cerebrospinal fluid homovanillic acid levels and a few studies have also been carried out following probenecid loading. The early studies reported normal (Shapiro et al, 1978) or even raised baseline levels (van Woert et al, 1976), but more recent papers have recorded low levels (Butler et al, 1979; Cohen et al, 1979). Butler and colleagues studied nine children (mean age 9.9 years) and 39 controls. All medication was stopped three weeks before lumbar puncture, baseline and post-probenecid samples were obtained in the patients and baseline samples in the controls. Analysis revealed a lower baseline homovanillic acid level and a trend towards lower levels of 5-hydroxyindoleacetic acid with normal 3-methoxy-4-hydroxy phenyl glycol levels. Cohen and colleagues measured CSF monoamine metabolite levels in 10 children (mean age 10.6 years). Results revealed lower homovanillic acid/log probenecid ratios and 5-hydroxyindoleacetic acid/log probenecid ratios compared with controls although no baseline homovanillic acid or 5-hydroxyindoleacetic acid differences occurred. These two studies hint at the possibility of a reduction in brain dopamine and possibly also 5-hydroxytryptamine. Several possible explanations exist including reduced central dopamine turnover, secondary effects following neuroleptic withdrawal or long-term adaptation to super-sensitive receptors. Singer et al (1982) have claimed that there is an exaggerated pharmacological response to small doses of haloperidol in patients with Gilles de la Tourette syndrome and a marked rise in CSF homovanillic acid levels, favouring the notion that Gilles de la Tourette syndrome might be caused by hypersensitivity of a subpopulation of dopamine receptors. The measurement of prolactin levels, however, as an index of dopamine receptor activity has failed to reveal any abnormalities. Shapiro et al (1984) have reported raised platelet monoamine oxidase and plasma amine oxidase levels.

Most studies have failed to detect any disorder of central noradrenaline although Ang et al (1982) have reported low urinary methoxyhydroxy phenyl-glycol levels in 25 cases, some of whom had never received medication. An elevation of red cell choline levels has also been reported but its significance is obscure (Comings et al, 1982). No abnormalities of whole blood or cerebro-spinal fluid gamma aminobutyric acid have been found (van Woert et al, 1982).

Van Woert et al (1976) were impressed by the vague clinical similarities between Gilles de la Tourette syndrome and the inherited disorder of purine metabolism, the Lesch-Nyhan syndrome. In a survey of 111 severe ticqueurs, a family history of gout was obtained in 24% and self-destructive behaviour plus a family history of hyperuricaemia was recorded in 13%. Moldofsky et al (1974), however, reported normal serum uric acid levels and red cell purine phosphoribosyl transferase levels in Gilles de la Tourette syndrome. Van Woert et al (1977), while confirming these findings, noted that the hypoxanthine guanine phosphoribosyl transferase levels from haemolysates of patients with Gilles de la Tourette syndrome were less stable and that on purification multiple enzyme peaks could be separated by isoelectric focusing, closely resembling the peaks seen in the enzyme fraction in patients with the Lesch-Nyhan syndrome. No consistent abnormalities of copper or calcium metabolism have been found in Gilles de la Tourette syndrome and acanthocytes are absent in the peripheral blood. Cerebrospinal fluid protein glucose and cell counts are normal.

NEUROPHYSIOLOGICAL DATA

A high frequency of electroencephalographic abnormalities have been reported in many of the series of patients with Gilles de la Tourette syndrome. Fernando (1967) in his review of 67 cases in the Anglo-Saxon literature reported abnormalities in about a quarter of patients and Abuzzahab and Anderson (1976) recorded an even higher figure of 44% in their review of 102 cases. Shapiro et al (1978) reviewed 11 separate studies; 82 (66%) of 127 cases were reported as having electroencephalographic abnormalities. In their own study of 79 patients, 71% of the children had EEG abnormalities compared with 25% of the adults. If only the children without associated hyperactivity and with moderate or marked abnormalities were included, the figure fell to around 45%. The abnormalities were usually of a non-specific sort including slowing and disorganisation of background activity, paroxysmal features with sharp waves, and an occasional patient with frank epileptic activity. Seven (23%) of the 39 patients with abnormalities were receiving neuroleptics. Many of the patients also had soft neurological signs.

In other studies, however, a much lower incidence of EEG abnormalities has been found. Bergen et al (1981) excluded patients with obvious signs of neurological dysfunction, and when those taking neuroleptics were also eliminated only four of 23 (17%) had abnormal records and these were of an inconsistent sort. From the United Kingdom study (Lees et al, 1984) only eight patients (13%) had EEG abnormalities and in two of these the excess slow wave activity may have been due to concurrent neuroleptics. Krumholz and colleagues found abnormalities including central spikes, generalised and paroxysmal slow wave activity in only 12.5% of 40 cases with a mean age of 14 years.

Different thresholds for defining epileptiform activity, and differing populations, some with a higher incidence of associated brain damage or drug effects, may explain some of these discrepancies. The frequency of muscle artefact on many of the records also makes interpretation difficult and some of the finer muscular discharges are identical to those reported in hyperactive children with Prechtl's choreiform syndrome (Prechtl and Stemmer, 1962) (Fig. 3–2).

It seems safe to conclude that no characteristic EEG abnormality exists which might reflect the pathophysiological basis of the movement disorder. Taken as a whole the findings would be most in keeping with some of the patients having additional heterogeneous central nervous system damage. Visual brain-stem and somatosensory evoked potentials have also so far failed to reveal any consistent abnormality (Krumholz et al, 1983).

NEURORADIOLOGICAL DATA

Air encephalography performed on a small number of patients has revealed no definite abnormalities, although dilatation of one lateral ventricle has been reported in two of seven cases. Two studies have failed to find any abnormalities on computerised axial tomography of the brain (Fog and Pakkenberg, 1980; Lees et al, 1984). A further study reported some sort of abnormality in six of 16 patients including mild asymmetrical dilatation of the lateral ventricles and prominent sylvian fissures or cortical sulci; four of these patients also had EEG abnormalities (Caparulo et al, 1981). Careful controlled studies are needed to evaluate the significance of these relatively minor findings.

CLINICAL PHARMACOLOGY

THE DOPAMINE HYPOTHESIS

As a result of the therapeutic effects of centrally acting dopamine antagonists on the symptoms of Gilles de la Tourette syndrome, it has been proposed

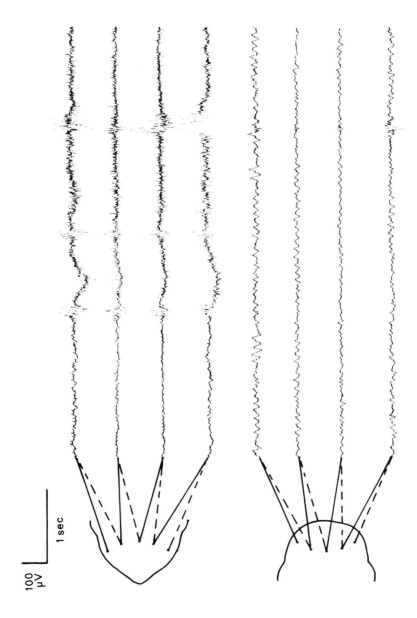

***Figure* 3.2** *Electroencephalographic recording showing unilateral muscle activity corresponding to tics.* (*By kind permission J. Neurol. Neurosurg. Psychiat. 1984, vol. 47, p. 5.*)

that excess dopaminergic activity might underlie the symptoms of this disorder. Available clinical pharmacological studies, however, provide no confirmation for this although it remains the most attractive of the currently proposed neurochemical hypotheses.

Dopamine receptor antagonists Shapiro et al (1978) reviewed 41 publications on the use of haloperidol in 144 patients. 112 (77.8%) benefited but the authors drew attention to the lower success rate (67.5%) in the studies after 1974 compared with the 89.7% success rate in the early investigations. They also examined the reasons for therapeutic failure which included premature withdrawal because of adverse effects, poor compliance and failure to titrate the dosage to obtain maximum benefit and minimum side-effects. Recasting the data using only those patients in which outcome could be accurately evaluated, 91.2% of cases were improved. In their own extensive studies 86% of patients were substantially improved by a mean dose of 4 mg/d (2–150 mg) of haloperidol for at least one year. The remainder discontinued treatment because of side-effects. A further follow-up study by the same authors on 78 patients given haloperidol between 1965 and 1973 revealed that four had spontaneously remitted, 59 were still on medication with an average improvement of 79% and the others who were on either no medication or other drug treatments had an average improvement of 25%. The original severity of tics did not correlate with the therapeutic response. The degree of improvement, however, seemed to correlate directly with the duration of therapy.

Pimozide (2–30 mg/d) has also been demonstrated in a number of studies to be equally efficacious (Debray et al, 1972; Ross and Moldofsky, 1978), producing improvement in 70% of 42 patients in one study (Shapiro and Shapiro, 1982). Fluphenazine (8–24 mg/d) and trifluoperazine (10–25 mg/d) were as effective as haloperidol in a double-blind placebo controlled study (Borison et al, 1982). Other phenothiazines such as chlorpromazine (Levy and Ascher, 1968) and penfluridol (Shapiro and Shapiro, 1982) produce beneficial effects although a review of 81 patient trials of neuroleptics other than haloperidol and pimozide by Abuzzahab and Anderson (1976) suggested they may be less effective. In my own experience, the substituted benzamide sulpiride, a D2 receptor antagonist, also markedly attentuates tic frequency.

Dopamine synthesis inhibitors and dopamine depleting drugs Alphamethylparatyrosine (3000 mg/d), a dopamine synthesis inhibitor, was given to six patients in a single-blind placebo study and lessened tics appreciably in three. Two failed to respond and one withdrew from the study after a week because of fatigue and sedation. Crystalluria reversed by forced diuresis occurred in four cases and bradykinesia, akathisia and oculogyric crises occurred as other side-effects (Sweet et al, 1976). Tetrabenzaine, a dopamine depleting drug, given to 14 patients to a maximum dose of 300 mg/d led to a marked initial improvement in four but this was not always sustained and side-effects including sedation, akathisia and bradykinesia were common (Sweet et al, 1976).

Dopamine receptor agonists L-dopa in doses of 3 g a day combined with the peripheral dopa decarboxylase inhibitor, carbidopa (100–200 mg/d), led to a dose-dependent increase in tic frequency with the appearance of reversible chorea and dystonia. No effect, however, occurred in two other patients given lower doses (Sweet et al, 1976). Apomorphine (0.5–1.5 mg subcutaneously), and piribedil (3 mg intravenously) led to a mild decrease in tic frequency although side-effects such as nausea and drowsiness made interpretation of these studies difficult (Sweet et al, 1976). Amphetamines, which increase cate-cholamine release and inhibit reuptake, occasionally exacerbate tics, but more commonly in therapeutic doses for hyperactivity syndrome have no deleterious effects.

Drugs which modify noradrenaline transmission The alpha-2-noradrenergic autoreceptor agonist clonidine (0.05–0.9 mg/d) which inhibits presynaptic noradrenaline release has been shown to reduce tic severity by about 40% in a number of studies (Cohen et al, 1980; Bruun, 1982a) and to have a beneficial effect on the associated behavioural disturbances. Disulfiram, a dopamine beta hydroxylase inhibitor (1–1.5 g/d) given to two patients, produced inconclusive results (Sweet et al, 1976).

Drugs which modify central acetylcholine transmission The studies using drugs known to modify cholinergic transmission are conflicting but it has been claimed that cholinergic hypoactivity might be involved in the pathogenesis of Gilles de la Tourette syndrome. Physostigmine (1 mg subcutaneously) produced no beneficial effects in five patients in one acute study (Sweet et al, 1976) but in another it was claimed to reduce tic frequency (Stahl and Berger, 1980a). Tanner et al (1982) demonstrated a consistent reduction in the severity of motor tics and an exacerbation of vocal tics after scopolamine injections (0.6–0.8 mg) and propantheline and the effect was reversed by physostigmine (2–2.4 mg). Choline produced benefit in only one of three patients and the unpleasant odour the drug produced led to its discontinuation. All three of these patients, however, derived sustained benefit from Lecithin (50 g/d) (Barbeau, 1980). 2 g/d of choline led to mild reduction of tics in another study (Stahl and Berger, 1980b) whereas in a recent double-blind trial lecithin 45 g/d produced no significant benefit (Polinsky et al, 1980). Deanol has also been reported to help individual patients in several studies (Finney et al, 1981).

Drugs which modify central 5-hydroxytryptamine transmission Van Woert (1982) reported no benefit in nine patients given 400–1100 mg/d of L-5-hydroxy-tryptophan and 200 mg/d of Carbidopa. In those with associated hyperactivity syndrome, there was a marked aggravation of behavioural difficulties with increased aggressiveness, floor pacing, head banging and agitation. L-trypto-phan (5.5 g/d) had no effect on tic severity in two patients (Sweet et al, 1976).

Methysergide, a 5-hydroxytryptamine antagonist (10 mg/d), also produced no effects in two patients treated for two weeks (Sweet et al, 1976) but Crosley (1979) claimed that cyproheptadine, another 5-hydroxytryptamine antagonist, aggravated tics and vocalisations in one boy with Gilles de la Tourette syndrome.

DIFFERENTIAL DIAGNOSIS

A combination of multiple abrupt stereotyped jerks with a predilection for the head and neck and unwanted vocalisations beginning in childhood presents a unique clinical picture. Diagnostic difficulties arise largely because of its relative rarity which means that most practitioners will never have encountered a case. Furthermore, the clinical distinction between chorea, myoclonus and tics may on occasions be extremely difficult. In the United Kingdom study there was (Lees et al, 1984) a mean delay of 11 years from onset before the correct diagnosis was made and most of the adult patients had received wrong diagnoses during childhood. Several patients had spent considerable periods in psychiatric institutions and received therapies as varied as behavioural treatment, eversion therapy, electro-shock and insulin coma treatment. The commonest misdiagnosis is Sydenham's chorea. This disorder is now probably rarer in the West than Gilles de la Tourette syndrome and the involuntary movements are less repetitive and more abnormal in appearance than tics. They almost invariably subside within a few months of their onset, although recurrences can occur and vocalisations are not part of acute rheumatic chorea. The rare condition, benign non-progressive hereditary chorea, may provide diagnostic difficulties although again vocalisations do not occur as part of the clinical picture. Some childhood myoclonic syndromes may resemble multiple tics but the movements are uncontrollable, more often in the limbs and often symmetrical. Acquired causes of Gilles de la Tourette syndrome also need to be excluded and enquiry about neuroleptic and psychomotor stimulant ingestion should always be made. Inexcusable mis-diagnoses include schizophrenia, obsessive compulsive psychoses, hysteria, epilepsy and personality disorders.

COURSE

Most cases begin between the ages of 5 and 7 with body and vocal tics and 90% of patients have presented by the age of 10 years. Onset as early as 2 years has been reported and occasionally the first symptoms appear in adolescence. It is a lifelong illness which is usually at its worst in adolescence and young adult life. Gilles de la Tourette regarded the condition as untreatable and commented *une fois ticqueur, toujours ticqueur*. In his original paper he wrote as follows about the course of the illness:

> The progression of this condition, as much as we can tell, is slow and insidious. There are times when each symptom appears to be exacerbated so that all three

symptoms increase simultaneously, the muscular jerks, the echolalia and the copro-lalia. In between periods of exacerbation there are times of remission or diminution. The cause of such remissions is poorly understood and they are quite variable among subjects. When they occur the muscular twitches become less frequent and less pronounced, the obscenities become only rarely audible and the echolalia disap-pears. Unfortunately these are not cures, since any remission is incomplete and never long lasting, the illness sleeps but does not disappear. Even during this 'somnolence' muscular twitches are still present and although they are diminished, one can still identify them perhaps only in an arm or more often in the face. These periods of remission may be prolonged for up to one year but at an unpredictable moment the problem reappears with the old symptoms as pronounced as before. These continue until the day when another remission finally comes. Could a patient eventually overcome the problem altogether after many episodes of remission? We cannot be absolutely certain but from our case histories we would conclude that the condition never completely disappears, hence there may be remissions but not cures.

This is in accordance with the findings of the United Kingdom study in which two patients remitted for more than a year only to relapse again and a further eight were virtually asymptomatic for several months before the disorder returned. Complete remissions, however, undoubtedly rarely occur (Dockner, 1959), and Fernando (1976) found that all three of his female patients followed for 10 years had adapted well to adult life and lost or virtually lost their tics in their late teens or early 20s. Milman (1976) also reported apparent complete remission of tics in male patients by the time they reached adult life. 3.3% of the patients in Abbuzahab and Anderson's International Registry spon-taneously remitted although the time period is not given. Coprolalia frequently remits and Shapiro et al (1978) give a figure of 19% remission for this symptom.

Most cases live out their full life-span and late psychosis is extremely rare. Nevertheless, personality scars are quite common and there is a high incidence of psychopathology. Lucas (1976) found that his cases who had attention defi-cits and hyperactivity as children tended to become isolated, socially inept young adults even when their tics had improved. Many had uncontrollable tempers and others had chronic anxieties or depression. Job records were often erratic and as a group they had difficulty accepting authority. Children who had not had behavioural disorders adapted much better and generally led normal lives, though they too tended to be somewhat withdrawn and introspective. In the United Kingdom study, most of the adult patients with moderate or severe tic disorders were severely socially disadvantaged and often in spite of consider-able natural abilities were repeatedly refused employment. A number, however, were holding down highly responsible prestigious professional posts and I have come across patients making successful careers for themselves on the stage as comedians or earning a lucrative living for themselves playing in rock or jazz bands.

Shapiro et al (1976) have suggested that there may in fact be several different or overlapping disease states concealed within the diagnosis of Gilles de la Tourette syndrome. They have delineated four small subgroups which probably together account for no more than 5–10% of the total cases. The first subcategory consisted of those cases with superadded dystonic features; the second, those with a more constant and stable pattern of tics and fewer vocalisations; a third group were characterised who had sexual preoccupations, fantasies and obsessional thoughts leading to marked behavioural disorders, and the fourth rare group were those in which self-mutilation was a prominent feature.

TREATMENT

No cure exists for Gilles de la Tourette syndrome and management therefore needs to be sufficiently flexible to adjust to an individual patient's needs. Many patients, especially children with mild disease, adapt reasonably well to their disability and do not require medication. Parents in particular need sensible advice and those who have often rebuked and chastised their children in an attempt to control the tics may feel guilty on learning that their child actually has a recognisable disorder which is beyond his or her control. Some parents then in fact over-react and become over-protective thus allowing the child to become spoilt and demanding. The best advice is to deal with the child as normally as possible and encourage him to perform to the best of his ability at school. Behavioural techniques have been used for many years but there is as yet little hard evidence that they do a great deal of good. In patients with severe chronic multiple tics, drug treatment probably offers the best hope of success. Therapy should probably be commenced with a small dose of a benzodiazepine and, if this is ineffective, a trial of clonidine is worthwhile. Undoubtedly the most effective medication is a dopamine receptor antagonist drug but side-effects are common and they should be prescribed only when the patient is severely handicapped and all else has failed.

PSYCHOTHERAPY

For the large majority of patients, structured psychotherapy has no role to play. Abbuzahab and Anderson (1976) reviewed 117 patient trials and found that only 12% obtained improvement for more than six months. However, in patients with associated severe emotional or behavioural problems, treatment of the child, rather than the tic, with sympathetic counselling and education may reap enormous benefits. Informal psychotherapy may also be helpful in motivated adolescents and adults as an adjunct to drug treatment. In common with simple tics, cases of remission have been reported following psychotherapy or family therapy (Ascher, 1948; Tiller, 1978) but these may reflect spontaneous variations in the natural history of the disorder rather than specific treatment effects. Group psychotherapy may also be of benefit and certainly much of the success of the American and United Kingdom Gilles de la Tourette Associations stems from their supportive role in counselling. Some patients, however, find the close proximity of other ticqueurs actually detrimental, leading to the occurrence of a new spectrum of undesirable movements. Carbon dioxide abreaction (Michael, 1957) and hypnotherapy (Lindner and Stevens, 1967) have a few advocates but the results are generally disappointing (Fernando, 1967; Abbuzahab and Anderson, 1976). Electroshock treatment, sleep therapy and bed rest are useless, although removal from an intolerable domestic stiuation by hospital admission may be valuable.

At best, psychotherapy can be said to reduce anxiety levels and provide often badly needed emotional support. At worst, intensive psycho-analysis in poorly motivated children can lead to long-standing disenchantment with the medical profession and feelings of alienation and insecurity.

BEHAVIOURAL THERAPY

The methodological inadequacies inherent in most studies make evaluation of behavioural treatments difficult. Most reports have been uncontrolled and carried out in patients often receiving concurrent alternative therapy, follow-up periods have been short or non-existent and methods of assessment have been unreliable. Massed or negative practice was the earliest and probably still the most widely used treatment. It is based on Hullian learning theory and relies on the repetitive voluntary evocation of the offending movements ultimately building up reactive inhibition and a negative habit. A comprehensive review of the available literature suggests that massed practice is occasionally effective for simple tics but rarely helps Gilles de la Tourette syndrome (Turpin 1983).

Contingency management has also been popular and relies on operant conditioning and the differential use of techniques such as aversion shocks and time out punishments. Good short-term results in individual patients have been reported by some authors but long-term maintenance of this improvement has proved difficult (Canavan and Powell, 1981).

Habit reversal, in which a competing behavioural response is introduced gradually and systematically, has shown promise in a few studies but controlled evaluation is needed. Friedman (1980), for instance, trained a patient to substitute a neutral word for an obscenity and Azrin et al (1980) reported similarly promising results with muscle tics. Temporary reduction in tic frequency has also occurred using self-monitoring techniques but long-term follow-up studies are unavailable (Thomas et al, 1971).

Relaxation techniques designed to diminish anxiety have been shown to be of some limited use in reducing the tics during the period of treatment but no carry-over effect has been demonstrated. Desensitisation to specific triggers has also been tried. Relaxation techniques based on the theories of Bliss (1980) in which patients are required to relax individual affected muscle groups in a controlled relaxation programme are also under evaluation (Turpin, 1983).

DRUG TREATMENT

The benzodiazepines, diazepam and clonazepam, undoubtedly help some patients probably by reducing anxiety levels. However, habituation and withdrawal effects may become serious problems with chronic use. Tricyclic anti-depressants, monoamineoxidase inhibitors, barbiturates, anticonvulsants and amphetamines are ineffective. Corticosteroids have also been reported to be beneficial in one study but this remains unsubstantiated.

Cohen and his colleagues in a series of open studies have reported worth-while improvement with clonidine in about 50% of cases (Cohen et al, 1980) and these findings have been supported by a further controlled study in which seven of 12 patients showed improvement at doses of 0.25–0.9 mg/d (Borison, 1982). Other reports, however, have been less enthusiastic and Shapiro et al (1983) concluded that although, there may be a small subgroup of patients who respond well to clonidine, the results are in general considerably inferior to those obtained with dopamine antagonists. There is, however, a suggestion from the available literature that the associated behavioural disturbances (compulsive behaviour, attention deficits, frustration and intolerance) may respond better than the tics. Side-effects are relatively uncommon but include transient orthostatic hypotension, sedation, dry mouth and diarrhoea. Toler-ance to the drug may occur with long-term use and withdrawal symptoms may follow abrupt discontinuation.

Haloperidol was the first dopamine receptor antagonist to be shown to be effective in controlling tics and as a result it is still the most widely prescribed. There is little evidence to suggest that it is more efficacious or better tolerated than any of the newer antipsychotic preparations. For example, pimozide in one study in doses of 2–30 mg/d produced marked improvement in 76% of 42 patients and was judged more effective than haloperidol in about two-thirds, as effective in a quarter and less effective in only about 12% of patients (Shapiro and Shapiro, 1982). Sulpiride, the selective D2 receptor antagonist, may prove to be even more effective with fewer long-term side-effects and chlorprothixene has also shown promise in my own hands.

A starting dose of 0.25–0.5 mg of haloperidol is usually advocated with increases of 0.25–0.5 mg every seven days. To obtain the optimum results patients must be thoroughly primed about potential adverse reactions and given detailed instructions about titration of dosage. 0.5–4.5 mg/d is usually adequate in children but occasionally adults require doses of up to 100 mg/d. Treatment, however, is empirical and has to be constantly titrated over time to achieve the best effects. The dose should be kept to the lowest possible which produces tolerable suppression of symptoms. A good early prognostic sign is when patients observe that although they may feel a tic about to occur, they are able to suppress it. A rapid change from day to day in the type and pattern of tics is also claimed to be a favourable early sign that the drug is working. Coprolalia is often the first symptom to disappear followed by vocal tics and finally muscular tics. Some patients, in fact, despite obtaining a dramatic relief of their tic frequency and severity, feel worse in themselves and it has therefore been recommended that these patients take medication whilst at work during the week but have a drug holiday at weekends.

Unacceptable side-effects frequently mar the therapeutic response and necessitate withdrawal despite careful titration. Acute dystonic reactions, particularly oculogyric crises, are common and akathisia is another distressing early complaint. This subjective motor restlessness may be difficult to distinguish from the discomfort felt by many patients on attempting to suppress their tics. Other patients develop Parkinsonian features with slowness of movement and stiffness. These reversible extrapyramidal side-effects can be improved by the concurrent administration of centrally acting anticholinergic drugs and, in order to improve compliance, some authorities actually recommend prophylactic treatment with these for the first few weeks of therapy. Tardive dyskinesias are rare but can occur (Caine and Polinsky, 1981). The relative frequency of acute dyskinesias and the comparative rarity of tardive dyskinesia in neuroleptic treated patients with Gilles de la Tourette syndrome is probably due to the young age of most patients. Autonomic side-effects due to the inherent anticholinergic properties of many dopamine antagonists are frequent and include dry mouth, blurred vision, constipation and nasal congestion. Agranulocytosis, photosensitive skin rashes and jaundice are uncommon allergic effects. Commoner problems are decreased libido and weight gain and potentiation of the effect of alcohol and sedatives, again leading to poor compliance. Sedation, apathy and mild cognitive blunting are other important causes of drug intolerance. Subtle problems with attention, memory and concentration also occur, all of which appear to be dose-dependent and quite distinct from any associated bradykinesia. A considerable number of patients also develop dysphoric symptoms with depression or anxiety on starting low dose therapy. This often leads to work and school avoidance phobias (Mikkelsen et al, 1981; Bruun, 1982). Finally, Shapiro et al (1978) have used the term 'fog state' to describe dose-dependent episodes of depersonalisation, mental slowing and paranoia associated with rushing thoughts and thought fixation lasting variable periods of time from hours to days.

SURGICAL TREATMENT

Hassler and Dieckmann (1970) have carried out bilateral stereotactic thalamolysis, ablating the rostral intralaminar and medial nuclei of the thalamus in three patients with excellent results. Hassler presented a cine film showing these cases at the First International Symposium in New York. In fact the operations were carried out primarily for severe associated obsessional conpulsive neurosis, but both the tics and the psychological disturbance improved. Bilateral coagulation of the cerebellar dentate nuclei reduced myoclonic facial and diaphragmatic movements and abolished a barking noise in a further patient (Nadvornik et al, 1972). Frontal lobotomies have also been reported to produce sustained relief (Baker et al, 1962; Stevens, 1964). None of these drastic procedures can be recommended except perhaps for the most severely incapacitated case, refractory to other treatments and with marked associated behavioural disorders.

METHODS OF ASSESSMENT OF TIC DISORDERS

The variability and high rate of production of tics lead to considerable difficulties in their accurate measurement. Most research groups have relied on direct observation, sometimes supplemented by a second observer, and video recording to obtain estimates of reliability (Billings, 1978). In these studies, however, it is essential to distinguish clearly tics from other more complicated manneristic movements and fidgetiness. The high degree of situational specificity of tics (Surwillo et al, 1978) also presents problems which necessitate the observation of ticqueurs in a variety of structured and real life situations. Shapiro et al (1978) used daily rating scales made by the patient of the frequency, intensity and distribution of tic movements and Cohen et al (1980) devised a check list, which contained 29 items each rated in terms of their severity, for assessing patients with Gilles de la Tourette syndrome. Self-monitoring procedures have also been recomended (Ciminero at al , 1977), but the very act of self-monitoring may lead to substantial decreases in tic rate (Hutzell et al, 1974). A self-monitoring-only control group, therefore, should be included in any trial in which this approach is used to assess new treatments. Another difficulty which arises out of most of these methods is the difficulty in assessing a reduction in intensity of tics without necessarily any change in tic frequency. A number of authors have attempted to employ more objective methods often using time-consuming and sophisticated instrumentation. These include EMG recordings, telemetry, time lapsed photography and the frequency of EMG activity on the electroencephalographic record (Sainsbury 1954; Moldofsky, 1971, Trimble et al, 1980).

The relative rarity of Gilles de la Tourette syndrome coupled with the occurrence of spontaneous remissions, and more especially fluctuation of symptoms over time, make it virtually impossible to design clinical trials to assess new treatments which would fulfil all statistical objections. A control group and long-term follow-up with as many patients as can be marshalled are clearly mandatory and it is probably important, particularly where small numbers of patients are being used, to include a record of intercurrent life events which could markedly affect the severity of the disorder. Finally, improvement needs to be assessed not only on the basis of a reduction of tic severity but more importantly with respect to the patient's degree of social adjustment and quality of life. It has been recommended, therefore, that process measures designed to distinguish between specific and non-specific treatment effects should be incorporated in any study design, examples being the use of subjective anxiety rating scales during the course of a study or the measurement of drug metabolites.

4

Some Celebrated Ticqueurs

The undoubted social stigma imparted by the presence of tics has not impeded the rise to fame and fortune of many great men. Meige and Feindel reported that Napoleon, Molière and Peter the Great all had tics and Claudius, the Roman emperor, as well as stammering, had a number of distasteful habits:

> Claudius had a certain dignity of presence, which showed to best advantage when he happened to be standing or seated and expressing no emotion. This was because, though tall, well-built, handsome, with a fine head of white hair and a firm neck, he stumbled as he walked owing to the weakness of his knees; and because, if excited either by play or serious business, he had several disagreeable traits. These included an uncontrolled laugh, a horrible habit, under the stress of anger, of slobbering at the mouth and running at the nose, a stammer, and a persistent nervous tic – which grew so bad under emotional stress that his head would toss from side to side. (Svetonius)

James Collier, the British neurologist, would hunch his shoulder, grimace and emit a loud noisy sniff when using hyperbole to illustrate an important clinical point. Mozart appears to have suffered from both coprographia and coprolalia, and Fog has suggested he may have had Gilles de la Tourette syndrome. André Malraux was also afflicted with a number of curious tics and gesticulations.

In fact, mannerisms and to a lesser degree tics are ubiquitous, affecting all races and social strata. Many public speakers develop an eye blink, a sniff or snort or a shoulder jerk particularly when under pressure. Many professional snooker players have ritualistic stereotyped movements before making a shot and a few of the top tennis players emit loud cries before serving. Recently an American tennis player developed the habit of jerking his head round to look behind him two or three times before each serve. A Welsh rugby international second row forward would unintentionally disrupt line-outs with his involuntary head jerks and capricious extension of his arm towards an opponent. However, it is in the field of music where tics flourish most. Music has a particular fascination for many ticqueurs and some find their speed of reaction, wild movements, and yodels and cries can serve them to great advantage in the world of popular music and modern jazz. In the award-winning American documentary film about Gilles de la Tourette syndrome called *The Sudden*

Intruder, a young man finally found his *métier* playing the marimba in a Tijuana brass band, and a vocalist in a British rock duo has a repetitive eyeblink tic which he uses to great advantage in his stage performance. Some classical musicians, especially pianists, embellish their playing with flamboyant shouts or curious grimaces. Swaying back and forth, twitching of the face and shoulder or head jerking are sometimes seen in violinists. Foot tapping is an extremely common habit and a few musicians raise or lower their eyebrows, open and close their lips or gnash their teeth during a performance. In the world of classical music these habits are generally frowned upon and may be positively detrimental to the musician's career.

SAMUEL JOHNSON

The large number of diaries, letters and biographical accounts published by Dr Johnson's admirers have provided fertile source material for those physicians interested in his complicated medical history. Excellent descriptions of his childhood scrofula, his recurring melancholy and the stroke that left him dysphasic but able to write up until his death are available. He was also observed by his friends to have incessant tics and gesticulations, constant compulsive mannerisms, and to make occasional involuntary noises. The best original accounts of these movements are to be found in Frances Reynold's *Recollections* and in Boswell's *Life of Johnson*. Lord Brain frequently referred to these peculiar movements in his writings on Johnson and further details are to be found in the papers by McHenry (1967) and Murray (1979).

According to Johnson himself, he was the product of a difficult and dangerous labour and apparently did not cry for some time after birth. In childhood he suffered from scrofula which undoubtedly lowered his physical resistance and left him with poor vision. It is unclear at precisely what age his abnormal movements began but there are frequent descriptions of awkwardness as a child and at the age of 7 his appearance was described 'as little better than that of an idiot'. A teacher's description while he was at Lichfield Grammar School was of 'a great over-grown boy, rolling clumsily about on his form as his body in some peculiar way responded to his mental efforts'. At the age of 20, on coming down from Oxford University for the holidays, he experienced his first bout of severe depression which then recurred throughout his life leaving him with a deep-seated fear of insanity and of death. The first clear accounts of his convulsive starts and odd gesticulations appear in the diaries of his friends when he was a young man. Johnson himself hardly ever referred to his tics either in public or in wrting. Most people on meeting him found it quite impossible to reconcile his superb intellect and eloquence with his slovenly appearance. Hogarth, for instance, on visiting Samuel Richardson and being unaware that Johnson was in the house was reported by Boswell to have reacted in the following way:

> While he was talking, he perceived a person standing at a window in the room, shaking his head and rolling himself about in a strange ridiculous manner. He

concluded that he was an idiot, whom his relations had put under the care of Mr Richardson as a very good man.

Most of the best descriptions of his movement disorder in fact are recorded when his subsequent friends first met him, and, although it seems clear that the disorder continued throughout his life, it was largely ignored in the later writings of those who came to love and respect him. In his early twenties he was refused several jobs as a teacher because of what was described as a haughty, ill-natured manner and facial grimacing. It was considered that his bizarre movements might become the subject of ridicule by the school children. It is also reported that his gestures at this time were so extraordinary that mobs would gather round him laughing and jeering. As a result he was forced to open his own school and was fortunate enough to have David Garrick, later to become the great actor, as one of his early pupils. Johnson's oddities of manner and gesture were the subject of great amusement to Garrick who would imitate them to the immense delight of the other pupils. Even when the two grew to be close friends in later life, Garrick would continue to mimic his old master much to Johnson's annoyance.

Johnson's tics included grimacing, mouth opening, eye blinks, lip twitching and shoulder, arm and leg jerks. Relatively few detailed descriptions of these are available.

> In contrast he was alive with grotesque repulsive mannerisms and antics which became both a source of social embarrassment and amusement to all those around him. He was particularly fond of moving his hands up and down in rhythmical jerky fashion with his fingers twisted as if in a cramp. On other occasions when thinking or bored his body and head would rock rhythmically up and down. His gait was most remarkable appearing often as he weaved from side to side along the pavement as if he was locked in chains. As he lurched along his head rolling from side to side he would be at particular pains to avoid treading on any pavement crack and insist on touching every post in his path.

One of Johnson's most extraordinary habits, however, occurred at doorways as Boswell describes:

> He had another peculiarity of which none of his friends ever ventured to ask an explanation. It appeared to me some superstitious habit, which he had contracted early and from which he had never called upon his reason to disentangle for him. This was his anxious care to go out or in at a door or passage by a certain number of steps from a certain point or at least so that either his right or left foot (I am not certain which) should constantly make the first actual movement when he came close to the door or passage. Thus I conjecture: for I have, upon innumerable occasions, observed him suddenly stop, and then seem to count his steps with a deep earnestness; and when he had neglected or gone wrong in this sort of magical movement I have seen him go back again put himself in a proper posture to begin the ceremony and having gone through it break from his abstraction, walk briskly on and join his companion.

One of his most alarming habits would be when in the parlour of his lady friends or at dinner to suddenly stretch out his hand in front of him holding a full cup of tea. Upon another such occasion when at the dinner table a lady jokingly put her foot in front of Johnson's hand which was moving up and down as he sat down. This led to her shoe being knocked off to the great hilarity of the assembled guests. Johnson responded as follows:

> I know not that I have justly incurred your rebuke. The motion was involuntary and the action not intentionally rude.

When standing he would often place his feet in the most remarkable positions sometimes with both heels touching one another at angles as if trying to make some curious geometrical shape. He was also fond of repetitively twirling his fingers, rubbing his left knee with his palm or stretching his leg out in front of him. Indeed Lord Chesterfield wrote:

> His figure (without being deformed) seems made to disgrace or ridicule the common structure of the human body. His legs and arms are never in the position which according to the situation of his body they ought to be in. They are constantly employed in committing acts of hostility on the graces.

From childhood Johnson had been fond of talking to himself and was often to be heard whispering lines of Shakespeare or extracts from the Bible. On occasions, however, he would also utter audible involuntary vocalisations the commonest of which were a half whistle, a clucking sound, blowing deep respirations, moaning, humming and a curious 'too, too, too' noise. On a few occasions he would make pious ejaculations but he was never known to swear and had a low opinion of those who did. Mrs Thrale records one possible example of echolalia. Johnson had in fact spoken roughly to her and she had replied by saying, 'Oh dear, good man'. Another lady who had heard Johnson's remarks also rebuked him repeating the same phrase. Later, while lying in his chair, Johnson was heard to repeat these words over and over again in a whisper.

In the engraving by Finden of Samuel Johnson, based on a miniature painting by an unknown artist said to have been painted in 1736, and in the portrait by Joshua Reynolds in 1756 it can be seen that Johnson tended to hold his head on the right. Boswell also recorded that when Johnson was talking or thinking in a chair his head would drift over towards his right shoulder. It is not clear whether this was a persistent deformity suggestive of associated spasmodic torticollis or simply a recurrent mannerism. However, it is also reported that he would frequently bring his left hand across his chest to support his chin as a *geste antagonistique*.

Sir Joshua Reynolds, along with many other of Johnson's friends, believed his movement disorder to be psychogenically determined and not convulsive in nature.

> These motions or tricks of Dr Johnson were improperly called convulsions (which imply involuntary contortions). He could sit motionless when he was told to do as well as any other man.

And:

> When in company where he was not free or when engaged earnestly in conversation he never gave way to such habits which proves that they were not involuntary.

Johnson himself also considered them to be merely bad habits triggered by his constant state of internal turmoil. Sir Joshua Reynolds who appears to have been the most astute observer of Johnson's movements and personality provides further revealing comments:

> My opinion is, that it proceeded from a bad habit, which he had indulged himself in, of accompanying his thoughts with certain untoward actions, and those actions always appeared to me as if they were meant to reprobate some part of his past conduct. Whenever he was engaged in conversation, such thoughts were sure to rush into his mind; and for this reason any company, any employment whatever he preferred to being alone. The great business of his life (he said) was to escape from himself. This disposition he considered as a disease of his mind which nothing cured but company.

The medical profession at the time, however, believed him to be suffering from Sydenham's chorea and subsequent authorities have raised the possibility of epilepsy or athetoid cerebral palsy. It seems likely, however, that Johnson did in fact suffer from Gilles de la Tourette syndrome and would fit best into that group of patients in whom the presentation is dominated by obsessional compulsive behavioural rituals and mannerisms with relatively few tics and vocalisations.

'O'

In their book on tics, Meige and Feindel provide a fascinating biography of a 54-year-old man with Gilles de la Tourette syndrome whom they interviewed in 1901. This patient's intimate confessions helped to reinforce their view that a psychical element precedes the motor reaction in tic and that most sufferers have a fickle, impressionable childish nature. O's grandparents were consanguineous, his grandfather having had tics of the face and head and also having suffered with a stammer; his brother, sister and daughter all had tics and his brother also stammered. Meige recorded that when O was examined he appeared to be in excellent physical health, looked younger than his years and was of high intelligence being devoted to sport and physical exercise. O recalled a propensity to imitate from a very early age but dated the onset of his tics to the age of 11 when he noticed a man with a curious grimace of the eye and face which he started to mimic. Ultimately he continued to carry out these facial movements involuntarily. Some years later he observed two boys with long hair tossing their hair back and he immediately picked up the habit which slowly converted into a head jerk. A snowflake entered his nose and catalysed a sniffing tic which his sister was foolish enough to imitate and she rapidly succumbed to an identical tic herself. He soon contracted a multitude of other tics affecting the shoulder, neck and limbs, the most persistent, however, being a twisting of his chin to the right or left. O considered many of his tics to stem from ordinary visual impressions; for example, he blamed his facial tics on his nose constantly impinging on his field of vision. The acquisition of a pince-nez spawned a host of new mannerisms and the discovery of a 'crack in his neck' led to habitual neck twisting:

> One day as I was moving my head about I felt a 'crack' in my neck and forthwith concluded I had dislocated something. It was my concern thereafter to twist my head in a thousand different ways, and with ever increasing violence, until at length the rediscovery of the sensation afforded me a genuine sense of satisfaction speedily clouded by the fear of having done myself some harm. The painlessness of the 'crack' induced me to go through the same performance many and many a time and on each occasion my feeling of contentment was tinged with regret. Even today notwithstanding that I ought to be persuaded of the harmlessness of the occurrence and the insanity of the manoeuvre I cannot withstand the allurement or banish the sentiment of unrest.

When out walking, O had developed, over a number of years, the habit of clasping his hands behind his back, crouching forward and holding his chin up in the air. This habit was believed by Meige to have fostered his tonic neck deviation, but when this was pointed out to him instead of attempting simply to correct the bizarre posture he resorted to a whole series of convoluted manoeuvres, which he termed 'para tics', to try to overcome it. First he used the curved handle of his cane to pull on his hat and then he modified this by actually supporting his chin on his cane and pressing down. Finally he resorted to slipping his cane between his jacket and overcoat so that his chin found support on the knob. All these movements were temporarily successful but, as he walked, his chin was constantly searching for the tip of his cane and this eventually led to a new side to side movement. Attempts at fixing his chin with increasingly absurd *gestes antagonistiques* ultimately resulted in the development of corns on his chin and bridge of his nose. The constant retrocollis also led to an apparent distaste for looking down despite normal eye movements.

Other favourite tics included a shoulder twitch which also appeared to have originated from a cracking noise, the striking of his right heel against the left ankle which finally led to the development of a painful wound, constant nibbling of the inside of his mouth leading to bruising, and alternate protrusion and retraction of his jaw in an attempt to produce a clicking sound. His vast repertoire of ever-changing antics and tics also included scratching movements, biting of pencils and even the habit of shaking his teeth in their sockets which finally resulted in his incisors, canines and first molars being removed. The dentures with which he was supplied were nearly swallowed on several occasions and several sets were broken within a short period of time.

O had also suffered with a vocal tic dating back to the age of 15 and had an impulse to use slang at every possible opportunity, although there was no suggestion of overt coprolalia or echophenomena. O's explanation of his vocal tics is as follows:

> We who tic are consumed with a desire for the forbidden fruit. It is when we are required to keep quiet that we are tempted to restlessness; it is when silence is

compulsory that we feel we must talk. Now, when one is learning his lessons, conversation is prohibited, the natural consequence being that he seeks to erode the galling interdict by giving vent to some inarticulate sound. In this fashion did my 'cluck' come into being. More over, we abhor a vacuum and fill it as we may. Various are the artifices we might employ, such for instance as speaking aloud; but that is much too obvious, and does not satisfy; to make a little grunt or cluck, on the other hand — what a comfort in a tic like that.

O was able quite effectively to conceal his tics in company for up to an hour or two but would at times, when overcome with a compulsion to tic, be forced to excuse himself for a moment or two and in blissful solitude relieve himself with a veritable carnival of gesticulations and muscular jerks. When cycling he would sit motionless but holding his head up to the sky and during his other favourite sports of billiards, fencing and rowing he would be quite free from tics. When fishing he would tic away furiously until he had a bite when he would become quite still and engrossed in landing the catch. Sleep also abolished his movements but restlessness on reclining forced him to sleep at the very edge of the bed with his head hanging over the side. Often he would wake after an hour or so with severe abdominal spasms during which he would stagger histrionically about opening his buttons, loosening his tie, sobbing and pretending to faint. During this time he would be awash with multiple body tics. Physical examination at these times was otherwise normal.

Despite O's impulsiveness and impetuosity he was able to lead a successful business career undertaking important commercial negotiations which demanded both initiative and alertness. He also had a remarkable facility for grasping what was needed in a given situation which served him well in his enterprises and assured him of a prosperous living. He was also a warm and loving father, adoring his children but tending, according to Meige, to spoil them to some degree.

O provided a number of fascinating insights into what actually seemed to make him tic:

I find myself seeking a knot in every bullrush. I experience a sensation of pleasure only to tax my ingenuity in discovering some danger or blame therein. If a person produces an agreeable impression on me I cudgel my brains in the attempt to detect faults in him. I take it into my head to ascertain how anything from which I derive enjoyment might become an aversion instead. The absurdities of these inconsistencies is perfectly patent to me, and my reflections occasion me pain; but the attainment of my end is accompanied with a feeling of pleasure.

In conversation O would continually take off at tangents, never completing his train of thought, with new disconnected ideas constantly flooding into his mind. This impatience and flight of thought was also evident in his writing:

It has often happened that I have commenced a business letter in the usual formal way, gradually to lose sight of its object in a crowd of superfluous details. Worse still, if the matter in hand be delicate or wearisome, my impatience is not slow to assert itself by remarks and reproaches so pointed and violent that my only course on reperusal of the letter is to tear it up.

Failure to immediately gratify his wishes would cause marked irritation and an increasing aggressiveness in gestures and speech, but this was always short-lived. O was also plagued by a whole variety of obssessional fears such as a dread of passing certain streets, a fear of breaking fragile objects coupled with a temptation to let them fall, and also a fear of contracting syphilis, ataxia and rabies.

Although O was initially indifferent to the arrest of his tics, intent only on gratifying the sense of anguish he associated with the movements in his limbs, he agreed to treatment. Meige used the fashionable treatments of the time which included behavioural techniques of immobilisation, Pitres respiratory exercises and mirror drill to great effect:

> I am conscious of very material gain. I do not tic so often or with such force. I know how to keep still. Above all, I have learnt the secret of inhibition. Absurd gestures that I once thought irrepressible have succumbed to the power of application. I have dispensed with my para tic cane, the callosities on my nose and chin have vanished; and I can walk without carrying my head in the air. This advance has not been made without a struggle, without moments of discouragement; but I have emerged victorious, strong in the knowledge of the resources of my will. To tell the truth at my age I can scarcely hope for an absolute cure. Were I only fifteen such would be my ambition, but as I am so shall I remain. I very much doubt whether I shall ever have the necessary perseverance to master all my tics and I am too prone to imagine fresh ones; yet the thought no longer claims me. Experience has shown the possibilities of control, and my tics have lost their terror. Thus have disappeared half my troubles.

Meige and Feindel are at pains to point out that O's introspective observations were not conditioned by the currently held psychological theories. O in fact had a fear of medical literature and his busy job, according to his family, precluded him from having the time to delve too much into the nature of his condition.

JOSEPH BLISS

At the age of 67 Joseph Bliss, an American citizen who had suffered from Gilles de la Tourette syndrome for 62 years, recorded his inner experiences and thoughts in an article published in the Archives of General Psychiatry in 1980. His tortured self-examination over 35 years finally led him to the conclusion that sensory tensions, springing up in different body areas, were the underlying stimulus for the apparent motor manifestations of his tic. Having discovered this he was able through self-control to abolish the sensory disturbance before it converted into a tic and obtain considerable release from his symptoms. This personal view coincides perfectly with the earlier views of the Chicago physician Patrick (1905) who wrote as follows:

> In nearly every case of tic the original cause is sensory. Not only that; very often it is the sensory element which perpetuates the spontaneous movement and makes it hard to cure. Even though each movement be not the direct response to a sensation one is pretty sure to find that the execution of the movement gives the

patient a certain sense of relief or satisfaction which shows a sensory foundation for the trouble.

Bliss developed tics at the age of 5 and his motor habits over the years included hissing, teeth grinding, eye blinking, neck jerks, nose twitching, brow lifting, back arching, touching, paper tearing, trunk twisting, picking at clothes and stabbing movements with the point of a pencil. Around the age of 40 he began to appreciate an unsatisfied feeling requiring relief at the site of each tic and then in 1976, while driving his car, he became acutely aware of sensory impulses in his head which he could direct voluntarily from site to site by shifting his attention. He noticed that as one site flared up another died down, no two ever occurring together, and that all this time no build up of tension occurred and no overt muscular jerks were seen. This revelation enabled him over the next few years, by subsequent endless practice, to develop a form of relaxation which allowed him to suppress symptoms at source rather than, as he had done previously, by masking them through inner tensing or manneristic alternatives.

Bliss believes that each tic symptom begins with its own sensory signal which builds up into a demanding and uncompromising urge. He is also aware of a less easily defined delicate sensation which actually initiates and then fuels the desire to tic. The movement of the body he believes is a voluntary capitulation to these sensations which build towards an unattainable climax. Concentration on the site where the sensation originates may precipitate the action so that he advises that attempts at improving awareness can be actually detrimental. If, however, the urge can be recognised before it becomes too strong, inner surveillance and delaying techniques may be used to prevent its emergence. He also points out, however, that if the mind is not constantly on its guard then symptoms may break through.

> The earliest sensory signals are incredibly subtle sensations that appear singly in endlessly varied sites and forms on or in the body or partly or even entirely in phantom imagery. Isolation of the earliest Tourette syndrome signal is further complicated by (1) site irritation and muscle tension soreness (2) emotional stress (in many forms) (3) competing and close by movement demands (such as normal involuntary eye blinks) and (4) the sense of inevitability which precedes overt action, the feeling of disaster which occurs when every nerve is trembling and muscular anarchy seems imminent. All these phenomena entangle the Tourette syndrome signal and make its isolation difficult.

Bliss also draws a parallel with a fleeting itch, the moment before a sneeze or the touch of a feather on the tip of the nose, but stresses that in most instances the muscular tic occurs before it is allowed to progress as far as these sensations. He believes a tic is a grotesque extension of a normal motor activity which is sudden because the underlying sensory urge is so intolerable. The feeling after a tic or vocalisation is also fleeting varying in severity but always conveying some sense of relief. Unlike normal motor activity when two willed movements may occur simultaneously, the attention targeting which dictates the localisation of a tic precludes multiple movements occurring at the same time.

Many tics may occur over a very short period of time, however, as a result of the rapid shift of attention from one point of the body to another. Bliss also invokes the possibility of phantom sensations occurring as a result of mental projection on to inanimate objects, thereby explaining such complicated behaviours as compulsive touching. He also considers that ticqueurs are extremely efficient in laying down new motor programmes and that little or no practice is needed to produce what appears to be a semi-automatic ingrained motor habit.

Bliss originally found that attention targeting to particular body areas was helpful in the control of his own tics. This he employed together with substitution techniques where different, often more acceptable, motor behaviour replaced the usual tic and, with successive substitutions, the sensation underlying the tic was finally inhibited. Later, instant recognition with denial of the sensory signal was used and ultimately found to be more satisfactory. Bliss describes his self-treatment as a kind of half-life between constant vigilance and divided attention, and stresses the need for intensive and prolonged training with strong motivation.

WITTY TICCY RAY (THE TICCER OF LITTLE NECK PARKWAY)

Sacks (1981) has provided an interesting account of a man who when aged 24, contacted him following an article in the *New York Times*. Previously undiagnosed, Ray had recognised himself in the newspaper's description of Gilles de la Tourette syndrome and begged for a consultation. He had been severely incapacitated by tics since the age of 4 and when examined by Sacks was having volleys of muscle jerks every four seconds affecting particularly his head and face but also his trunk and limbs. His tics disappeared consistently only in sleep or after sexual intercourse and were also improved following deep involvement in his work or when playing music. In spite of ostracisation and rebuke throughout childhood, his natural wit, intelligence and determination had enabled him to graduate from school and college. However, since leaving college he had been sacked from at least a dozen jobs always because of his tics rather than incompetence and his marriage was now threatened by his cries of 'shit' and 'fuck me' at times of sexual arousal. Much of his weekend was spent as a talented jazz drummer renowned for his impromptu improvisations which would germinate from a tic or compulsive involuntary drum strike. His astonishing speed of reaction also made him a gifted table tennis player, some of his shots, described by him as 'frivolous', being so unexpected as to be quite unreturnable. On the surface Ray appeared as a court jester, a master of witty repartee, impatient, pugnacious and emotionally explosive, but as Sacks got to know him better he unearthed a darker side of deep-seated hopeless despair. Despite his tics Ray was a competent motorist and swimmer, activities he found helpful in suppressing the intruding movements.

When learning of the possibility of treatment with haloperidol Ray's initial reactions were a mixture of excitement and anxiety. Nevertheless, he agreed to be treated and in the first instance Sacks administered a single injection of haloperidol which was strikingly effective, almost abolishing Ray's tics for up to two hours. He was then given a small dose of haloperidol by mouth. Within a week Ray returned with a black eye and broken nose screaming obscenities It transpired that the medication had damped down his normally quick reflexes and upset his timing so that his familiar antics such as dodging in and out of revolving doors had become impossible and resulted in injury. Many of his tics had also slowed down and had extended so that he would become as he put it 'suspended in mid tic'. Even on this minute dose of medication he presented a picture of psychomotor retardation, blocked and ambivalent about life. It was at this time that his early reservations about treatment came to a head and he began to question Sacks in the following way:

> Suppose you could take away the tics, what would be left? I consist of tics — there would be nothing left.

It seemed that he was unable to envisage life other than as a ticcing, clownish freak and it became clear that he was exploiting his illness in an almost exhibitionistic way. He did, however, agree to explore his inner self with Sacks' help over a three-month period during which time all manner of normal human desires and potentials came to light, finally resulting in him beginning to see 'a life beyond Tourette'. At this stage Sacks decided to reintroduce haloperidol, on this occasion with excellent results. Within a short period of time he was virtually free from his impulsive obscenities and his tics were markedly reduced. For the first time he began to enjoy social gatherings as a normal person and within a short time was leading a moderate staid life working on Wall Street. His marriage stabilised and he became a loving father. New friends appeared, admiring him for himself rather than his former buffoonery and life generally became much more tolerable. However, he had lost his impetuosity, killer instinct and sharpness and with these went his enjoyment of table tennis. Even his dreams changed, being stripped of the 'elaborate Tourette extravaganzas'. More upsetting, however, was that his music which had previously been so important to him had become dull, predictable and uncreative. Soon after the response to the drug became clear, Ray made a conscious decision that he would live during the week on haloperidol as a responsible calm business man, husband and father, but at weekends he would become his old frenetic self off haloperidol. This double life worked well for him over the next few years and according to Sacks Ray found an inner security and resilience brought about by his self-realisation. In Ray's own words:

> Having Tourettes is wild, like being drunk. Being on Haldol is dull, makes one square and sober and neither state is really free. You normals who have the right transmitters in the right places at the right times in your brains have all feelings, all styles available all the time — gravity, levity, whatever is appropriate. We Touretters don't; we are forced into levity by our Tourettes and forced into gravity when we take Haldol. You are free, you have a natural balance, we must make the best of an artificial balance.

STEVE THE MOD

Following a chance meeting at a church social with a ticqueur who attended the National Hospital, Steve, a 20-year-old unemployed delinquent, appeared unannounced in the early evening to the out-patient department of the National Hospital for Nervous Diseases. His belligerent manner, explosive movements and mental restlessness made initial contact extremely difficult but after two or three lengthy interviews it was possible to obtain a few details of his previous history. As far as he knew, his birth had been normal and there was no delay in his motor milestones. As a young child he recalled nail biting, school refusal and vivid nightmares. His natural father, who was Irish, abused alcohol and was prone to violence, working most of his life as a floor manager at the Ford's car factory. His mother worked as a secretary and had received treatment for depression. He remembered his relationship with both his parents as being strained from an early age and following their deaths he was adopted at the age of 10. Two years after this he developed a head tossing tic and this was soon to be followed by a number of other abnormal movements. As an adolescent he played truant frequently from school, had his first sexual experience at the age of 13 and became involved in petty crime, stealing cars and ending up in street fights. He left school at the age of 14 and qualified as a painter and decorator but was unable to keep any job for long, working successively over a short period of time as a painter, labourer and warehouseman. After a short period as a 'plastic skin head' he joined the mod subculture and abused a wide range of drugs including barbiturates, amphetamines and LSD 25. He glue-sniffed and on a few occasions took heroin. At the time of his attendance he was unemployed without a National Insurance number and had been living in squats with his Yugoslavian punk girl-friend for seven months.

On examination, he had coarse pugilistic features with cropped hair and tattoos on his forehead reading 'K, K, K'. He had the words 'fuck off' inscribed on the side of his neck and 'fuck' tattooed on the metacarpals of his fingers. Despite his hostile appearance he was cooperative and there was no evidence of psychotic behaviour. He was, however, below average intelligence with an extremely poor attention span. The variety and severity of his abnormal movements were quite astonishing. Within a brief interview period he displayed eye blinking, eye rolling, facial grimacing, snarling, wide smiling and mouth opening, jerky obscene palm back V signs, tightening of neck muscles, shoulder shrugging, head shaking, arm jerking, tongue protrusions, striking of his chest with his arms, moving his jaw forwards, kissing his clothes and simulating masturbation. Vocalisations included 'ee', throat clearing, sniffing, 'zzz', 'sss', 'zing', 'Tottenham', 'Sieg heil', 'mod' and 'monkey'. His repertoire of obscenities was equally extensive with 'fuck', 'fuck off', 'fucking wanker', 'oral sex', 'Suki's crutch', 'tits', 'knickers' and 'cunnilingus' being shouted in an aggressive voice. Alcohol, orgasm and fever all temporarily reduced the severity of his symptoms and arguments with his girl-friend or boredom exacerbated them. He agreed to take small doses of diazepam and haloperidol and undoubted improvement occurred in both tic frequency and severity over the first few weeks. At the same time he felt more relaxed and less aggressive but his attendances continued to be erratic. Within two months of his first clinic appointment he was arrested for assaulting someone and forging prescriptions for barbiturates. He also claimed to have been charging himself up with amphetamines to avenge himself on a rival punk group who had slashed an old lady with a knife. Dialogue remained strained and it was impossible to determine much about his inner feelings or desires. When reviewed nine months after his original attendance he was living with his girl-friend at the home of another patient with Gilles de la Tourette syndrome. A new tattoo printed by his girl-friend on the inside of his lip had appeared and he had apparently been increasingly violent, smashing down doors and attacking people. According to his girl-friend, amphetamines actually seemed to calm him down and reduce his tic frequency. One year after he was first seen he demanded admission to hospital, having parted from his girl-friend and claiming that he had gone mad. On examination his tics were less obvious than when he had first been seen. A further tattoo reading 'ein Volk, ein Reich, ein Führer' had appeared and he now had a new girl-friend. When last seen he was taking his treatment regularly, had been reconciled with his Yugoslavian girl-friend and had just come out of jail for burglary.

5

Tics Occurring in Association with Neurological Disorders

There are a handful of poorly documented and often unconvincing anecdotes describing tics in association with neurological disease. Lack of precise definition and differing cultural terminologies make many of these hard to evaluate but infections such as viral encephalitis and neurosyphilis, intoxications including manganese and coal-gas poisoning, cerebrovascular disease and head trauma have all been claimed to unleash tics.

The occurrence of tics, sometimes with coprolalia, in encephalitis lethargica survivors is one line of evidence used to support the belief that tics are generated as a result of damage to the corpus striatum. Despite a tendency of the tics to occur together with extrapyramidal signs, the diffuse inflammatory involvement of the whole neuraxis in most reported cases of encephalitis lethargica makes precise pathological localisation of tics to the basal ganglia on these grounds alone unjustifiable. Nevertheless, these reports are of some interest and will be described in detail. Respiratory dyskinesias, oculogyric crises and post-encephalitic speech disorders including palilalia will also be considered.

EPIDEMIC ENCEPHALITIS LETHARGICA (VON ECONOMO'S DISEASE)

It is now more than half a century since the last epidemic of encephalitis lethargica. Nevertheless, this 'experiment of nature' as it was called by Jelliffe continues to fascinate neuropsychiatrists, and the numerous case reports provide abundant examples of psychopathology attributable to structural brain damage.

Although the pandemic of 1916–1927 burst forth unrecognised as an 'obscure disease with cerebral symptoms', in hindsight it was obvious that this was not a new disorder. Accounts of febrile somnolent illnesses followed by lethargy, tremors, chorea and ophthalmoplegias abound in the early literature. Sydenham's febris comatosa of 1672–1675 in which hiccough was a prominent symptom, the Schlafkrankheit which devastated Tubingen in 1712–1713 and the dreaded Italian nona of 1889–1890 are but three of a large number of potential predecessors. None of these, however, compared in severity with the devastation of the 'sleepy sickness' which left in its wake five million dead or disabled. Indeed, sporadic cases still occur to remind contemporary physicians of its undisputed virulence and it would be foolhardy to believe that one had seen the last of this malignant sleeping giant.

The clinical manifestations of the first outbreaks in France and Vienna in 1916 were so protean and unlike any other currently recognised disease that it was at first believed that a whole host of new disorders had erupted simultaneously. Chaos continued to reign until Constantin von Economo, using his clinical acumen reinforced by childhood recollections of his family's description of nona, showed that they were in fact confronting a single polymorphous infection. He was also able to demonstrate that the disease could be transmitted to monkeys by a filter-passing agent and that at post-mortem the brain was riddled with scattered foci of non-purulent inflammation with a particular predilection for the central grey matter of the brain-stem, the hypothalamus, substantia nigra and limbic system (Von Economo, 1931). Even the application of modern virological and neuro-epidemiological methods has failed as yet to uncover the underlying infective agent, although it is now believed that the disease may have been brought to Europe by French soldiers returning from the Chinese province of Yunnanfou. Currently popular theories incriminate the swine influenza virus or a normally innocuous virus such as herpes simplex rendered virulent at the time by the coexisting outbreak of Spanish flu.

After early sporadic outbreaks in several European cities, the disease really took off from London in 1918 spreading virtually throughout the world within three years. Some of the helpless bewilderment within the medical profession at the time may be captured by reading the incredible report published by His Majesty's Stationery Office and the editorials and correspondence in the *Lancet* and *British Medical Journal* of that year. Heterogeneity continued to be a perplexing feature, each fresh outbreak often running close to form but differing markedly from others close by. The only unifying features seemed to be the tendency for each new rash of notifications to occur in winter and for young adults to be most vulnerable.

Gradually, however, three main types of the acute disease were distinguished, the most usual being the somnolent-ophthalmoplegic variety. After a prodromal influenza-like illness lasting a few days, increasing drowsiness and delirium appeared. If recovery then failed to occur deterioration to virtually permanent sleep and subsequent coma resulted. An external ophthalmoplegia often with pupillary involvement or nystagmus occurred early and signs of upper motor neurone, basal ganglia or cerebellar damage were sometimes also seen. A mild leucocytosis with slightly elevated protein and 15–40 lymphocytes/mm^3 in the cerebrospinal fluid were the only recorded laboratory abnormalities. A smaller number of patients presented from the outset with bradykinesia, rigidity and sometimes catalepsy and mutism. This Parkinsonian variety sometimes subsequently transformed into the somnolent-ophthalmoplegic type. Intense motor unrest reminiscent of that seen during impulsive crises in catatonic schizophrenia characterised the onset of the disease in a further group of patients. These individuals tossed about in bed, sat up repeatedly, clicked and hissed, jerked and twitched with frequent wild jactitations and often manifested florid visual hallucinations. It was from this hyperkinetic form that abnormal involuntary movements most frequently sprouted in the convalescent phase. Some of these patients also experienced hypomania, schizophreniform psychoses or even fell into a melancholic stupor.

In all forms, rapid debility occurred with marked weight loss. Convalescence was always prolonged and often punctuated by recrudescences. Sleep disorders, depression and apathy sometimes persisted for years. In fact about one-third of the patients died in coma in the acute stages, a further third survived with a multitude of incapacities, the more severe being exiled to special colonies, long-stay wards and homes for the incurable. The remainder appeared to recover completely, although a fair number subsequently succumbed to the delayed ravages of the disease.

The most destructive residual sequela of epidemic encephalitis lethargica was the frequent emergence of Parkinson's syndrome. This usually occurred in adults and developed either acutely, insidiously during the convalescent phase, or even months or years after apparent full recovery. A reactivation of the initial inflammatory process was reported in some of these late onset cases. In children, personality disorders and repetitive motor phenomena were more frequent and some were left with severe chorea, myoclonus or dystonia. Many of the disorders labelled tics at the time, such as oculogyric crises and respiratory dyskinesias, would not now be classified as such but bona fide examples undoubtedly occurred.

POST-ENCEPHALITIC TICS

Von Economo (1931), Wilder and Silbermann (1927), Stern (1936) and Marie and Levy (1920, 1922) provide the fullest descriptions of tics occurring either acutely or more usually as post-encephalitic sequelae. These accounts make reference to eye blinks, limb jerks, grimaces, head tossing, clicking and sucking sounds, sniffing, licking and spasmodic coughing. Children seemed to be particularly at risk and many of the most severe examples also had personality disorders. As a generalisation, post-encephalitic tics tended to be more stereotyped and less ephemeral than those occurring in Gilles de la Tourette syndrome and an even greater proportion were localised to the face and neck. In a few patients they appeared as part of a short-lived eruption of a whole host of extraordinary motions and notions which seemed to herald the Parkinsonian strait-jacket.

Sacks, in his book *Awakenings*, vividly describes the rekindling of tics and other dyskinesias by L-dopa in the group of post-encephalitics at Beth Abraham Hospital in the New York suburbs. His case histories include an acount of Hester Y who contracted encephalitis at the age of 30 after which she became catatonic, speechless and akinetic. Within 10 days of therapy she had regained her mobility and independence, exhibiting remarkable pressure of speech and palilalia. Three days later darting head movements, compulsive touching, akathisia and screaming appeared. From then on new tics, or modifications of existing ones, appeared daily, often a dozen or two proceeding simultaneously each with its own rhythm and melody. As Sacks (1982a) relates, 'It gave the impression of a clock-shop gone mad with innumerable clocks all ticking in their own time and tune.' Gasps, pants, sniffs, finger-snaps, throat clearing, pinching, scratching and occasional ballistic movements so extreme as to throw her to the ground occurred over the ensuing weeks. Irrepressible compulsions and gestures so comical and vigorous as to defy description also erupted finally forcing withdrawal of L-dopa. Similar tic phenomena occurred in many of the other patients, 17 of the 25 developing what Sacks terms 'acquired Tourettism'. In seven of these patients, tics and impulses already present were increased, in the others they emerged *de novo*. In his writings he also draws attention to the odd elfin humour, swiftness of association and invention and a tendency to frivolity inherent in the personality of many of these patients.

RESPIRATORY DYSKINESIAS

The commonest respiratory event occurring during the acute stages of the disease was a profound tachypnoea, often up to 100 breaths per minute without a change in heart rate. When present, this usually pointed to a fatal outcome. Encephalitis lethargica also left in its wake an astonishing collection of respiratory dyskinesias in the many crippled survivors. The majority of these abnormalities seemed integrally related to sleep disturbances and could clearly be influenced by emotional factors. Indeed all the stimuli which are known to aggravate simple tics were found to operate in the same way with respect to post-encephalitic breathing abnormalities. Aldren Turner and Critchley (1925) divided respiratory dyskinesias into three broad groups; disorders of respiratory rate, disorders of respiratory rhythm, and respiratory tics. The commonest disturbance of rate seen was a continuous or paroxysmal tachypnoea. The breathing was usually shallow, occasionally jerky, and voluntary control was usually possible for short periods. Myoclonic twitches of the arms were seen in some patients and tetany was a rare complication. In contrast, bradypnoea with a respiratory rate falling as low as 6 breaths per minute was much rarer.

Deep inspiratory sighs followed by a compensatory expiratory apnoea were common particularly in post-encephalitic Parkinson's syndrome. Some patients would exhibit a synchronous tic-like grimace, open their mouths or shrug one shoulder. Sleep apnoea, prolongation of the inspiratory phase of respiration during the waking state, alternating deep and shallow breaths (bigeminal respirations) and rarely Cheyne-Stokes breathing were the reported rhythm disturbances. Breath holding in full inspiration was another unusual phenomenon not uncommonly seen in the early evening or during sleep. These attacks were often ushered in by deep inspiratory efforts and noisy expirations during which time complaints of dizziness might occur. The inspiratory breath would then be maintained for up to 30 seconds and, during this time, limb chorea, throwing back of the head or running the fingers through the hair might be seen. Cyanosis was unusual and the attack usually terminated with a series of loud noisy respirations.

Respiratory tics seemed to occur most often in children and included repetitive mouth opening, yawning, hiccough and the expiration of air through the nose as if to dispel a foreign body (soufflement). Spasmodic coughing and throat clearing were other tic-like post-encephalitic manifestations.

In her monograph, Levy (1922) describes a boy of 10 with paroxysmal blowing and sniffing paroxysms which brought on such exhaustion that he would drop off to sleep. This child's conduct deteriorated so badly that he was transferred to a psychiatric hospital, his tics then remaining unchanged for at least two years.

In a follow-up study of 29 patients with respiratory dyskinesias carried out over a two- to three-year period, it was found that about half the cases spontaneously remitted, this most usually occurring in those with a progressive Parkinson's syndrome (Aldren Turner and Critchley, 1928).

OCULOGYRIC CRISES

These were other characteristic post-encephalitic sequelae nearly always associated with Parkinsonism and often with compulsive motor behaviour and palilalia. They were reported to occur in at least 20% of post-encephalitic Parkinsonians. Tonic, paroxysmal deviation of the external ocular muscles was the pathognomonic feature. This usually occurred in the vertical plane often slightly to one side or the other, but down gaze, horizontal and even convergence attacks were sometimes seen. Brief correction by voluntary effort was often possible but usually occurred at the expense of increasing anguish. Many attacks were heralded by compulsive thoughts or panic attacks and some patients were beleaguered with thoughts of impending disaster, depression and suicide (Jellife, 1929). Fugue-like states sometimes with surges of paranoia occasionally accompanied the attacks and Schwab et al (1951) described a patient whose paranoia was restricted to one side of the body during the crisis. Although many of the attacks were monosymptomatic, others would be associated with retrocollis, eye blinking, jaw spasms, respiratory dyskinesias and palilalia (Van Bogaert, 1934). Malaise, vertigo and headache were common and occasionally life-threatening rises in blood pressure tachycardia and sweating were recorded. The duration of an oculogyric crisis varied from a few seconds to several hours and the latent interval between attacks was equally unpredictable although usually longer than 24 hours except for occasional attacks of 'status'. The cause is unknown and, although they share many of the features of tic, the movements are more tonic and prolonged. Damage to the midbrain is probably important in mediating their occurrence.

PALILALIA

Palilalia is a disorder of speech characterised by the compulsive repetition of a word, phrase or sentence with increasing rapidity and indistinctness. It was first described by De Renzi (1879) and subsequently by Brissaud (1899) as auto-echolalia and then by Souques (1908). Most of the cases described in the literature occur in association with either post-encephalitic Parkinson's syndrome or diffuse bilateral cerebrovascular disease with pseudo-bulbar palsy (Critchley, 1927) but there are reports of it occurring in Alzheimer's disease (Frey, 1914), idiopathic Parkinson's disease (Pick, 1921), post-traumatic encephalopathy and multiple sclerosis (De Renzi, 1879) and in association with dysphasia (Benson, 1979). Boller et al (1973) have also described a familial disorder with chorea, dementia and extensive symmetrical intracerebral calcifications, in which pali-lalia was a striking feature. Emotional lability and cognitive impairment are commonly associated features.

Palilalia occurs equally during spontaneous speech and in response to questions, but is rare during preformed speech automatisms, such as recitals and singing. With succeeding repetitions the words tend to be clipped and abrupt, the rate of speaking accelerates and the voice becomes progressively less audible. Sometimes the lips may be seen to continue forming additional but inaudible repetitions (palilalia aphone). Palilalia also appears during emotional speech; oaths and exclamations exceptionally being repeated up to 20 times in post-encephalitics. As a generalisation, the shorter the phrase the greater the number of repetitions and, if the patient's spontaneous diction is longer than a sentence or two, it is almost invariably the last few words which are reiter-ated. In post-encephalitics, palilalia is often associated with oculogyric crises and respiratory dyskinesias and characteristically varies in intensity from time to time. If the patient's attention is drawn to the disturbance, will power can temporarily improve it but fluctuations seem to correlate more closely with the patient's general physical state. Paligraphia (writing repetitions) are rarely associated (Boller et al, 1973) but palipraxia (palikinesis) has not been reported.

Palilalia should be distinguished from a number of other speech disorders which may be acquired in post-encephalitic Parkinson's syndrome. Stammering is more explosive and involves repetition of syllables, not words or phrases. Verbal perseveration is the repetition of the same word as though the orig-inal idea was persisting. This distinctively may lead to the same reply being proffered for different questions. The progressive change in pitch, speed and amplitude noted in palilalia is also absent. Logoclonia and verbigeration are the meaningless repetition of words or jargon most often seen in dements and schizophrenics. Echolalia in which the patient repeats statements or questions put to him is extremely rare in post-encephalitic syndromes but may be seen with palilalia in diffuse cerebrovascular disease.

Many patients with palilalia are loathe to start speaking, exhibiting a sort of mutism. Once started, however, they find it extremely difficult to stop, thus mirroring closely the gait abnormalities of Parkinson's disease with start hesi-tation, festination and propulsion. Once into the flow of things, palilalia rarely occurs and its appearance seems to coincide with the mind going into neutral on completion of the concepts the patient was attempting to express.

Boller et al (1973) have proposed that palilalia may be due to bilateral lesions of inhibitory motor circuits and reported improvement coincident upon the amelioration of chorea by chlorpromazine. In post-encephalitic Parkinson's syndrome, anticholinergic drugs may also be of modest benefit. More promising, however, would appear to be the use of delayed auditory biofeedback techniques and pacing boards.

KLAZOMANIA

This term was introduced by Benedek in 1925 to describe the extraordinary attacks of compulsive shouting sometimes seen during oculogyric crises. Horrifying macabre wailing and spine-chilling cries reminiscent of the caged screams of a menagerie were not uncommon in the post-encephalitic wards of long-stay hospitals. Wohlfart et al (1961) have reported a 47-year-old postman who at the age of 12 had encephalitis lethargica and at 22 developed oculogyric crises and orofacial dyskinesias. At the age of 44 years he began to have frenzied screaming attacks which would begin with him becoming dazed and vacant and responding only in monosyllables. His eyes would then tonically deviate upwards for 10 minutes during which echolalia often occurred. About 15 minutes after the onset, jerky limb movements appeared with large irregular circular arm movements, his face reddened and he would unintentionally strike himself. At the same time he would grunt and bark like a dog, pant, shout, scream and utter obscenities uncontrollably, whilst at the same time remaining aware of his surroundings. Profuse sweating and salivation accompanied an attack and the electro-encephalogram remained normal throughout. I have also seen a middle-aged woman who, on recovering from a severe encephalitic illness, developed severe verbigeration with a marked scatological and salacious component. This was associated with some echophenomenena, a compulsion to put things in her mouth and severe impairment of short-term memory. These sort of attacks have been likened to the sham rage of animals with posterior hypothalamic lesions.

CHOREA, MYOCLONUS AND DYSTONIA

About half to all the encephalitis patients in Munich in 1920 exhibited chorea in the acute phases of the illness and similar high figures were reported in a number of other local epidemics. The movements were often exceptionally violent, largely confined to the limbs and trunk without much facial grimacing and often occurred in conjunction with a toxic delirium. Some authors used the term choreatic to distinguish them from Sydenham's chorea but in truth there were no distinctive features. A post-mortem study conducted on a child dying in the acute stage with severe chorea revealed severe damage in the head of the left caudate nucleus, but the whole of the basal ganglia and cerebral cortex were affected to some degree (Greenfield and Wolfshon, 1922). In many instances the chorea present in the opening phase disappeared but chronic cases did occur. In some of these there seemed to be a tendency for the movements to become more and more rhythmical and stereotyped as time went on (Sigwald and Piot, 1953).

Powerful and often painful myoclonic jerks of the face, neck, shoulders, limbs, diaphragm and abdomen were seen commonly between 1919 and 1920. These often prevented sleep and occurred together with refractory hiccoughs, pupil dilation and severe sweating bouts. The jerks were occasionally rhythmical but more often they appeared haphazard and paroxysmal. These myoclonic forms resembled descriptions of the electric chorea of Dubini described in 1846 which may well have been caused by a sporadic outbreak of encephalitis. Myoclonic twitches also presented as chronic sequelae. Individual muscles were occasionally singled out to become the seat of almost constant rhythmical jerks (myorhythmias). These contractions affected the lower jaw, limbs, platysma and face, occurred up to 60 times a minute and in some patients alternated regularly between different muscle sites.

Dystonic syndromes were rare in the acute illness but generalised torsion with opisthotonus and gait disturbance occurred in some children as a late event. Torticollis, oromandibular spasms and segmental dystonia were also reported.

POST-ENCEPHALITIC PSYCHIATRIC SEQUELAE

Examples of almost every known psychiatric condition occurred in the aftermath of von Economo's disease but personality disorders, paranoia and a spectrum of devastating compulsions were particularly frequent (Jelliffe, 1927). Children and adolescents seemed to be most at risk, many also having signs of Parkinsonism or hypothalamic damage.

About one quarter of the children became impulsive, destructive, hyperactive and distractable. Over-exuberance led to unreasonable mischievous excesses and even petty theft or sexual misdemeanours. Despite preserved intelligence, poor concentration often resulted in profound learning deficits, many of the worst cases being banished to institutions as ineducable moral degenerates. Capricious emotional swings were common, surges of callous maliciousness exploding out of states of mawkish tearfulness or panic. Parents found these transformations incomprehensible. Docile, well-behaved little boys were changed by the illness into irascible, importunate querulous monsters, unresponsive to even the harshest of punishments. Improvement did occur eventually in some, although usually at the expense of progressive Parkinsonism; in others the mental scars remained. Fairweather (1947) described the characteristics of 278 post-encephalitics admitted to Rampton, a state institution for patients of a violent and dangerous disposition. About 25% of the men and 12% of the women experienced paranoid delusions and almost twice as many were schizoid. Most had been referred from other institutions such as mental hospitals, prisons and orphanages and many had signs of Parkinson's syndrome. The most horrific crimes, however, had been committed in those with no severe Parkinsonian features, their neurological abnormalities being restricted to ophthalmoplegias, palilalia, coprolalia, tics and myoclonus. Serious damage to property was the commonest offence but sexual perversions of every imaginable kind were also common. Many of the patients appeared mentally retarded and indulged in a variety of self-injurious behaviours.

Endless ruminations on futile and restricted themes also occurred in many post-encephalitics, driving them to complex manneristic rituals, erotomanias and erethisms which, once commenced, could only be stopped with the greatest of difficulty. One individual would jump up and run around the room because of a strange feeling in his head, another carried out stereotyped trouser-hitching movements. Another patient I have seen, once prompted to recite Gray's 'Elegy', would monotonously reiterate the whole poem over and over again despite imprecations to cease. Claude et al (1927) reported patients with overwhelming compulsions to tear clothes, pull out teeth and even strangle cats.

Upon recovery from the acute stages of the disease, hypochondriasis, depression and paranoid hallucinatory states were by no means rare. In a careful review of the literature, Davison and Bagley (1969) found that 10% of those patients admitted to mental hospitals had paraphrenia and even more had transient and variable paranoid hallucinatory states. Affect was claimed to be 'sticky' or 'viscous' like epileptic psychoses and some authors claimed a better preservation of rapport and lack of personality deterioration when compared with schizophrenics. Of the 40 cases reviewed by Davison and Bagley (1969) only one had a schizoid premorbid personality and only two had family histories of schizophrenia making an inherent predisposition unlikely. Many of these patients had Parkinsonism and a few also displayed catalepsy.

ACANTHOCYTOSIS AND NEUROLOGICAL DISEASE

Three distinct neurological syndromes have been described in patients with an excess of circulating acanthocytes. Bassen-Kornzweig disease is an autosomal recessive disorder of childhood often presenting in the first year of life with steatorrhoea and failure to thrive. Atypical retinitis pigmentosa and a progressive spinocerebellar degeneration appear in late childhood and there is a reduction in serum lipids, abetalipoproteinaemia and negligible vitamin E levels. An autosomal dominant condition presenting in adult life with progressive cerebellar and pyramidal deficits and sphincter involvement has also been reported. These patients also have lipid abnormalities and acanthocytes were demonstrable in vitro, but not in routine, blood studies.

In 1967 a third neurological syndrome was described in a New England family. Abnormal involuntary movements and proximal limb weakness were the characteristic clinical features and it appeared to be inherited as a dominant condition (Levine et al, 1968). In this disorder, lipid abnormalities are absent but circulating acanthocytes comprise 5–50% of the total red cell count. Since then 10 further detailed clinical reports have occurred (Critchley et al, 1968,

1970; Aminoff, 1972; Bird et al, 1978; Kito et al, 1980; Sakai et al, 1981), and there are two post-mortem studies (Bird et al, 1978; Sakuta et al, 1980). No clear model of inheritance has emerged, both autosomal recessive and sporadic cases having been described.

The underlying cause for the abnormality of red cell morphology is unknown in these patients but the biophysical data of Betts et al, (1970) suggests that the outer membrane of the misshapen cells is not significantly abnormal. Aminoff (1972) considered an unidentified serum factor to be responsible, and increased sensitivity of platelets to adenine diphosphate (ADP) has also been regarded as a possible underlying factor (Betts et al, 1970). Kito et al (1980), however, favoured an intrinsic red cell defect as normal red cells incubated with the serum of a patient did not change shape and conversely no restoration of normal morphology occurred when the acanthocytes were mixed with normal serum.

The disorder usually presents in the third or fourth decade of life with orofacial dyskinesias. Stereotyped tongue protrusions, grimacing, lip movements and champing are particularly characteristic, the movements bearing a close resemblance to those seen in tardive dyskinesia. Vocalisations are common and include grunts, clucks, sucking sounds, hiccoughs, snorts and sniffs. Echolalia but not copralalia has been described (Kito et al, 1980). Tongue, lip and cheek biting is the most distinctive abnormality. In one of the cases of Critchley et al (1968) this became so severe that the patient was obliged to walk around with a protective rag stuffed between his teeth to avoid further laceration to his tongue and lips. Choreiform limb and trunk dyskinesias are usual and some patients have dystonic postures. The condition is distinguished from Huntington's disease by the presence of limb wasting and weakness due to anterior horn cell and peripheral nerve damage. Dysarthria is also a prominent early symptom whereas intellectual decline is not invariable and, when it appears, tends to do so late in the course of the illness. Life expectancy is probably reduced and psychiatric morbidity is high.

In a recent neurophysiological study comparing three patients with choreoacanthocytosis and three with Huntington's disease a number of clinical distinctions were noted. Mental arithmetic, holding the tongue out for fixed periods of time, and requests to voluntarily suppress the dyskinesias all led to a considerable reduction in the abnormal movements in the patients with choreoacanthocytosis. In contrast, these manoeuvres tended to aggravate the disabilities in the patients with Huntington's disease. Surface EMG recordings over limbs and trunks in both groups revealed unpredictable motor discharges lasting 100 ms to 1 s. However, using EMG triggered back-averaging techniques to record pre-movement cortical events, differences were again apparent between the two groups. Two of the three choreo-acanthocytosis patients had a typical negative Bereitschafts potentials maximal at the vertex (5–6.5 μv) and starting 1 s before the averaged EMG discharge whereas this was not evident in any of the patients with Huntington's disease. This suggests that some of the abnormal movements in the choreo-acanthocytosis syndrome may be voluntary and self-paced (Shibasaki et al, 1982).

Both post-mortem studies demonstrated neuronal loss and gliosis in the caudate and putamen indistinguishable histologically from the abnormalities found in Huntington's disease (Bird et al, 1978; Sakuta et al, 1980). In the report by Bird et al (1978) cortical atrophy was absent, correlating with the lack of dementia in life, and there was also no spinal cord or peripheral nerve degeneration. One interesting finding was the normal activities of glutamic acid decarboxylase and choline acetyltransferase in the corpus striatum despite the presence in life of severe chorea, a finding which contrasts with the depressed levels usually present in Huntington's disease.

SYDENHAM'S CHOREA

Although the opportunities for misdiagnosis are appreciable, a number of patients with a past history of rheumatic chorea have been reported to develop post-choreic tics (Straus, 1927a; Ossipowa, 1930; Krauss, 1934) and coprolalia (Straus, 1927b). In fact Osler in his monograph on chorea described a 21-year-old baker who developed jerky movements of the head and limbs and whistling inspiratory noises. When examined two years later the movements seemed to more closely resemble tics (Osler, 1894). Creak and Guttmann (1935) reviewed the case notes at the Maudsley Hospital between 1932–35 and found 14 cases in which tic was noted in the diagnosis, six of whom had a previous history of Sydenham's chorea. All six of these cases had grunts or barks as well as bodily tics and case 5 had copralalia. Although some of these cases sound quite convincing examples of Sydenham's chorea, no mention of cardiac involvement is made and it is conceivable that they in fact represent examples of Gilles de la Tourette syndrome. Recently Behan et al (1981) have reported five cases of Sydenham's chorea in which grunts, tics and copralalia were present. Three of these cases were over 65 years old and treatment with tetrabenazene alleviated both the involuntary movements and coprolalia.

HUNTINGTON'S DISEASE

Sniffing, snorting and grunting are not uncommon in patients with Huntington's disease. Sacks (1982b) has also reported cases in which tics, coprolalia and arithromania occurred. In one of these patients extensive damage to the medial thalamus as well as the corpus striatum was found at autopsy.

CEREBROVASCULAR DISEASE

Sacks (1982b) has reported an elderly hypertensive woman who presented with a *grand mal* fit and subsequently developed a variety of abnormal movements on the left side of her body. Some of these were simple rhythmical repetitive jerks diagnostic of epilepsia partialis continuans but in addition finger snaps, touching of the nose and eye, grunts and curses with a tendency to wisecrack appeared. All her movements were accentuated by stress and diminished by relaxation. The electroencephalogram showed high voltage spikes and sharp waves on the right side, and anticonvulsants effectively eliminated both the tics and the seizure activity. A number of other cases are also reported in less detail in which Sacks describes tics down one side of the body immediately after a stroke or alternatively appearing following a latent interval. Obeso and Marti Masso have also reported a patient with coprolalia associated with hemiballismus.

Bleeker (1978) has described a 43-year-old man who developed sensory symptoms in the limbs and right upper motor neurone signs. Following a vertebral angiogram he became blind and lost the power and sensation down the right side. These disabilities improved but he was left with visual hallucinations, emotional lability, hyperaesthesiae of the right side of the face, a right palatal weakness and right-sided cerebellar signs. Snorting, sticking out of the tongue, clonic eye blinks, sniffing, grimacing and rocking also appeared for the first time. Compulsive touching and tapping, rubbing of the forehead, pinching of the cheeks and knee pounding were also seen. Thumb and lip sucking and violent jerks of the head and limbs were other additional features and his speech was characterised by severe echolalia, palilalia, tongue clicks and stereotyped 'eeh, eeh, eeh' noises. These symptoms persisted for 18 months and were then helped considerably by haloperidol treatment.

A further case of Gilles de la Tourette syndrome in a mentally retarded boy who died at the age of 9 years has been described in which the pathological changes suggested congenital vascular malformations and status lacunaris. The changes were extensive, however, and most could be attributed to previous infection and mental retardation. This boy had a number of tics including eyebrow raising, mouth opening, spitting, verbal tics, eye blinking and coprolalia. In addition, however, he body rocked, head banged, ground his teeth and had rhythmical tremor movements. An EEG was severely abnormal and an air encephalogram showed marked dilatation of one lateral ventricle. Bilateral thalamotomies had also been performed (Borak and Osetowska, 1976).

SENILITY

Critchley (1931), in his lectures on the neurology of old age, drew attention to the frequent occurrence of stereotyped rubbing, touching, stroking and patting movements in the elderly. Palipraxia is also common and occasional demented individuals can be seen parcelling up imaginary objects.

At the First International Gilles de la Tourette Syndrome Symposium held in New York from 27th–29th May 1981, Sutula, Stackman and Hobbs showed a video film of an 81-year-old black man with atherosclerosis and treated syphilis who had recently developed grimaces, rocking head movements, belching and barking noises and stereotyped repetition of a word sounding like 'boogie'. Onset of this illness was gradual and there was no history of neuro-leptic administration. The CAT scan of the brain showed cortical atrophy and the EEG diffuse slow wave activity. Haloperidol completely suppressed the vocal and motor tics and reduced his involuntary spitting (Sutula and Hobbs, 1983).

TRAUMA

Fahn (1982) reported the case of an 18-year-old youth who was struck in the face by a steel girder and thrown backwards striking his head against a wall. He was unconscious for two minutes and remained in hospital for two weeks complaining of confusion, dizziness and tinnitus. Within six weeks, however, he had returned to work but shortly afterwards began to experience involuntary asymmetrical facial twitching. Shortly after this he lost his job because of an inability to concentrate. About a year later compulsive behaviour appeared which was treated briefly with neuroleptics and then diphenhydramine. Grunt-ing appeared six months after this and, when seen four years after the accident, he had facial tics, eye blinks, sniffing and snorting and mild dystonic neck move-ments. Treatment with both clonazepam and neuroleptics was unsuccessful.

Eriksson and Persson (1969) mentioned a child who developed tics, loud bellowing noises, and attacks of opisthotonus and cyanosis following a skull fracture at 3 years. Symptoms had decreased at the last follow up nine years later.

METABOLIC ENCEPHALOPATHIES

There are two well-documented examples of tics occurring as a consequence of hypoglycaemic fits. Wilder (1946) reported a patient who following a hypo-glycaemic episode developed a dancing tic lasting three days. This patient also had tics, myoclonic jerks and chorea. At post-mortem, pituitary and pancreatic, tumours were demonstrated as well as extensive neuronal loss in the corpus striatum. Weingarten (1968) described a further case due to an insulinoma in which mannerisms, tics, myoclonic jerks and athetosis occurred. Both these cases showed megaphonia with an inability to lower their voices to request.

Pulst et al (1983) described a 58-year-old man who developed head and neck tics, vocalisations, palilalia and echolalia, fits of shouting, hypersexuality and coprolalia following carbon monoxide poisoning. He was also moderately demented and the CAT scan showed lesions in the medial parts of the basal ganglia.

6

The Hyperekplexias

Synonyms Startle-induced myoclonus, startle disease.

The startle response is a polysynaptic alerting reflex common to all mammals. In response to an unexpected stimulus a rapid eye blink occurs followed after 100 ms by a characteristic facial grimace, head flexion, raising and drawing forwards of the shoulders, forward bending of the trunk and flexion of the elbows, hips and knees. Mild left-right asymmetry is usual and on rare occasions a short cry may be emitted (Landis and Hunt, 1939). Tachycardia, elevation of systolic blood pressure and transient apnoea followed by overbreathing are autonomic accompaniments and there are alterations in the psychogalvanic skin response (Gastaut and Villeneuve, 1967). During the startle which lasts 0.5–0.8 s all other motor activity is suspended (Wieser, 1958). The reflex makes its appearance at around 4 months of age around the same time as the extensor Moro reflex. In contrast to the Moro reflex, however, it becomes more apparent with time. Its tendency to habituate with repeated stimulation makes it a difficult reaction to study but it is now believed to originate in brain-stem structures. For example, it is present in anencephalic children and Buser et al (1966) have demonstrated that the jump engendered by a noise in the cat is elaborated within the inferior colliculus. They have also shown that this subcortical startle reflex is under considerable cortical control. For instance, the cortical area specific for the startle stimulus can, depending on its degree of excitation or inhibition, alter the amplitude of the jump. When directly stimulated, however, the subcortical centre frees itself from higher centres and consistently gives rise to a non-fatiguable reflex of maximum intensity. In their original study in which the test stimulus was a .22 calibre pistol fired behind each subject, Landis and Hunt concentrated almost entirely on the first 0.5 s but noted in passing that other much less logical responses which were not obviously directed to the stimulus occurred. For example some changed their positions, others smiled aimlessly or addressed some remark to the experimenter.

Jumping with fright is a commonplace emotional response which may serve some crude protective function. In normal individuals excessive startle usually occurs as a result of tension or sleep deprivation. Chronic anxiety states, benzodiazepine withdrawal and catatonic schizophrenia also cause exaggerated responses. It is likely that a genetic predisposition exists to startle in the general population which follows a normal biological distribution. An interesting observation supporting this notion of constitutional susceptibility has been made by Humphrey and Warner (1934) who, while attempting to breed more robust strains of German police dogs, came across 'gun shy' or 'stick shy' animals who were impossible to train because of an excessive sensitivity to gun-sound or physical contact with sticks.

Thorne (1944) has described a syndrome of 'startle neurosis' which he estimates to occur in about one in 2000 healthy males. In his post as a civilian neuropsychiatric examiner at a United States Army Induction Centre he encountered three individuals with excessive startle reactions to unexpected stimuli, vague hyperaesthesiae and associated personality disorder. A recent newspaper advert harvested 12 of these individuals, some of whom reported throwing or dropping objects, uncontrollable vocalisations and occasionally uttering inappropriate embarrassing obscenities (Simons, 1980).

At the end of the last century a number of exotic, apparently culturally-determined, abnormal responses to startle were described by anthropologists, floklorists and travellers to distant climes. These included the jumpers of Maine, miryachit or Arctic hysteria and the latah reaction. As an intern Gilles de la Tourette translated some of these reports into French and his interest in these strange disorders stimulated his search for similar cases. This culminated in his description of the disorder, which, thanks to Charcot, earned him eponymous fame, and which he likened to latah and the jumpers (Table 6.1).

More recently a further group of closely related disorders characterised by grossly exaggerated startle reactions have been described in which falls, hypnagogic myoclonus and a hesitant staggering gait may be seen.

Table 6.1. A COMPARISON OF STARTLE SYNDROMES AND GILLES DE LA TOURETTE SYNDROME

	Latah	Hyperekplexias	Miryachit	Jumpers	Gilles de la Tourette syndrome
Exaggerated startle reaction	+ +	+ + +	±	+ + +	±
Echophenomena	+ + +	0	+ + +	+	+
Automatic obedience	+ +	0	+ +	+	0
Coprolalia	+ +	0	±	±	+
Tics	0	0	0	0	+ + +
Stimulus-induced aggressive outbursts	+ +	0	0	+ +	0

+ + + — invariable; + + very common; + common; ± may occur; 0 absent.

The latah reaction, miryachit and the jumping Frenchmen of Maine These phenomena, although traditionally considered as discrete entities, have much in common. All three occur in response to startle and may be conceived as conditioned habits in suggestible individuals. They appear to be particularly prevalent in unsophisticated peasant communities and, with the possible exception of miryachit, are regarded as odd behavioural quirks rather than illnesses. Although it is probable that these are regional variants of the same basic disorder, available accounts do suggest some differences and consequently they will be considered separately.

THE LATAH REACTION

Latah was first mentioned in Malay literature in the Hikayat Koris, a 15th-century manuscript which refers to a queen 'falling into a fit of latah and behaving like a lunatic not knowing what she was doing'. The word conveys to the Malays a clownish conduct which is often inherited and may be metaphorically translated as 'ticklish', 'love madness' or 'the creeps'. The commentary by O'Brien in 1883 in a local Malaysian journal was the first to attract the medical profession's attention and this was soon followed by a number of other excellent non-medical descriptions.

The essential feature is a frequently comical, stereotyped reaction to an unexpected stimulus such as a sharp command or tickle (Aberle, 1952). Echolalia, echopraxia and automatic obedience are commonest but the latah may also jump, freeze or become violent (amok) and sometimes shouts uncontrollably or utters a train of obscenities. No fixed pattern exists for this remarkable disturbance and admixtures of the imitative and startle varieties are common. The behaviour appears to be commoner in women and when it appears in men seems to single out those of a timid, submissive and retiring disposition. Affected individuals usually have no overt psychopathology and it is exceptional to find a latah in a psychiatric hospital.

Some of the best accounts are to be found in Sir Hugh Clifford's book *Studies in Brown Humanity* where he confirmed the earlier observations of precipitation by startle and added:

> While in this condition they appear to be unable to release their own identity, or to employ any but imitative faculties though they very frequently, nay almost invariably make use of villainously bad language without anyone prompting them to do so.

Clifford first became interested in latah when he discerned that his cook suffered from the condition and he relates with amusement an incident in which a small boy decided one day to have some fun with this cook and the cook's friend who was also latah. The two men were in the kitchen chewing betel nuts when the young rascal suddenly made a loud noise with a rattan.

> Each of the latah gave a sharp cry and jump and since there was nothing to distract their attention from one another, fell to imitating each others gestures. For nearly

half an hour so far as I could judge, from what I learned later, these two men sat opposite to one another, gesticulating wildly and aimlessly using the most filthy language and rocking their bodies to and fro. They never took their eyes off one another for sufficient time for the strange influence to be broken and at length utterly worn out and exhausted first sat and then the Trengganu man fell over on the platform in fits foaming horribly at the mouth with thin white flakes of foam.

In considering the cause of this remarkable response, Clifford also made the prophetic statement:

> Anyone who desires to really account for this affliction must, I am convinced, begin by analysing and examining and explaining the pathology of the common start or 'Jump' to which we are all in a lesser or a greater degree subject.

These lay descriptions were ultimately substantiated by medical men who were struck by the resemblance of latah states to hysterical somnambulism and hypnotic trance. Yap (1952) studied several middle-aged Malay women and concluded that it may represent a culturally-determined form of fright reaction.

Simons (1980) has made a recent study of latah in Malaysia and the Phillipines and distinguished three types of latah. The first he has termed immediate response latah which consists merely of a strong response to startle that others find amusing, violent body movements, assumption of habitual defensive postures, throwing or dropping objects and coprolalia. In Malaysia the commonest words were 'puki' (cunt), 'butoh' (prick) and 'buntut' (arse) and nearly always appeared as the first word in a series or preceded by an 'oh' or an 'ah.' Sometimes attempts were made to conceal the obscenity so that one mali-mali would shout 'utes' instead of 'uten', the Tagalog word for penis. Another ploy to lessen embarrassment would be to downgrade the oath by adding an animal reference as for example 'uten kabayo' (prick of a horse). Most of these swear words appeared to be automatically triggered verbalis- ations and other latahs would often repeat the last thing said or respond with the name of the object which elicited the startle. A second form, attention capture latah, was also common in the Malay villages of Negri Sembilan and Melaka. This took the form of matching, echophenomena and obedience. Simons has suggested that with increased arousal as occurs in latah, excessive compliance may occur. An audience, the improper nature of the commands or the presence of people of higher status all increased arousal and hence vulner- ability to this capture of attention. On questioning the latahs and mali-malis, he found that most when alone exhibited only a brief startle response and it was only after a volley of very strong and flustering startles following teasing by villagers that they would repeat and execute forcefully presented commands. Simons makes the interesting suggestion that a possible neurophysiological equivalent in the West might be the occasional report of a startled person driving a car straight into rather than away from a suddenly appearing danger.

Finally, he describes role latah which involves the practice of selecting behaviours from the other two types and elaborating them idiosyncratically into intentionally amusing performances. These might occur after the slightest stimulus such as a gentle nudge, and some latahs during a performance would self-stimulate themselves with abrupt jerky turns of the head away from the audience and sharp 'eh' noises. Among the Malays this often socially rewarding comical behaviour was only seen in women or homosexual males.

On the basis of these observations Simons concluded that these forms of latah were culture-specific exploitations of a constitutionally exaggerated startle reflex.

Reports of similar phenomena have since appeared from all parts of the world and it is clear that the latah reaction of the Malays is but a local name for a condition referred to as 'imu' by the Japanese Ainu, 'mali-mali' in the Phillipines, 'Yaun' in Burma, 'Bah-tsche' in Thailand, 'ramenajana' in the Malagasy Republic, 'olanism' in Siberia and 'ikota' by the Samoyedes. Identical reactions are also seen in the Kaffiers of South Africa, the Dayaks of Borneo and the Laplanders (Lapp panic) and occasional cases have also been reported in Western Europe and the United States of America.

MIRYACHIT (TO ACT FOOLISHLY)

This was probably initially described by the voyager Steller in 1774 but the first clear narration comes from William Hammond, former United States Surgeon General. He had been struck by an unusual report from three naval officers on a journey from the Pacific through Asia and considered that their account, published by the US Navy Department, merited being drawn to the attention of doctors (Hammond, 1884). The incident in question occurred on a boat journey up the Ussuri River near its junction with the Amur in Eastern Siberia and is quoted by Hammond as follows:

While we were walking on the bank here, we observed our messmate, the captain of the general staff (of the Russian army) approach the steward of the boat suddenly, and without any apparent reason or remark, clap his hands before his face; instantly the steward clapped his hands in the same manner, put on an angry look, and passed on. The incident was somewhat curious, as it involved a degree of familiarity with the steward hardly to have been expected. After this we observed a number of queer performances of the steward, and finally comprehended the situation. It seemed that he was afflicted with a peculiar mental or nervous disease, which forced him to imitate everything suddenly presented to his senses. Thus, when the captain slapped the paddle box suddenly in the presence of the steward, the latter instantly gave it a similar thump; or if any noise were made suddenly, he seemed compelled against his will to imitate it instantly, and with remarkable accuracy. To annoy him some of the passengers imitated pigs grunting, or called out absurd names; others clapped their hands and shouted, jumped, or threw their hats on the deck suddenly, and the poor steward suddenly startled, would echo them all precisely, and sometimes several consecutively. Frequently he would expostulate, begging people not to startle him, and again would grow furiously angry, but even in the midst of his passion he would helplessly imitate some ridiculous shout or motion directed at him by his pitiless tormentors. Frequently he shut himself up in his pantry, which was without windows, and locked the door, but even there he could be heard answering the grunts, shouts or sounds on the bulkhead outside.

On questioning the captain of the boat about the affliction of his steward the naval officers were informed that it was quite common around the Yakutsk region and was more often seen in men than women.

This report sparked off an international debate, Italian and subsequently Russian authors claiming precedence for its description. Yankovsky claimed that in 1876 at Novokievsky he had observed an epidemic of miryachit amongst 14 soldiers following the ingestion of hemp oil supplied by a Korean who was also latah. All of them exhibited striking echolalia, euphoria, dilated pupils, hyperkinesic and mirror movements. He also described four children from Vladivostock who, in response to startle, repeated words and actions.

Miryachit is characterised by uncontrollable echolalia and echopraxia. Automatic obedience may occur but there is no startle reaction or copralalia. It is said to be commoner in females and Yap (1952) is of the view that it is identical to latah. Hammond described this group of conditions as follows:

> They are analogous to reflex actions and especially to certain epileptic paroxysms due to reflex irritation. It would seem as though the nerve cells were very much in the condition of a package of dynamite or nitroglycerin in which a very slight impression is sufficient to effect a discharge of nerve force. They differ, however, from the epileptic paroxysms in the fact that the discharge is consonant with the perception which in these cases is an irritation.

THE JUMPING FRENCHMEN OF MAINE

In 1878 at the Fourth Annual Meeting of the American Neurological Association, Dr George Beard announced that he was about to carry out a study on a new endemic disorder restricted to a group of lumberjacks, mainly of French-Canadian descent, who lived in the Moosehead Lake region of northern Maine. Three years later he reported his findings on 50 individuals including 14 cases from four families. The condition was familial, usually began in childhood around the age of 4 or 5, and was uncommon in females. The cardinal feature of the disorder was a marked involuntary jump occurring in response to a loud noise, sharp command or startle. Many cases also displayed echolalia and automatic obedience even to the extent of performing acts that might be dangerous to themselves. For instance, Beard observed cases who would strike their best friend to command and others who would be prepared to place their hands in a burning fire. Some were commanded to repeat lines from Virgil verbatim and were able to accomplish this with a facility that belied their rather low intellectual capacities. These extraordinary behaviours would usually be preceded by a shoulder shrug or more often by a jump several inches off the ground, the severity of the response bearing a direct relationship to the degree of unexpectedness in the command or startle. Beard also commented that most of the afflicted men had shy, retiring, rather simple personalities.

Although the jumpers received no further medical attention for more than 50 years they continued to be recognised and accepted as part of the folk-culture of northern New England. The regional bard Holman Day, in his poem 'The Jumper', describes a man who startled violently at the whistle of the passing train each night and would thereby unintentionally strike his wife. Rabinovitch (1965) records that during his boyhood in rural Quebec, a popular childhood game was based on recognition of these jumpers. To play it the unsuspecting victim was followed silently, preferably at twilight, and was surreptitiously poked from behind in the ribs. At the same time the child doing the prodding would let out the cry of a kicking horse which would cause the boy who had been poked to jump into the air and echo the cry. He would then turn about and for a few seconds shout, grimace and give vent to his anger. The game was believed to have its origin in the old custom of lumberjacks of scaring their friends when they entered a horse's stable.

Chapel (1966) also recalls being in contact with a number of jumpers when working as a miner in the Porcupine district of Ontario. These friendly, witty and gregarious men were constantly harassed by fellow miners who would delight in startling them by shouting commands or obscenities which inevitably produced a jump, echolalia, and automatic obedience. Stevens (1965) reported a further case of a 59-year-old man of French-Canadian extraction living in northern Maine who was admitted to hospital for anorexia and weight loss. When struck by the patellar hammer in the course of a routine medical examination he would jump 10 inches off the bed. A passing nurse, sudden flashes of light or unexpected noises were equally potent stimuli. When standing, rapid flexion of the limbs and trunk would often accompany the jump leading to falls. Electroencephalography was normal even during a jump and anticonvulsants were ineffective. In Stevens' report two other related cases of Protestant Scottish-Irish extraction were adumbrated. At the presentation of this paper at the American Neurologists' Association, a Dr T. Fitch recalled being taken by a fisherman of French-Canadian extraction to see his five children in Wedgeport, Nova Scotia, all of whom manifested the syndrome.

Kunkle (1967) carried out a field study in Maine and was able to trace a considerable number of jumpers and examine 15 cases personally. Thirteen were males, most of whom were employed in manual trades and could recall the disorder starting in early childhood. Automatic obedience was present in seven but only two had echophenomena. Many of these individuals had incorporated an involuntary aggressive gesture into their jump and there were a few known as 'killer jumpers' whom it was considered extremely dangerous to 'goose' when they were carrying weapons as they would strike out uncontrollably at whoever was nearby. Four secondary jumpers were also described whose jumps appeared to begin in adult life after an illness. Kunkle considered the response to be a socially-conditioned reflex serving to release concealed hostility. Further cases of aggressive jumpers sensitive to tickle or goosing have been reported from North Carolina (Hardison, 1980).

Recently, video-taped interviews have been made with several jumpers from the Beauce region of Quebec by Dr Saint-Hilaire and his daughter. This is probably the area of origin of the lumbermen of Moosehead Lake which is linked to the Beauce directly by a main road. These individuals startled excessively, had a history of suggestibility and when surprised would often exclaim or swear.

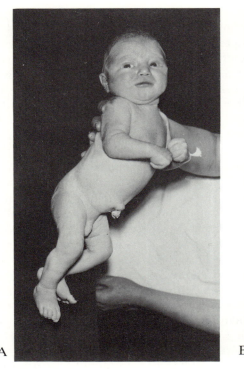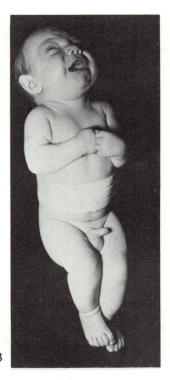

A   B

Figure 6.1. *A child with familial hyperekplexia.*

Finally Marsden et al have cast doubt on Beard's maxim 'once a jumper always a jumper'. They described a young woman with jumps whose movements were shown by neurophysiological back-averaging techniques to be voluntary and who, when confronted with this knowledge, ceased jumping altogether.

PRIMARY HYPEREKPLEXIA

This rare disorder usually occurs as an autosomal dominant condition with two phenotypic expressions. In its severe form it presents in infancy with severe transient hypertonia, associated poverty of spontaneous movement and slightly delayed motor milestones (Fig. 6.1). An exaggerated startle response with muscular stiffness usually begins in early childhood causing frequent falls with injury and a reactive insecure hesitant gait. Multiple hypnagogic myoclonic jerks and increased brain-stem and stretch reflexes are other features. In its minor form excessive startle triggered by acute febrile illnesses in childhood or stress in adult life is the only feature. Sporadic cases have also been recorded.

Suhren et al (1966) studied 25 individuals spanning five generations of a family of German-Dutch origin. They reported a mother who knew, immediately her child was born, that he was affected because of the stiffness of his muscles. The child's fists would clench tight and could not be opened without a great deal of force. As a result of severe adductor, spasm nappy-changing could only be achieved by the mother putting her head between the infant's knees. In early childhood many of the affected patients began to freeze on startle causing them to fall. As soon as they hit the ground, however, they were able to get up immediately without any disturbance of awareness. Some found that if they held on to a small object this could attenuate the response. These authors also commented that if the child had normal muscle tone then an excessive response to startle without falls would be the only symptom. In the hypertonic individuals, a slowness and stiffness of movement was also seen but if the child was examined while asleep muscle tone would be normal. If awakened suddenly, severe flexion hypertonia would immediately appear. Many of the cases also had exaggerated head retraction, palmomental and orbicularis oris reflexes and inguinal umbilical and epigastric hernias. The severity of the disorder throughout life varied, some individuals being most affected in youth then remaining the same or improving, others waxing and waning unpredictably. A number of cases stated that their symptoms were worse in winter. Four of the patients also had fits.

Andermann et al (1980) have described a similar family of French-Canadian extraction. Two sisters are described in detail with the major form of the disease. The 22-year-old proband had been considered to suffer from spastic quadriplegia at birth. Shortly after she began to walk at 13 months her mother had observed that loud noises would cause her to become stiff and fall to the ground without loss of consciousness. These episodes became so frequent that she returned to crawling until the age of 5 years. At the age of 5 she developed nocturnal myoclonus, mainly affecting the legs and lasting several minutes. At 14 years of age she again began to startle easily and fall. Her younger 13-year-old sister developed intermittent stiffening of the limbs and urinary incontinence two days after birth and was believed to have epilepsy. In common with her sister, although capable of walking at 18 months, she continued to crawl until the age of 5 because loud noises made her stiffen and fall. Nocturnal myoclonus was an additional prominent feature. Andermann also reported a further apparently sporadic example in a 12-year-old Italian boy who, when fishing at the age of 10, stiffened and fell over when a small fish he was attempting to land suddenly flipped against him. Another day a grasshopper landed on him causing him to jump, stiffen and collapse. A bizarre hesitant gait was the most confusing sign in all of these cases, occurring as a direct response to fear of falling.

A third family is described by Kurczynski (1983) in which nine cases were found over five generations. During the first few months life-threatening apnoeic episodes occurred in the proband, an observation which might also explain the sudden death of one affected infant at 6 months in the original family described by Suhren et al (1966). Tapping the tip of the nose was found to be a consistently specific stimulus for startle in the proband whereas forehead tapping, noted to be effective by Andermann in his patients, had no effect. An umbilical hernia was also present in the proband. Saenz-Lope et al (1984) have reported five (three boys, two girls) of seven children with the condition and Markand et al (1984) identified 15 members of five generations, six of whom had congenital hip dislocations, four hernias and one a subdural haematoma from falls.

Gastaut and Villeneuve (1967) described 12 seemingly sporadic cases with similar clinical features to the minor form. Nine were females and three males, most presenting in the second and third decades. The clinical picture was dominated in all of them by stimulus-triggered jumps and nocturnal myoclonus. The stimulus had to be unexpected and was most commonly auditory such as slamming a door, clapping hands, the sound of a car horn or telephone. Jumps were provoked by loss of balance in nine cases, unexpected touching such as a drop of water falling on the hand in eight cases and visual stimuli such as a lightning flash or witnessing a bicycle swerve in six. Five patients emitted a shout at the onset and four were slightly incontinent of urine. The frequency of jumps ranged from 10–100 per day, they were aggravated by stress or worry in all cases and in five of the females were worse at the time of the menses. Accidents and injuries were common due to falls or biting the tongue if startle occurred when the patient was eating. Vasomotor symptoms followed the jump in three cases. The nocturnal jerks were sometimes triggered by noise or movement but more usually occurred on falling asleep. One patient had epilepsy and four were regarded as mildly mentally deficient. Most of the patients also appeared to have personality problems, some exploiting their illness in order to get special attention.

The most striking electroencephalographic correlate of startle in primary hyperekplexia is the occurrence of a few fast spikes followed by a positive sharp wave of 80–100 ms duration, then one or more delta waves with desynchronisation of background alpha rhythm for several seconds which occurs bilaterally and is maximal fronto-centrally (Fig. 6.2). In contrast to the physiological response habituation is poor allowing up to 20–30 recordings in some patients. Andermann et al (1980) believed that the spike was a cortical potential evoked by the sensory stimulus but Markand et al (1984) were unable to demonstrate a cerebral potential either by conventional electroencephalography or back-averaging techniques and concluded that the spikes were muscle artefact and the sharp wave due to eyeball retraction. Suhren et al (1966) found frank epileptic discharges in four of their cases and abnormalities more in keeping with a deep midline disturbance than a cortical event in others. One of the patients of Andermann et al (1980) also had an active spike and wave discharge and another a parietal sharp wave abnormality. Using high-speed filming Suhren et al (1966) demonstrated a marked increase in the amplitude of the head retraction reflex which was considered an integral part of the startle response. The startle response was also excessive in amplitude and in some lasted for longer than 800 ms.

It has been proposed that the abnormalities underlying hyperekplexia may be due to a delay in the maturation of control of brain-stem centres by higher inhibitory mechanisms leading to the discharge of an uninhibited primitive

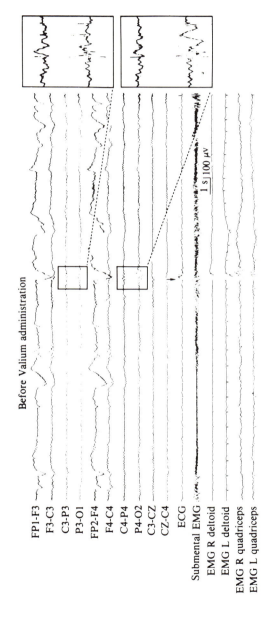

Figure 6.2. *Polygraphic recording illustrating a pathological startle response induced by noise (arrow) before intravenous Valium administration. The EEG response (insert) consists of an initial spike recorded from both centro-parieto-occipital regions followed by a short train of slow waves and desynchronisation of background activity. (By kind permission of Dr Andermann and colleagues, 1980. In: Brain, vol. 103. Oxford University Press pp. 985–997.)*

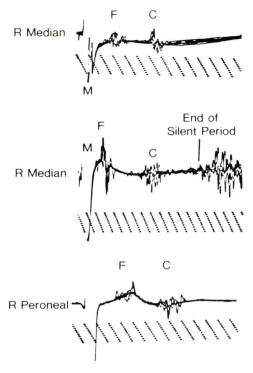

Figure 6.3. *C response recorded in a patient with hyperekplexia. Top —
stimulation of right median nerve at wrist, with thumb in rest position.
Centre — stimulation of right median nerve with thumb in 'hold' position.
Bottom — stimulation of right common peroneal nerve at knee with foot in
rest position (cal. 10 ms 0.5 mv). M = motor response; F = F wave. (By
kind permission of Dr Markand and colleagues, 1984. Arch. Neurol., vol. 41,
pp. 71–4.)*

nociceptive reflex (Suhren et al, 1966). Gastaut and Villeneuve also considered
functional hyperexcitability of the rhombo-mesencephalic reticular formation
to underlie the disorder. Recently a case was reported of a man who developed
hyperekplexia at 37 and then experienced full resolution eight years later.
Twenty years later he sustained a posterior thalamoperforate artery occlusion
leading to the reoccurrence of severe hyperekplexia. Somatosensory evoked
potentials revealed an increased voltage of the N_2–P_2 wave recorded from the
right somatosensory cortex but the left cortical potential overlying the thalamic
lesion was normal. On the basis of this finding, interruption of the rubro-
thalamic pathway at the level of the red nucleus has been claimed to disinhibit
the startle reflex (Fariello et al, 1983). Markand et al (1984) have demonstrated
a prominent C response in both the rest and hold position after median nerve
stimulation in six patients. This occurred following the F wave response and
before the end of the silent period with a latency of 48–65 ms. Similar results

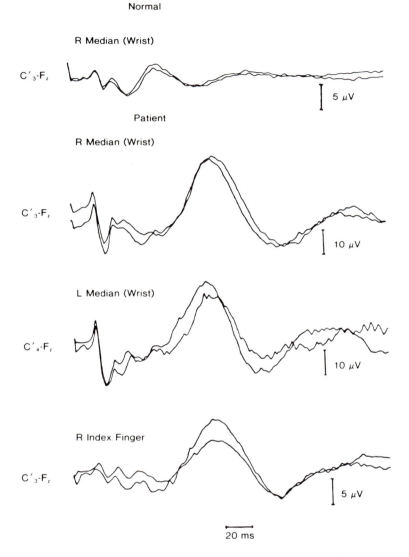

Normal

R Median (Wrist)

C′₃-F₂

5 μV

Patient

R Median (Wrist)

C′₃-F₂

10 μV

L Median (Wrist)

C′₄-F₂

10 μV

R Index Finger

C′₃-F₂

5 μV

20 ms

Figure 6.4. *High amplitude scalp somatosensory evoked responses after stimulation of right and left median and interdigital nerves of right index finger in a patient with hyperekplexia. The top tracing shows a normal response. (By kind permission of Dr Markand and colleagues, 1984. Arch. Neurol.,vol. 41.)*

occurred with interdigital and common peroneal nerve stimulation, the C response being more prominent in the hold position (Fig. 6.3). Somatosensory evoked responses were obtained in seven patients with median and posterior nerve stimulation and in most of these large amplitude early and later responses

were found similar to those seen in cortical myoclonus and progressive myoclonic epilepsy (Fig. 6.4). On the assumption that the enhanced long loop reflexes were of cortical origin, these authors suggested that increased cortical
neuronal hyperexcitability is the basic pathophysiological mechanism underlying the hyperekplexias.

Clonazepam, a long-acting benzodiazepine with effects on central 5-
hydroxytryptamine metabolism, seems to be the treatment of choice but this
is not consistently effective. Phenobarbitone, 5-hydroxytryptophan, chlordiaze-
poxide, sodium valproate, primidone and piracetam have also been reported
to be beneficial.

SECONDARY HYPEREKPLEXIA

Excessive startle occurs commonly in Little's disease (Marsh, 1965) and
athetosis (Foley, 1983). It is also seen in patients with magnesium deficiency
(Fishman, 1965) and startle myoclonus occurs in Creutzfeldt-Jakob disease. In
startle epilepsy (Alajouanine and Gastaut, 1958) a startle reaction is
accompanied by a tonic seizure with impaired consciousness lasting 5–10 s and,
according to Gastaut and Villeneuve (1967), in contrast to hyperekplexia it may
be accentuated by pentylene tetrazol and not by strychnine.

Many of these cases have infantile hemiplegia, the fit being restricted to the
paralysed side and associated with epileptic discharges on the electro-
encephalogram. Myoclonic jerks, indistinguishable from hyperekplexia clini-
cally and triggered by noise, also occasionally occur, the EEG showing slow
polyspikes or polyspike waves (Gastaut and Tasinari, 1966).

Hyperekplexia must be distinguished from cataplexy in which there is a
sudden loss of muscle tone with a fall, in response to emotional stimuli. This
usually occurs together with narcolepsy as part of Gelineau's syndrome. Falls
may also occur in post-traumatic cortical reflex myoclonus, and startle enhances
myoclonic jerking in post-anoxic or familial reticular reflex myoclonus. In these
conditions, however, widespread action myoclonus is also present. However,
in both hyperekplexia and cortical reflex myoclonus, enhanced long loop
reflexes have been described. Drop attacks due to reflex epilepsy or vertebro-
basilar ischaemia of the reticular formation also lead to unpredictable falls but
do not occur in response to specific startle stimuli. Finally, some patients with
myotonia become stiff on startle but this is quite long-lasting and not associated
with falls.

7

Hyperactivity Syndrome

Synonyms Hyperkinetic syndrome, Prechtl's choreiform syndrome, Strauss syndrome, clumsy child, minimal brain dysfunction, minimal brain damage, attention deficit disorder.

Definitions *The hyperactivity syndrome* is a childhood behavioural disorder in which an unusual degree of purposeless motor restlessness interrupts concentration and impairs attention leading to difficulty in the completion of structured tasks.

Minimal brain dysfunction is a disorder of learning and attention in children of normal or near normal general intelligence which leads to scholastic under-achievement. It may be associated with subtle neurological abnormalities including perceptual, language and memory deficits. About two-thirds of these children are hyperkinetic.

Attention deficit disorder is a selective defect of attention span leading to abnormal distractability.

The abundant natural exuberance of young children renders them all hyperactive when compared with adults. Economy of movement and the acquisition of kinetic melody are learned slowly over the first five years of life and a degree of fidgetiness, particularly in response to emotional stress, lingers in most of us into adulthood. It is also common experience that constant restlessness may occur as a constitutional peculiarity in some youngsters. Winnicott, in his *Clinical Notes on Disorders of Childhood* (Winnicott, 1931), describes these individuals as follows:

> Such a fidgety child is a worry, is restless, is up to mischief if left for a moment unoccupied, and is impossible at table, either eating food as if someone would snatch it from him, or else liable to upset tumblers or spill tea . . . sleep is usually restless. . . . These children are over-excitable or 'nervy' rather than nervous (of things, people, the dark, being alone). However, these children are often happy, though irritable if restricted in activity. Picturing such a child one remembers countless children of between five and ten years old, thin and wiry, quick in the uptake and eager.

Sydenham's chorea may be simulated by some of these children and there is an old aphorism that a choreic child is punished three times before the diagnosis is made; once for fidgetiness, once for breaking crockery and finally for making faces at his grandmother. Over a century ago the German physician Heinrich Hoffmann first described hyperactivity in *Struwelpeter*, a book for children in which he related the humorous tale of 'Fidgety Phil' in pictures and doggerel (Hoffmann, 1845). In the late 19th century, Ireland (1877) described a group of 'mad idiots' who were prone to violent motor outbursts and destructiveness. Tuke (1892) believed hyperkinesia to be a symptom of impulsive insanity and the younger the affected child the more likely it was that the child would be restless and distractable. It is only in this century, however, that the concept of hyperkinesia as a behavioural disorder with educational repercussions has emerged and it has been claimed by cynics that the whole notion of the disorder is an artefact based on changing concepts of education and the consequent inability of some children to adjust to a structured environment.

Large numbers of sociopathic hyperkinetic children began to be described after the outbreak of von Economo's disease in the 1920s (Bond and Smith, 1935) and in 1932 Kramer and Pollnow described a condition of motor unrest in children aged 2–4 years in association with epilepsy or mild brain damage (Kramer and Pollnaw, 1932). These children were slow to develop intellectually, although intelligence ranged from high average to borderline defective. They were distractable and had a marked tendency to put objects in their mouth and chew them. Lewin (1938) studied 279 restless subjects and concluded that cerebral lesions were responsible in large part for the production of severe forms of motor restlessness and mild forms were due to disturbed parental relationships. In the last 20 years a veritable epidemic of presumptive cases has appeared, leading to prodigious social problems and sensational newspaper cuttings claiming that large numbers of disruptive elementary school children were being placed on psycho-stimulant drugs at the request of teachers without parental consent. In the United Kingdom, attention has always been given to its occurrence in brain-damaged populations (Ounsted, 1955) and only when overactivity is severe and associated with distractability is the diagnosis made. In America, in contrast, a broader definition is used embracing conduct disorders and impulsive behaviour and excluding cases with marked neurological impairment.

EPIDEMIOLOGY

The prevalence of the syndrome varies greatly depending on the diagnostic criteria used, the methods of investigation and the population studied. For example, in the Isle of Wight Study in the United Kingdom Rutter et al (1976) found only two hyperkinetic children in a total population study of 2199 10- and 11- year-olds and only 1.6% of all disturbed children in this investigation were labelled hyperkinetic. Thorley (1984) identified 73 children and adolescents in a total children clinic population of 5923 seen at the Maudsley Hospital between 1968 and 1980. In contrast Huessy (1967) found a 10%

prevalence in Vermont second-grade children and Stewart et al (1966) reported a 4% prevalence in St Louis children aged between 5 and 11. General agreement exists that there is a marked predilection for male children with the sex ratio ranging from 3:1 to 9:1 in different series.

AETIOLOGY

It is probable that the hyperactivity syndrome is in fact a heterogeneous group of conditions with different aetiologies. Certainly it may occur as a result of structural brain damage but this is not inevitable. Thorley (1984) for example found 51% of his cases were of normal intelligence. Furthermore, the large majority of brain-damaged children do not exhibit hyperactivity. Attempts to visualise the brain by computed axial tomography have provided limited but inconsistent evidence for variations in normal hemispheric widths and asymmetries (Rosenberger and Hier, 1980). Neurophysiological investigation has also failed to reveal any electroencephalographic abnormalities specific to the syndrome although the use of newer techniques such as discriminant analysis and computer-assisted analysis of brain bioelectrical activity have at least succeeded in separating learning disabled children from normal controls (John et al, 1977; Duffy et al, 1980). Evidence for a neurochemical abnormality is also lacking at present, although a functional depletion of central catecholamines has been mooted.

Some evidence also exists to support a genetic factor, although many of the available studies have been criticised on methodological grounds. A high concordance rate has been reported in the available twin studies (Willerman, 1973) and clinicians have long noted familial clustering with an apparent increased prevalence among siblings and parents. In one study Safer was able to locate 14 minimally brain-damaged children whose siblings or half-siblings had been reared in foster homes. This study showed that 50% of the full siblings and 14% of the half-siblings were characterised by short attention span repeated behaviour problems and hyperactivity (Safer, 1971).

PATHOLOGY

Only two post-mortem studies on patients with minimal brain dysfunction have been carried out. Drake (1968) studied a 12-year-old boy with fits and severe reading disability who died suddenly from a haemorrhage from a cerebellar arteriovenous malformation. Abnormalities of gyrus formation were noted in both parietal lobes and the related areas of the corpus callosum were thinned. The cerebral cortex in the affected regions showed disorganisation of structure and ectopic neurones in white matter.

An autopsy on a 20-year-old boy with a history of fits and developmental dyslexia who died from a fall showed a consistently wider left cerebral hemisphere, an area of polymicrogyria in the left temporal speech area and evidence of cortical dysplasia in limbic primary and association areas (Galaburda and Kemper, 1979).

CLINICAL DESCRIPTION

The hyperactivity syndrome is best regarded as a symptom complex of which the cardinal features are excessive fidgetiness, distractability, impulsiveness and emotional instability. Parents usually complain that the child has always appeared to have excessive energy, needing far less sleep than his siblings and wearing his clothes out more rapidly. In retrospect mothers often state that the child was unduly fretful as a baby, proving difficult to soothe and constantly crying. Parents and teachers observe a never-ceasing restlessness and an inability to sit still even when watching a favourite television programme. The child is constantly in motion, into everything, whistling, chattering, annoying siblings and classmates and compulsively touching anything that comes within his reach. It remains unclear, however, whether hyperkinetic children actually have a greater amount of daily motor activity or a different type. At least three-quarters of the children exhibit a marked clumsiness and dyspraxia, are forever tripping over things and may be described as having two left feet. They are also inordinately slow at mastering dextrous activities. Many find it difficult to learn to ride a bike and are woefully bad at ball games.

The most incapacitating disability, however, is the short attention span with difficulty in concentrating. Teachers complain that the child never listens and, because of his difficulty in grasping concepts and completing projects, he is often labelled as an 'underachiever'. Some of these children develop compensatory perseverative behaviour and others day-dream for long periods, incapable of even absorbing a short story. Reading seems particularly difficult for them to master but arithmetic and writing also usually present problems. Many are quite fearless, jumping into the deep end of swimming pools without knowing how to swim or running into the street in front of cars. They also fail to respond to normal disciplinary measures, being described as always wanting their own way or as being bossy and domineering. Some seem quite incapable of thinking ahead and making plans. Temper tantrums are frequent but response to pain is diminished, most of them being impervious to quite severe injuries. In stimulating situations or when with groups of other children, they become over-excitable and aggressive. When compared with matched psychiatric patients with conduct disorders, they have a higher frequency of motor disturbance, inattention and articulatory disturbance and a lower incidence of aggression, antisocial, emotional and psychosocial disturbance (Thorley, 1984).

Physical examination is usually normal, although defects of vision or hearing are sometimes present and mild speech disorders may also be found. Minor physical deformities such as widely-spaced eyes, a short incurved finger, adherent earlobes and abnormal skull shape are quite common. Major neurological abnormalities are not found although in one study minor deficits indicative of sensorimotor incoordination occurred (Werry et al, 1972). Similarly psychological testing has failed to reveal any specifically abnormal profile. Some studies have noted a greater range of variability on the WISC subtests than controls, whereas others have commented on mild right/left confusion, difficulty in auditory discrimination and auditory synthesis and problems transferring information from one sensory modality to another. In fact there is a considerable overlap with developmental dyslexia.

PRECHTL'S CHOREIFORM SYNDROME (Prechtl and Stemmer, 1962)

In the course of performing electroencephalograms on hyperactive children, Prechtl and Stemmer observed chorea-like twitchings in some cases which showed up on the EEG as characteristic spiky muscle artefacts. In a few the movements were sufficiently pronounced to suggest the possibility of rheumatic chorea but none had a past history of this disorder or residual evidence of rheumatic heart disease. Fifty of the children aged 9–12 years were then studied more extensively. The movements were slight and jerky, occurring irregularly and arrhythmically in different muscle groups particularly at times of stress. The tongue, face, neck and trunk were involved in all the patients. In about one-fifth of cases, however, the distal extremities were spared. Difficulties in ocular fixation during reading and hyperreflexia were common associated features. Most of the children were distractable and hyperactive, with poor attention span.

The EEGs revealed epileptic discharges in seven children, the remainder being normal apart from the striking muscle artefacts. Of interest in this regard is the occurrence of similar muscle artefacts on the EEG's of children with Gilles de la Tourette syndrome (Lees et al, 1984). 66% of the patients were found to have had foetal distress or post-partum asphyxia and minimal anoxic damage to the corpus striatum was postulated as the underlying cause. Wolff and Hurwitz (1966) recorded these choreiform twitches with the arms outstretched in 12% of normal children and 28% with hyperactivity, although Rutter, et al (1966) failed to confirm this.

COURSE

Hyperactivity, emotional immaturity and associated enuresis frequently recede as the child enters adolescence but the long-term outlook is frequently poor. Underachievement at school makes many of these children ill-equipped for the demands of modern society and many develop antisocial traits and delinquent behaviour. Parental rejection and difficulty in making close friends leads to low self-esteem and some of these children become overtly psychotic. Menkes et al (1967) studied the outcome of 14 children who had been hyperactive at Johns Hopkins 25 years previously. Four were institutionalised psychotics, two more were mentally retarded and in institutions and, of the remaining eight, one had been in jail, two more had been in institutions for juvenile delinquents and three were still hyperactive. Weiss et al (1971) followed their own patients for a mean period of five years and found that although hyperactivity diminished, disorders of attention remained and many children continued to be emotionally immature, aggressive and antisocial. In a further study the high incidence of sociopathic behaviour was emphasised. More than half had been involved in fighting, stealing and destructive behaviour and two-thirds were considered incorrigible by their parents. More than one third had threatened to kill their parents, 7% carried weapons, 15% were arsonists and 15% were excessive drinkers before the age of 16 (Mendelson et al, 1971).

No prospective studies into adulthood exist but indirect evidence suggests that the outcome is likely to be as poor as it is in adolescence. Increased prevalence rates for alcoholism, sociopathy and hysteria occur in the biological parents of hyperkinetic children compared with controls (Cantwell, 1972). Furthermore, 10% of the natural parents of hyperkinetic children were themselves hyperkinetic as children, and most of these were psychiatrically ill as adults suggesting that the hyperkinetic syndrome might be a precursor to the development of adult psychopathology (Morrison and Stewart, 1971). Retrospective studies of sociopathic adults and alcoholics have also revealed a high incidence of childhood hyperactivity (Shelley and Reister, 1972). No clear cut prognostic indications are available and there is no evidence that psychostimulant therapy improves the long-term outlook.

TREATMENT

Management guide-lines must be multifaceted, and medical treatment without parental counselling and remedial education has no long-term benefits. The physician, parent and teacher all have an important role to play in management, and behaviour modification therapy employing rewards may be helpful. Remedial teaching with special schools and individual tutors should be made available in severe cases. Parents are often stricken with guilt when the diagnosis is made and the disorder is probably best explained as a maturational delay in the nervous system brought about by some cryptic noxious factor. Living with a hyperactive child demands patience and considerable sympathy. Praising good behaviour, tolerance, tempered with consistent discipline, speaking quietly but firmly and the use of visual cues to reinforce verbal explanations are all of use. A well-structured calm and consistent routine for eating, play and bedtime are also important. The general principles for educating a hyperactive child include the use of multiple sensory cues and novel and creative ways to engage the child's attention, the avoidance of extraneous distractions and long periods of teaching which exceed the patient's short attention span. Basic principles should be overlearned before proceeding to more complicated problems, and instruction centres around maximising strengths rather than exposing weaknesses.

Central nervous stimulants should only be considered if these methods alone are inadequate. Indications for their use would include severe and persistent hyperactivity in a child of school age who is unable to function in a class room because of distractability and impulsiveness. Children with visual perception or eye-hand co-ordination problems and also other soft neurological signs do especially well. Hyperactivity caused primarily by anxiety, depression or psychosis and a history of fits are relative contra-indications. The commonly used drugs are dextro-amphetamine, methylphenidate and pemoline. Imipramine may also be tried if there is associated depression or enuresis. Treatment should be started at the smallest dose and increased gradually at weekly intervals. Drug holidays at weekends should be encouraged to avoid tolerance. Common adverse reactions include headache, anorexia, insomnia, dysphoria and weight loss. Stunting of growth may occur if large doses are given for long periods. Surprisingly, addiction problems in adolescence are rare. Amygdolotomies and other forms of stereotactic psychosurgery have been used but should probably be considered only in the severest intractable cases.

8

Habitual Manipulations of the Body

Definition Socially offensive co-ordinated movements which tend to occur particularly at times of boredom, fatigue, anxiety or self-consciousness.

In contradistinction to tics, habitual manipulations of the body are carried out at a much higher level of awareness. They can be interrupted at any stage by will power and are initiated more slowly than tics, sometimes requiring considerable preparation before they can be executed. There is also no limit to their duration. The commonest varieties are listed in Table 8.1. Chain smoking and the chewing of gum could be construed as adult equivalents and feeding disorders such as aerophagy and rumination also bear some similarities.

Finger sucking Finger or occasionally toe sucking is an everyday symptom regarded as a normal habit in early childhood. It has been estimated to occur in at least 80 % of all infants, and babies have exceptionally been born sucking their thumbs. The habit usually starts in the first two years of life and has often disappeared by the age of 3 or 4 years. Occasional finger sucking, however, still occurs in up to 30 % of 12-year-olds. There is some evidence to suggest that it may be slightly commoner in girls and white races. In essence it is a passive leisurely activity which is apt to occur when the child is unoccupied or getting ready for bed. Some children finger suck in a stereotyped way usually selecting one or other thumb for their attentions, while others attack any digit indis-

Table 8.1. A CLASSIFICATION OF HABITUAL MANIPULATIONS OF THE BODY

Oral:	thumb and finger sucking, nail biting or picking
Nasal:	nose picking, nose scratching
Hair:	trichotillomania
Head:	head or chin scratching
Manual:	fist clenching, finger clicking
Ocular:	eye rubbing
Aural:	ear touching, ear picking
Genital:	manipulation of genitals, thigh rubbing
Related disturbances: aerophagy, merycism, hyperventilation	

criminately. There is some evidence to suggest that finger sucking is used to provide relief from hunger in the early months of life and subsequently to assuage the pain of teething. If it persists in severe form much beyond the age of 9, it tends to be associated with general emotional immaturity and there may be an increased incidence of co-existing baby talk and enuresis. If the habit continues into adult life, shame and awareness of public ridicule may lead to its clandestine indulgence, and embarrassment may be such as to prevent help being sought. Constant thumb or finger sucking over several years occasionally leads to malocclusion of the anterior dentition or rarely to stomatitis or structural damage to the incisor teeth. The thumb may also become flattened or wrinkled and digital necrosis has been reported. The cause of finger sucking is unknown but its execution undoubtedly affords relief and any attempt to obstruct the habit leads to fractiousness and irritability. Regression to oral satisfactions, so called larval masturbation, at times of duress or fatigue is the explanation favoured by the Freudians. Incompleteness of the sucking phase of feeding is another popular theory supported by the observation that if the feeding of some domestic animals is interrupted before satiety, licking or sucking behaviour may ensue. There is also a heated debate concerning the relationship between inadequate or unsatisfactory breast feeding and the later development of finger sucking.

The notion that it was damaging to suck the thumb did not emerge until the end of the 19th century. Indeed some of the early Italian Masters depicted children sucking their thumbs in order to create a feeling of serenity. Based on the erroneous premise that finger sucking was detrimental to normal psychical development, all manner of barbaric mechanical devices including cuffs, muffs and strait-jackets were employed at the turn of the century, largely to no avail. In addition, foul-tasting ointments were smeared on the child's hands several times a day in a vain attempt to avert them being brought to the mouth. Modern management centres around distraction with some interesting activity as well as emphasis on reassurance and love, especially before going to bed. Behavioural techniques using positive reward systems are also successful in refractory childhood and adult cases.

Nail biting Nail biting occasionally starts as early as the first year of life but its incidence rises sharply between 4 and 6 years and reaches a peak at puberty, where figures of 40–55% have been recorded. It occurs equally in males and females and up to adolescence it is so commonplace as to be considered a normal habit. After that its frequency drops rapidly so that only one in five young adults continue to bite their nails. By the age of 60, possibly as a result of impaired dentition, the incidence falls to one in nine of the normal population. In contrast to finger sucking, nail biting occurs at times of anxiety or stress and tends to be most frequent in oversensitive, nervy children. In one study, 50% of nail biters carried out other manipulations of the body especially thumb sucking, a quarter had motor restlessness and insomnia and 19% had tics (Kanner, 1948). In another investigation, however, the incidence of nail biting was no higher in a group of psychiatric in-patients than in the normal population. Indeed a lower than normal incidence was found in mongols and high-grade mental defectives, whereas those mentally retarded individuals with an IQ above 65 had a significantly higher rate (Ballinger, 1970). No general relationship exists in the normal population, however, between its occurrence and intelligence.

Nail biting begins with the hand being moved close to the mouth. The finger may then be trapped against the front teeth and this manoeuvre is then followed by a number of quick bites with the nail pressed against the teeth. The finger is then removed from the mouth and palpated or inspected visually. During the procedure the facial expression is rather anxious and serious and if the biter becomes aware of being watched he usually shamefacedly brings the habit to an end. A few mentally disturbed people also bite their toe-nails.

It has been suggested that nail biting is simply a transfer from the thumb sucking habit but it is, in essence, a much more active process and occurs under different emotional circumstances. Most children ingeniously resist all parental demands to discontinue the habit, but somewhere around the age of 14 years censure by peer groups makes it expedient for other behaviours to be substi-

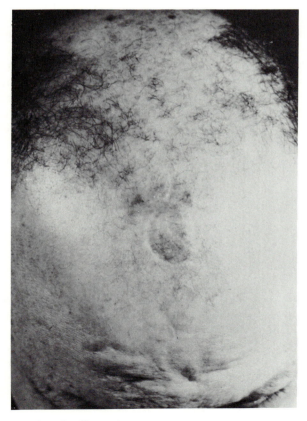

Figure 8.1. *A case of trichotillomania.*

tuted. Examples include pencil biting, hair twiddling or chewing gum. More surreptitious substitutes include lip biting, nail picking and nose picking.

Many people bite their nails in moments of stress and during the last war it was observed that nail biting occurred in soldiers either during tense emotional situations or more commonly at times of enforced inactivity. Children nail bite in moments of anguish and seek solace in their fingers when rejected. Twice as many children reared in orphanages nail bite as those fostered out, and tense home situations are a well-recognised predisposing factor. It is commonplace to observe adults shortening their nails through biting rather than using scissors but chronic nail biters reduce the nail tissue to a bare minimum often destroying the nail bed in the process and inducing bleeding and severe trauma. Many of these people are insecure and chronically anxious and treatment centres around reducing stress and building up feelings of self-importance and adequacy.

Trichotillomania Plucking and constant twiddling with the hair, often in response to scalp itchiness, may lead to patches of alopecia and occasionally, in severely disturbed individuals, to complete baldness (Fig. 8.1). On inspecting the head the disorder can be distinguished from alopecia areata by the differential growth of hair follicles within the bald patch. This disturbance is commoner in mentally defectives (Feré, 1906) but in mild degree occurs in many normal individuals at times of boredom or anxiety. Occasionally the hair is eaten leading to the formation of a trichobezoar in the stomach.

Nose picking This is a common habit which may be associated with conveying nasal contents to the mouth where they are chewed and swallowed. In chronic cases the nasal mucosa may become ulcerated and infected with recurrent epistaxes.

Lip biting or sucking This is common in the first year of life and consists of the passive thrusting of the lip between the upper and lower incisors, the lower lip being turned inwards and grasped by the incisors. In later life it is seen during acute emotional stress or intense concentration.

Tongue sucking This is a rare habit most often seen in the mentally retarded, especially in children with Down's syndrome.

Ear pulling This may be seen as an accessory manipulation occurring simultaneously with finger sucking. The ear is usually fondled or pulled slightly; picking or scratching the ears may indicate underlying otitis externa.

Aerophagy This fairly common disorder, characterised by excessive compulsive belching, bears some similarity to both tics and habitual manipulations of the body. The condition may begin with a feeling of tension in the epigastrium which is then followed by sighing movements which unintentionally introduce air into the stomach. This air is then emitted by belching which is followed by temporary relief. It is particularly likely to occur at times of boredom or stress and always disappears in sleep. In severe cases it may continue for hours until the sufferer is tired and his saliva flow exhausted. The head is bent forward, the chin lowered and air is imprisoned in the pharynx at the end of expiration. The individual then swallows and as air is driven down the oesophagus a clucking or low rumbling noise may be audible. The mouth is then opened and eructation of inoffensive air occurs. Gastric discomfort or left upper quadrant fullness (splenic flexure syndrome) may be the presenting complaint and acute gastric distension has occasionally resulted in death. Chronic anxiety, poor eating habits or occasionally actual/gastrointestinal disease may be the underlying causes. Intractable belching may also occur in extrapyramidal disorders.

Rumination (merycism) This was first described by Fabricius in 1687 and, curiously, several of the reported cases occurred in literary figures or eminent physicians. The neurologist Brown-Sequard, for instance, was a self-confessed merycole. The habit consists of the involuntary regurgitation of food without nausea, vomiting or retching and is not uncommon in small infants. The head is held back with the mouth wide open and sucking movements of the tongue with straining and back arching occur. The projectile expulsion of food appears to afford pleasure and in young children so much food may be lost that malnutrition with cachexia and fatality can result. A number of professional merycoles have been studied. One astonishing performer was able to drink 50 tumblers of water and expel the fluid in a stream, swallow nuts, handkerchiefs and other objects and return them in a set sequence as well as other equally implausible tricks (Long, 1929). X-rays have revealed that marked contraction of the abdominal musculature and the stomach combine to expel the gastric contents back into the oesophagus from where they are returned to the mouth by rhythmic contractions.

9

Disorders of Movement in the Mentally Retarded

Simple motor stereotypies and displeasing habitual manipulations of the body are a characteristic feature of the behaviour of many mental defectives (Table 9.1). Body rocking, head shaking, head banging and repetitive hand movements are particularly common and closely resemble the rhythmical body movements seen in many healthy infants. Self-injurious behaviour, tics and other seemingly irrational motor acts are encountered with great frequency. All these types of movement also occur with great frequency in the blind (blindisms) and in orphans raised in institutions.

The early alienists Pinel and Esquirol were fascinated by these abnormal movements and by studying them sought to gain insight into the mental life of

Table 9.1. ABNORMAL MOVEMENTS SEEN IN THE BLIND AND THE MENTALLY RETARDED

Stereotypies

Oral:	bruxism, lip movements, verbal perseverations, snorting, blowing, groaning, clicking, hooting, screaming, squealing, barking, singing
Head:	nodding, tossing, banging, bizarre posturing, weaving
Manual:	holding hand at arm's length and watching the fingers move, finger drumming, finger flicking before the eyes, hand to face, mouth or ear movements, pill-rolling movements, rubbing, pounding
Trunk:	body rocking, pelvic swaying or thrusting, twirling, circling, pirouetting
Leg:	lotus position, jumping, hopping

Habitual manipulations

thumb sucking, nail biting, lip biting, trichotillomania, masturbation, picking, grooming, smelling, finger licking, rag sucking, pica

Tics and Gilles de la Tourette syndrome

Echophenomena

Self-injurious behaviour

hurling against walls, hand biting, self-beating, eye poking and gouging, lip mutilation, krouomania, scratching imbeciles. Bourneville and his pupil Noir (Noir, 1893) working at L'Hôpital Bicetre attempted the first simple classification, drawing attention to the large number of intricate 'coordinated tics' to be found in idiots and *arrières*. Within this category, Noir included rhythmical movements such as balancing, head tossing and striking or beating oneself (krouomania). He considered all these activities provided a soothing effect on the individual, however brutal they might appear. In addition to simple tics and the occasional mentally retarded individual with Gilles de la Tourette syndrome, he also described a further group of abnormal movements by the epithet 'large tics'. These were restricted to those individuals without substantial motor deficits or spasticity where they often constituted the predominant external aspect of the patient's imbecility. Examples given included jumping, climbing, turning round and round or pirouetting as in Ros, affectionately known at Bicetre as 'the waltzer'.

Clark and Atwood (1912) distinguished the rhythmical, automatic behaviour seen in nearly all their institutionalised mental defectives from simple tics which astonishingly they noted in only three of 1100 residents. They remarked on the high incidence of finger and rag sucking in pre-pubescent idiots and re-emphasised the ubiquity of onanism in adults. They also viewed body rocking, head banging, tongue and lip chewing as auto-pleasurable acts leading up to, or substituting for, the act of masturbation.

In 1934 Earl described an adult disorder he termed 'the catatonic psychosis of idiocy'. None of his 38 patients had suffered from epidemic encephalitis lethargica and the illness was characterised by signs of progressive mental deterioration with emotional dissociation and catatonia. Eighteen cases exhibited hyperkinetic features including hand wringing, moving pieces of string constantly through the fingers, digit flicking, body rocking and violent, impulsive limb movements. Others exhibited echophenomena, monotypies, inexplicable protracted bouts of weeping and minor self-mutilation. Autistic children also manifest some of the phenomena associated particularly with the mentally retarded; rocking, hand flapping, curious body postures, hand movements to alter the light falling on the face, twiddling and flicking movements, jumping and spinning being a few of the most frequent autisms. Many of these children also have abnormal head and eye movements. For example, when shifting gaze, these children may seem unable to move the eyes without turning the head, and head movements in response to verbal commands are larger in amplitude and more erratic than normal. In general, however, the rhythmical stereotyped behaviour of the mentally retarded is easily distinguished from the more complex and bizarre motor acts of catatonic schizophrenics.

Attempts are now being made to identify specific clinical syndromes in the mentally retarded on the basis of particular forms of motor behaviour. The best example is the Lesch-Nyhan syndrome, a rare genetically determined disorder of purine metabolism affecting male children and causing severe compulsive self-multilation, spasticity, chorea and dystonia. The group of myopic, gosling mouthed, short necked, hand wringers reported by Engel (1970) may also prove to be a distinct disease with an underlying biochemical abnormality.

Epidemiological surveys confirm the high incidence of stereotyped behaviour in the mentally defective. Berkson and Davenport (1962) noted rhythmias in two-thirds of randomly selected male patients. Kaufmann and Levitt (1965) assessed the frequency of three different behaviours in 83 partially or totally mobile mentally retarded patients and found that 69% body rocked, 63% head rolled and 53% hand waved. The peak incidence for rocking and head movements was seen just before meal time and in the middle of the afternoon. Foley (1975) examined 751 children and young adults and found that in the 345 without focal neurological signs, 31.6% had stereotypies or mannerisms, the commonest being overbreathing, head banging, body rocking and hand movements. In the rest with neurological abnormalities, the incidence was surprisingly less at only 16.4%. In a series of studies by Corbett, about 40% of severely retarded children were found to have stereotypies and 18% of adults in contact with services for the mentally handicapped were similarly affected (Corbett and Campbell, 1980). Fischer-Williams (1969) examined 90 mental defectives for neurological abnormalities. One striking finding was the frequency of abnormal gaits which were inexplicable on the basis of abnormal physical signs. Perseveration was also very common. Of the 56 children examined, 23 were hyperactive, 18 body rocked, 15 finger sucked, eight head banged and six had tics, figures which, apart from hyperactivity and body rocking, did not differ greatly from the normal population. In the 34 adults, 11 body rocked, nine were hyperactive, seven had tics, three head banged and three finger sucked. Echophenomena occurred in about 10% of both adult and childhood groups.

Finally, in a recent detailed survey of every mental deficiency hospital in Scotland, in which all but one institution cooperated, 33% of residents were seen to carry out stereotyped behaviour (15% body rocked, 12% had repetitive hand movements and 12% manifested self-injurious behaviour). These activities occurred significantly more frequently in males, the young and those in the profoundly or severely mentally deficient category. This study also concluded that imitation, while still the most likely explanation for the acquisition of particular topographies of behaviour, might not be the only causal variable; staff patient ratios, ward dimensions and nursing practice were believed to be contributory (Tierney et al, 1981).

The *tic d'encenser* of horses in which the animal repetitively raises and lowers its head is a form of stereotypy, and body rocking has also been seen in chimpanzees reared in isolation in laboratories. Stereotyped cage pacing, seen particularly in the big cats but also in birds and primates, bears some resemblance to the repetitive motion sometimes seen in the depressed or anxious and although restriction of space has been considered the most important provoking factor, anxiety and early experience factors may also be relevant. The occurrence of rhythmias in normal infants, particularly at transitional points in motor development, has led to the view that they may represent a pathological fixation in motor programmes which are normally outgrown in childhood. The delay in the appearance of habitual manipulations of the body such as finger sucking in the mentally defective may also be apposite in this regard (Kravitz and Boehm, 1971). However, it is by no means certain if stereotyped behaviours are hangovers from an earlier developmental period as longitudinal studies have not been carried out.

Two principal theories have been put forward to explain the high incidence of stereotyped activity in the mentally retarded. The standard view for many years has been that they are self-stimulatory and comforting, providing an optimal level of arousal in under-stimulated individuals with a vestigial behavioural repertoire. Alternatively, it has been suggested that they occur at times of increased arousal from stimuli such as hunger, physical restraint, frustration, noise or bright light and as such may represent an expression of tension, discomfort or dissatisfaction.

Recent studies have shown that these behaviours can be reduced by the presentation of brightly coloured objects, playthings, the enforcement of alternative activity or the frequent administration of mini-meals. Body rocking was reduced in one investigation by giving a sweet every 10 minutes, interaction between nurse and patient being minimised (Tierney et al, 1981). Outdoor stimulation, particularly in parkland with rivers and waterfalls, has also been claimed to be beneficial. On the basis of current knowledge it seems no longer reasonable to consider stereotypies to be an irrevocable auto-erotic characteristic of the mentally retarded. In times of stress due to under- or over-stimulation they may be used to maintain arousal, but for the most part they are a functionless behaviour reflecting basic ultradian 90–110 min rest-activity cycles and impeding rehabilitation. Whether they are solely driven by intrinsic oscillators or maintained by sensory input from the movements themselves in unclear (Berkson, 1983).

HEAD NODDING

Synonyms Head rolling, head tossing, nodding spasms, head shaking, spasmus nictitans, gyrospasm, nutatio capitis spastica, eclampsia rotans.

Head nodding was looked upon by the Druids and priestesses of Bacchus as a token of ecstasy. Disciples of the Wesleyan revivalist sects frequently indulged in head shaking during particularly moving sermons and more recently mass rhythmical head rolling by an audience has been employed as a means of enhancing musical appreciation at rock concerts. The earliest medical reports are those of Ebert (1850) and Romberg and Henoch (1851). Up to 20% of normal infants below the age of two years toss their heads (Kravitz and Boehm, 1971), onset usually being between the ages of 3 and 12 months (Lourie, 1949). No marked sex differences exist although some series report a female preponderance. The movement consists of rhythmical, usually side to side, oscillations of the head on the pillow, sometimes up to 200 movements/min and usually stopping abruptly on lifting or sitting the child up. Affirmatory nodding, like a mandarin doll, is less common. A special nocturnal variety (tic de somneil, or jactatio capitis nocturna) is frequently seen either before the child dozes off to sleep or in heavy slumber. Side to side or rotatory oscillations often in synchrony with respirations occur lasting for up to two hours and sometimes associated with soft crooning noises. Usually the habit disappears in early childhood but it occasionally persists into adult life. It occurs when the head is unsupported and especially at times of excitement or on attempting fixation. In a few children it is superseded by head banging. Gresty and Halmagyi (1979) have analysed head nodding on the basis of its resonant frequencies and harmonic components and have shown it to consist of regular, sustained 2–4 Hz pendular oscillations looking like a series of tics or tremor and capable of brief, voluntary suppressions.

Many patients with congenital nystagmus have compensatory head nods which may persist throughout life. Onset is at birth and both eyes exhibit nystagmus. Spasmus nutans (Still, 1909; Osterberg, 1937) is now an uncommon disorder which usually appears between the fourth and twelfth month after birth. It always begins with inconstant or slow head bobbing, the movements being from side to side, up or down or occasionally rotational and varying in range and speed. Associated nystagmus occurs in most of the children usually appearing one to two months later, the eye movement being rapid and in the horizontal, vertical or rotational plane. Occasionally the nystagmus is monocular. Torticollis is a further symptom in about one-third of cases and involuntary limb and trunk movements are occasionally seen. Many children also develop a rather curious way of looking at things out of the corner of their eyes, a tendency to tilt their heads backwards and stare absent-mindedly. The prognosis is excellent with most cases recovering in about one year. It is commoner in malnourished, institutionalised children some of whom are mentally backward, and in one study appeared to start more often in the winter months. Contributory factors of doubtful validity are neurosis, being kept in dark rooms, visual defects and rickets. Gresty and Ell (1981) have analysed head nodding with abnormal eye movements and defined three subgroups. They described head movements which did not aid vision, others which acted as a compensatory conditioned response to nystagmus and finally a form of spasmus nutans in which head shaking suppressed nystagmus.

Other causes of head bobbing include labyrinthine fistulae and the slow regular backward and forward movements usually seen in the upright position in the bobble head doll syndrome. This is usually due to hydrocephalus from obstruction in the region of the third ventricle and occurs in early childhood. There may be additional involvement of the shoulders and pendular arm movements. They may be reduced by distraction and disappear in sleep.

Tremor of the head (titubation) also occurs in cases of essential tremor when it may be associated in young children with shuddering attacks. Sudden head nods may occur as salaam seizures and head flexion may be seen in Lennox-Gastaut syndrome.

HEAD BANGING

Rhythmical repetitive striking of the head against a solid surface is a more alarming but equally benign childhood disorder. It usually starts between the ages of 6 and 18 months, is probably commoner in male infants, and estimates of its incidence in the normal population range from 3–7% (Levy, 1944; Kravitz et al, 1960; De Lissovoy, 1962). It usually occurs at bedtime or during daytime naps but occasionally may appear on waking. Most children head bang on all fours with the elbows extended and the knees drawn up or alternatively with legs extended. Less commonly the prone or supine position is adopted or the child kneels or stands against the cot-side. It is the forehead which usually makes contact with the mattress or cot, but about 10% of cases are occipital head bangers. The rate of head-object contacts ranges from 19–121 per minute (de Lissovoy, 1962) and each session may last anything from a few minutes to four hours finally ending in exhausted sleep. Other rhythmical motor rhythms such as head tossing and body rocking are common but finger sucking is not seen to excess. Severe injury is rare and the children rarely cry whilst engaged in the activity. Fear that the child may injure himself, or the loud noise engendered by the activity disrupting family life are the common reasons for referral.

Neurological examination is generally normal and the majority of children have normal electroencephalograms. Occasionally, however, the autistic or mentally retarded child may be picked up at examination, particularly in older children who have continued to head bang after their fifth birthday. The prognosis generally is good, most cases remitting spontaneously within two years of onset. Some children, however, substitute other rhythmical activities such as bruxism, toe curling, scratching or stereotyped play activities. The cause of head banging is unknown but maternal neglect or deprivation and disturbed parent-child relationships have been implicated. Treatment should centre around reassurance to the parents that the disorder is self-limiting and close contact between mother and child at bedtime should also be encouraged. This variety of essentially auto-erotic head banging must be distinguished from tantrum head banging which usually starts around the time the child is learning to talk. The child throws himself to the ground with arms and legs extended, thrashing and kicking about and may also breath-hold. Head banging in mental defectives may be ferocious, non-rhythmical and apparently purposeful, seemingly in response to some obscure source of irritation.

BODY ROCKING

A slow, rhythmical backwards and forwards swaying of the trunk from the hips, usually in the sitting position, dominates the behaviour of many mental defectives. In most it is episodic but it can continue for hours and may be accompanied by masturbation. In children it usually begins between 6 months and 1 year and rarely persists in normal infants beyond the age of 4 years. It has been claimed that it usually begins at the time of shift from all fours to an erect posture. Accurate prevalence figures are unavailable but Lourie (1949) found in an unselected paediatric population that 15–20% of children had rocked, head banged or swayed. In a study of infants in institutions a much higher figure of 35% for body rocking was arrived at.

In infants, body rocking usually occurs at bedtime. the tempo of the to and fro movements often building up gradually to a crescendo and then declining. Boredom and excitement are potent triggers. In the mentally retarded, on the other hand, the amplitude and rhythm of the movement usually remains remarkably constant. It is of interest that musical rhythms can alter the speed of spontaneous rocking. Many children croon or hum at the same time attesting to the pleasure derived from the activity. The popularity of the nursery cradle, rocking horse and swing is in fact probably related to this infantile delight in rhythmical body movement. Developmental theories as to its nature stem from the belief that rhythmical motor programmes are normal during the acquisition of learned motor skills in infancy and if the child is developmentally disabled or emotionally disturbed these behaviours may persist. Psychological theories consider frustration, boredom and parental neglect to be potent triggers.

SELF-INJURIOUS BEHAVIOUR

Although self-injurious behaviour is seen to a mild degree in many mentally retarded individuals, severe persistent self-mutilation is relatively rare. Corbett found it to be present to a mild degree in 13% of patients (Corbett and Campbell, 1980), a figure almost identical to that reported in the recent Scottish survey (Tierney et al, 1981). Striking the head, banging against objects or scratching seriously enough to draw blood are the usual manifestations. Only one in 10 000 patients repeatedly and seriously injures himself with acts such as eye gouging, hand gnawing and wrist slashing (Corbett and Campbell, 1980). A particularly lurid description is given by Esquirol (1845):

> The insensibility of idiots is sometimes most remarkable. We have seen these wretched beings bite and lacerate themselves and sometimes tear out their hair. I have seen an idiot who with her fingers and nails has pierced through her cheek, play with a finger placed in the opening, and end by tearing it to the very commissure of the lips without seeming to suffer.

In the Lesch-Nyhan syndrome, in which a deficiency of hypoxanthine guanine phosphoribosyl transferase leads to over-production of uric acid, self-mutilation begins as soon as the teeth erupt and leads to loss of tissue around the lips and partial auto-amputation of the digits. An animal model of self-mutilation has been produced by the chronic administration of the 1:3 methyl-purine derivatives caffeine and theophylline to underfed rodents (Nyhan, 1973). Purine derivatives related to adenosine and guanosine are now also known to be released from brain cells and to influence the activity of other neurones. Furthermore, hypoxanthine and caffeine inhibit the binding of diazepam to its receptors making it tempting to suggest that the benzodiazepine receptor might be involved in some of the bizarre behavioural manifestations of the Lesch-Nyhan syndrome. The extrapyramidal features of the disease, however, have been attributed to a decrease in striatal dopaminergic function possibly as a result of a marked deficit in the terminal arborisations of dopaminergic neurones (Lloyd et al, 1981).

GILLES DE LA TOURETTE SYNDROME IN THE MENTALLY RETARDED

Although uncommon, this undoubtedly occurs and I have seen three cases. One 14-year-old mildly retarded boy with a history of cerebral anoxia developed facial tics, vocalisations, compulsive touching and coprolalia at 12 years. He was particularly remarkable in having an obsession with watches and clocks and a number of frontal lobe signs including utilisation behaviour. He responded poorly to haloperidol in high doses but another 16-year-old boy with severe rubella encephalopathy was greatly improved by 1–5 mg of haloperidol. Golden and Greenhill (1981) reported six cases aged between 5 and 11 years. Four of these children were mildly retarded, the other two more severely so; three were psychotic and two were hyperactive. Perinatal injury was the aetiological factor in four and congenital rubella in one. Three of these children had compulsive touching, two had coprolalia and one echolalia and the response to haloperidol was generally gratifying.

10

Disorders of Movement in Schizophrenics

Although eccentricities of movement are rife in many captive populations, those occurring in schizophrenia are distinctively grotesque and incomprehensible. A few of the movements bear a superficial resemblance to dyskinesias more usually associated with basal ganglia disease whereas others are much more complex and co-ordinated, acting as external symbols for delusional ideas. It has been suggested that much of this abnormal motor behaviour is an artefact of chronic institutionalisation but this seems improbable as schizophrenics living within the community also display oddities of posture and movement.

The catatonic syndrome, first described by Kahlbaum, comprises abnormal posturing, muscular rigidity and catalepsy (waxy rigidity). Profound mental withdrawal with negativism, mutism and stupor or conversely a state of psychomotor excitement is usually also present. Many catatonics exhibit stereotyped behaviour, mannerisms, perseveration, echophenomena and automatic obedience. Approximately 5% of schizophrenics in Europe and the United States of America manifest catatonic features at some stage and it is in this group that disorders of movement are most commonly seen. Catatonic states can also occur as sequelae to limbic encephalitis, frontal lobe or basal ganglia damage, or occasionally after the administration of high doses of phenothiazines or amphetamines (Gelenberg, 1976a). They may also be induced in animals by the alkaloid bulbocapnine which structurally resembles apomorphine and blocks dopamine receptors (De Jong, 1945) and by endorphins (Bloom et al, 1976).

Kraepelin (1919), Bleuler (1924), Reiter (1926) and Kleist (1960) have described the disorders of movement seen in schizophrenia in exquisite detail. For reasons which remain unclear, the incidence of catatonic schizophrenia appears to have fallen considerably in the West in the last 50 years. Inclusion of patients with structural neurological disease in the early reports may offer a partial explanation but a real decline may have occurred, and it is interesting to note that catatonic schizophrenia is still common in certain parts of the Third World.

Recent attempts to re-examine the movement disorders occurring in schizophrenia have been impeded by the ubiquitous prescription of neuroleptics. Furthermore, documentation of motor symptoms and medication in long-stay

Table 10.1. CLASSIFICATION OF MOTOR DISORDERS IN SCHIZOPHRENIA

1. Abnormal spontaneous movements
    stereotypies
    tics and other hyperkinesias
    eye movement disorders
    complex movements
2. Abnormal induced movements
    motor perseveration
    automatic obedience
    echophenomena
    mitgehen, mitmachen, gegenhalten
3. Disorders of execution of movement
    mannerisms
    blocking
    ambitendencies

psychiatric wings often leaves much to be desired. As a result even in those individuals who would appear from their drug charts to have never received antipsychotics, nagging doubts remain that parenteral medication may have been administered at times of acute psychotic excitement.

A modification of the classification proposed by Fish (1976) will be used here. Although artificial and lacking in pathophysiological substantiation it has the advantages of being reasonably pragmatic and simple to use (Table 10.1).

ABNORMAL SPONTANEOUS MOVEMENTS

1. STEREOTYPIES

A whole host of characteristic stereotypies can be seen in schizophrenics, ranging from the simplest tic-like movements to complicated symbolic gestures (Fig. 10.1). In one recent study 24% of 250 catatonic schizophrenics among a total population of 20 000 psychiatric in-patients exhibited stereotyped behaviour (Morrison, 1973). They are said to appear early in the course of the disease and as time passes to become more and more fragmentary and unintelligible.

In some individuals a single abnormal action is pursued for year after year without modification. Bleuler (1949) described a spinster who incessantly imitated the movements of a cobbler at his awl. Kraepelin looked after a patient who played the same weary refrain over and over again on the piano. He also noted that paths could be discerned carved through the long grass in the grounds of mental asylums by patients who were in the habit of taking the same unvarying stereotyped daily peregrination. Other examples include rubbing the right hand over the left thumb, running a finger constantly along

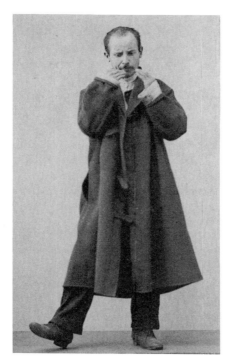

Figure 10.1. *A catatonic schizophrenic.*

the edges of hard surfaces, making bread pellets, tapping the foot in a certain plane or repeatedly touching the same part of a wall. Some patients handle and touch everything within reach; other stereotypies may be senseless and self-mutilating such as pulling hair out, ripping buttons off or scratching the face. Hoarding is another manifestation. Leonhard had a patient who stole bicycles even though he could not ride them. Verbigeration in which a patient endlessly reiterates a handful of meaningless words cr sentences is a commonly occurring verbal stereotypy. All these behaviours assume monotonous rhythmicity and may come to dominate the patient's life. Kraepelin's patients explained their motives as follows: 'I must shake my head or I am in terror'; 'I must turn round as when a magnet draws a needle'; 'I could not have rested until I had done that'. Kraepelin and Bleuler also believed that patients exhibiting this sort of repetitive activity tended to become progressively more maladroit and clumsy as the illness progressed.

In a recent investigation of 13 schizophrenics (mean age 49 years, mean duration of illness 25 years) (Jones, 1965). all but one of whom was receiving neuroleptics, walking backwards and forwards, rocking, biting, grimacing, tongue curling and verbigeration were seen. No close correlation between delusions and activity was detected nor was there any direct relationship between the severity of stereotypy and length of hospitalisation. The movements were less frequent during work or distraction. Withdrawal of medication for four months increased the stereotypies in all seven patients in whom it was carried out. Sustained neuroleptic therapy, however, may provoke stereotypies.

2. TICS AND OTHER DYSKINESIAS

Kraepelin observed distorted movements of the face and hands in some of his patients and associated them with a poor prognosis. The movements included wrinkling of the forehead, irregular movements of the tongue and lips, opening and closing the eyes and grimacing. Sudden sighs, sniffs, throat clearing, lightning lip movements and tongue smacking also occurred. Sprawling, irregular writhings of the limbs with extension of the fingers, so-called athetoid ataxia, was also noted. Continuous twitches, jerks and grimaces were recorded by Wernicke and termed parakinesias, and Kleist reported movements reminiscent of chorea, athetosis and dystonia. Another curious and well-recognised phenomenon was the schnauzkrampf which consisted of wrinkling of the nose with lip pouting reminiscent of a hog's snout. Bleuler also describes grimaces, shoulder shrugs, tongue and lip movements and sudden involuntary gestures but clearly distinguished these from chorea and regarded them as tics. Indeed, it is probable that many of the choreoathetotic signs described in the earlier literature were in patients with neurological disease such as Huntington's chorea. Recent studies suggest that chorea is extremely rare in chronic psychiatric populations who have never received neuroleptics (Mettler and Crandell, 1959). In a retrospective study by Jones and Hunter (1969) 45 untreated patients were found, in four of whom facial tics were noted. Two patients had body rocking movements and another two had stereotyped movements. Many of these cases, however, were post-encephalitics.

In a retrospective study in which the charts of patients admitted to the Iowa City Psychiatric Hospital between 1935 and 1945 were reviewed, 200 patients who met the Feighner criteria for schizophrenia were identified and, of these, 103 met research diagnostic criteria for hebephrenic schizophrenia. The majority of these patients also exhibited motor symptoms more traditionally associated with catatonic schizophrenia. Of these hebephrenic/catatonic cases adequate longitudinal data over at least 12 years was available on 52 who had a mean age at onset of disease of 21 years. Thirty-one (60%) had mannerisms and 24 (46%) tics and grimaces but none displayed chorea. The mannerisms appeared on average five years after the onset of the schizophrenia whereas the tics appeared somewhat earlier. There was also a suggestion that tics and grimaces tended to remit spontaneously during the course of the illness although it is possible that they were just not subsequently recorded in the notes (Pfohl and Winokur, 1982).

Yarden and Discipio (1971) have documented 18 young untreated schizophrenics who had abnormal involuntary movements including chorea, athetosis, tics, stereotypies and mannerisms. Compared with schizophrenic controls without movements, the patients had an earlier onset, a steadily progressive course and early and profound mental deterioration. Owens et al (1982) also believe that spontaneous dyskinesias may be a feature of severe chronic schizophrenia and go even further in considering that neuroleptics are not responsible for most of the persistent dyskinesias now seen in psychotic patients. In a recent study of 411 chronic schizophrenic in-patients, 47 of whom had apparently never received antipsychotic drugs, they were unable to find significant differences in the prevalence, severity and distribution of abnormal movements in the treated and unmedicated groups. Patients were evaluated blind on two occasions, at least one year elapsing between the first and second assessments. Using the AIM and Rockland scales, 53.2% of the untreated patients received a score of at least two on one or more item of the AIM scale with a comparable figure of 76.6% on the Rockland scale. Orofacial dyskinesias were most common, indistinguishable from those seen in tardive dyskinesias. Tongue tremor, limb chorea, head nodding, body rocking and other perioral movements were also recorded. The mean age of the untreated cases was 67 years, somewhat older than the drug-treated majority. All these patients had been under the care of a physician who practised a dynamic, family-orientated approach to management and avoided physical treatments of all kinds. Co-existent encephalitis lethargica, associated neurological disorder or senile idiopathic orofacial dyskinesias were considered inadequate explanations for these findings.

Despite these two recent investigations, the consensus remains that most of the dyskinesias seen in untreated schizophrenics are best categorised as tics, mannerisms or stereotypies.

EYE MOVEMENT DISORDERS

A number of extraocular movement disorders occur in schizophrenia including staring, an abnormal blink rate, absent glabellar tap reflex and an increase in horizontal eye movements (Stevens, 1978).

COMPLICATED MOVEMENTS

Occasional patients perform bizarre spontaneous motor behaviour. Somersaulting, cartwheeling and circling resembling the acts of circus clowns, jumping in the air, genuflecting, skipping and hopping are but a few of the multitude of antics seen in long-stay psychiatric wards.

ABNORMAL INDUCED MOVEMENTS

Most of these movements result from an excessive compliance on the part of the patient. Perseveration is persistence of a goal-directed activity after the need for it has ceased. It may take the form of repetition of a word, act or thought process and may lead to a rigidity of thought resulting in great difficulties in switching concepts (Freeman and Gathercole, 1966). It can be distinguished from stereotypy in that it is triggered off by a specific goal-directed act. Bleuler observed that one of his patients, a talented pianist, would invariably get stuck on a particular note and repeat it over and over again like a broken record. A stage-prompter had as his first symptom of schizophrenia the inappropriate reiteration of the same phrase during a theatrical production. Perseveration is a striking feature in many patients with particular types of frontal lobe damage raising the intriguing possibility that this area of the brain may be abnormal in schizophrenics.

Automatic obedience is still seen occasionally in catatonic schizophrenia. It may occur at any stage of the illness and exceptionally is the only remaining symptom after all the other features of the illness have regressed. Waxy flexibility or catalepsy is another uncommon phenomenon in which a patient will preserve whatever position he is put into for lengthy periods of time. The best-known manifiestations are the psychological pillow where the patient reclines with his head some distance off the pillow and the curious rigid, statuesque poses adopted by some catatonics. Patients with this disturbance will continue to protrude their tongue when commanded to do so even when warned that it will be pricked with a pin each time. This is not simply a reflection of pain indifference as patients grimace each time the noxious stimulus is directed.

In the Iowa 500 study, eight of the 52 hebephrenic/catatonics developed waxy flexibility usually at least five years after the onset of their illness and interestingly in seven of these subsequent resolution of the symptom occurred (Pfohl and Winokur, 1982).

Mitgehen is another related disturbance in which an individual moves his body in response to the lightest of pressures by the examiner. For instance, light pressure applied to the underside of the forearm will cause the arm to levitate as if it had been triggered by clockwork. This effect occurs even after a patient is instructed to resist and is distracted by conversation. Some patients acquiesce to every passive movement, but immediately the examiner removes his hand the body returns to the resting position — mitmachen. Forced grasping and magnetic apraxia are other occasional findings as is gegenhalten (paratonia) in which there is forced resistance to all passive movements. Many of these phenomena are also observed in patients with severe frontal lobe damage.

ECHOPHENOMENA

Echolalia may occur in transcortical motor dysphasia and is also a common feature in the early stages of normal speech development. Stengel (1947) has claimed that in these groups echolalia occurs usually only in response to remarks addressed to the patient and, remarkably, in dysphasia, if a part, sentence is delivered the patient may complete it. Difficulty in understanding with an attempt to relate with the interlocutor may underlie this disturbance in dysphasias and mentally retarded children.

Echolalia and echopraxia are now rare in schizophrenia but still occur occasionally. These disturbances may appear early in the disease in a transient and controlled form, often emerging when verbal communication is beginning to disintegrate.

Chapman and McGhie (1964) describe a particularly severe example in a mute institutionalised catatonic who, whenever he perceived any change in position or action in another group member, would automatically move into an identical pose no matter how uncomfortable. This occurred constantly with mimicry of different patient's actions up to 30–40 times an hour. Another hebephrenic schizophrenic in the same group who also displayed echopraxia explained the disorder as follows:

> I'm sitting here body snatching. I keep picking up fresh bodies, nobody else can make them work.
> (How do you work them?)
> I just sit in them and they work.
> (You sit?)
> You don't sit you imagine or realise it. You can go in or out of any mind.

Echolalia in schizophrenia tends to be more automatic than in other conditions in which it occurs and although often present for years cannot be elicited with regularity and may disappear overnight (Stengel, 1947). It has been suggested that it may occur as a primitive attempt to maintain a tenuous dialogue with the outside world.

COPROLALIA

This is relatively common and, when it occurs, usually has a compulsive element to it. In contrast to its occurrence in Gilles de la Tourette syndrome, where obscenities are released without any appropriate underlying stimulus, in schizophrenia underlying paranoid delusions are often the catalyst.

DISORDERS OF EXECUTION OF MOVEMENT

MANNERISMS

Many normal people possess a mannerism or two which may be regarded as no more than a quirk or slight eccentricity. However, mannerisms may be used to attract attention, particularly in insecure individuals who wish to appear more than they actually are. Their artificiality and pompousness immediately strike the eye as affected, ostentatious and contradictory. In schizophrenics an astonishing plethora of odd, senseless caricatures are seen, the underlying rationale in many cases being incomprehensible.

Bleuler relates the case history of a catatonic schizophrenic who aped Bismark even down to his handwriting and speech and another who adopted the pose of Napoleon, running around with his arm crossed on his chest. Some patients grasp everything with their fingers outstretched, others whenever they shake hands utter grunts or smack their lips and Kraepelin mentions a patient who lifted his legs like a stork when walking. One male patient walked everywhere with his shirt lifted in the air whilst a female inmate always played the piano with gloves on. Most patients, however, content themselves with imitating a facial expression, another's clothing or speech or a style of handwriting. In a few individuals mannerisms remain constant for years whereas others are constantly stepping out of their roles and assuming new behaviour. Watching schizophrenics eat, one is immediately struck by the number of unnatural, affected flourishes incorporated into their table manners. One may grasp his spoon tightly at the tip and eat from the handle, another may strike the plate three times before eating, a third may stir the food between each mouthful and yet another may divide his vegetables into tiny heaps. Some of these mannerisms may be so extreme as to actually frustrate the underlying action. Schizophrenic speech is also often riddled with manneristic tic equivalents. Telegrammatic jargon, adding 'ism' to the end of every word or speaking in rhyme are just a few examples. Expressive gestures may also be distorted and shaking hands may be done stiffly with only the little finger being extended. Extra-ordinary tongue and lip movements, finger play and curious gesticulations are also apparent. In fact it is these often repugnant ludicrous antics which first strike the lay person on entering a psychiatric hospital and are at the root of the popular picture of a lunatic.

BLOCKING AND AMBITENDENCIES

In blocking, a movement is initiated correctly at first but is suddenly curtailed before it is completed, the body returning to the neutral position. Alternatively, the movement is completed after a pause. This can be regarded as the motor equivalent of thought blocking. Ambivalence occurs when a patient desires and simultaneously does not desire to execute a specific action. For example, if commanded to shake hands he may start to do so then retract then start again and so on.

11

The Adult Onset Focal Dystonias

Meige and Feindel used the term 'tonic tic' to describe disorders such as spasmodic torticollis, tonic contraction of the masseter muscles (mental trismus) and blepharospasm. They considered these disorders to be characterised by abnormal, abrupt, excessive tonic contraction limited to one part or segment of the body and they were convinced that most of such patients showed overt psychiatric disturbance. Occupational cramps and other bizarre spasms were subsequently considered in a similar light, the consensus being that all were of psychiatric origin. This view was fortified by the extraordinary appearance of many of these dyskinesias, their acute sensitivity to stressful events and their occurrence often on certain specific tasks only. Most damning of all appeared to be the absence of histological abnormalities in the few available post-mortem studies. However, a psychogenic origin for these disorders implies that the dyskinesia is part of the clinical picture of an underlying psychiatric illness. Despite a large amount of anecdotal evidence suggesting that psychoneurosis is commonly associated with these conditions, no convincing controlled studies exist to show that psychiatric illness occurs more commonly in these patients than in age-matched controls. Indeed many of the patients appear extraordinarily well balanced and in others successful treatment of associated mental illness has had unpredictable effects on the motor symptoms.

The currently fashionable view is that spasmodic torticollis, writer's cramp, Meige syndrome and spasmodic dysphonia are caused by abnormal function of the basal ganglia. The evidence in favour of this is circumstantial but persuasive. All these disorders may be provoked by neuroleptic drugs in susceptible individuals and all occur rarely as unwanted effects of sustained L-dopa therapy in patients with Parkinson's disease. They may also be seen as part of a more generalised movement disorder in conditions with known basal ganglia pathology such as Hallervorden Spatz disease and Wilson's disease. They may be found as part of the clinical picture of idiopathic generalised torsion dystonia and, with the exception of blepharospasm, they may be its presenting feature. All of them also have the clinical and electrophysiological characteristics of dystonia, and segmental spread occasionally occurs to involve adjacent parts of the body. Finally, they are slowly progressive or non-progressive, a feature characteristic of idiopathic adult onset generalised dystonia. The fact that this group of conditions is acutely influenced by proprioceptive inputs and emotional stresses, which may be crucial in disrupting the normal sequencing of motor programmes within the brain, would not be incompatible with dysfunction of the basal ganglia.

SPASMODIC TORTICOLLIS

Synonyms Dystonic torticollis, spasmodic wry neck, spastic torticollis, attitude tic, mental torticollis, rotatory tic.

Definition An idiopathic focal dystonia in which tonic and jerky involuntary movements of the cervical musculature cause intermittent or sustained deviation of the head and neck.

The caput obstipum referred to in early medical texts is probably an early observation of congenital wry neck, while dystonic twisting of the neck has also been described in fossil dinosaurs (Kaiser, 1954). Rabelais is believed to have used the word 'torty colly' to describe a neck deformity and Paul Scarron, a crippled 17th century dramatist described the malady in an autobiographical poem:

Mon pauvre corps est raccourci
Et j'ai la tete sur l'oreille;
Mais cela me sied a merveille
Et parmi les torticollis
Je passe pour des plus jolis.

Isaac Minnius, a German army surgeon, is reputed to have attempted surgical correction by dividing the contracted neck muscles in 1641 but the first medical descriptions on the subject are those of Wepfer in 1727, who described the condition as 'convulsio particularis', and Jaeger who published a thesis in 1737. A peak of interest in this uncommon condition occurred in France at the turn of the century with Brissaud, Meige, Redard and Cruchet all writing extensively on the subject. In his 800-page tome Cruchet (1907) collected the 350 or so documented cases and distinguished seven clinical subtypes. Like the rest of the French school he regarded the majority of cases as psychologically determined. Brissaud (1895) differentiated two main groups: mental torticollis and torticollis spasm. The former, which in his experience contributed the majority of cases, was analogous to tic developing from a co-ordinated purposive act; frequent repetition ultimately leading to its involuntary reproduction. Weakness of the will, often associated with signs of mental instability, was considered to be the triggering factor in most instances. Torticollis spasm on the other hand he considered to be due to irritation of the peripheral reflex arc, the contraction being painful, uncoordinated and sometimes persisting into sleep. Gowers (1893) also distinguished a 'hysterical form' most often seen in women under 30 and a 'true form' caused by overaction of lower brain centres whereas Kinnier Wilson, who was strongly influenced by Cruchet, regarded psychogenic factors as paramount in the pathogenesis of spasmodic torticollis. Critchley (1938) felt able to distinguish four types — psychogenic, post-encephalitic, torticollis associated with an extrapyramidal disorder and a progressive intractable spasm of uncertain cause.

In contrast to most of his contemporaries, Babinski (1900) favoured an organic cause for most cases of spasmodic torticollis, describing it as *un syndrome strié*, a view which was later championed by Foerster (1933). Foerster postulated that in some cases the corpus striatum might be congenitally weak or diseased causing a predisposition to torticollis often unmasked by emotional stress. Cases were reported in association with rheumatic fever, encephalitis lethargica, neurosyphilis, malaria and multiple sclerosis, and Patterson and Little (1943) concluded that the majority of their large series of 103 cases were due to degenerative, inflammatory or toxic lesions in the extrapyramidal or vestibular pathways. The realisation that identical neck deformities could occur as a side-effect of neuroleptics further helped to consolidate the swing away from the notion of spasmodic torticollis as a psychogenic disorder. Herz and Glaser (1949) referred to the disorder as dystonic torticollis and Cooper (1964) suggested that it might represent a specific type of adult onset dystonia. Most authorities now consider a derangement of basal ganglia function as the underlying pathophysiological mechanism but the cause is unknown and as yet no supportive histological or neurochemical abnormalities have been detected.

EPIDEMIOLOGY

Spasmodic torticollis is an uncommon disorder and no accurate figures are available as to its prevalence. It occurs equally commonly in the two sexes and has a peak incidence in the fourth decade. At least two-thirds of cases present between 30 and 50 years but it may appear in childhood or old age. Paterson (1945) estimated that it contributed to one in 1200 psychiatric referrals and most of the large series from hospital centres have averaged a collection rate of about 8–10 new cases a year. Ninety-eight cases were seen at the National Hospital for Nervous Diseases between 1918 and 1926 and 52 were admitted between 1977 and 1982.

ANIMAL MODELS

A syndrome that simulates torticollis can be produced in monkeys by lesions in the brachium conjunctivum and mesencephalic tegmentum (Carrea and Mettler, 1954). Foltz et al (1959) found that a unilateral lesion of the medial mesencephalic raticular formation, caudal and dorsal to the red nucleus at the level of the brachium conjunctivum, produced torticollis in the monkey. As in man, anxiety and agitation brought out these adventitious movements which were hardly noticeable when the animals were at rest.

Jung and Hassler (1960) induced rotatory head movements by stimulation of the nucleus interstitialis and Koella (1955) produced similar responses by stimulating the midline cerebellar nuclei. Interruption of ascending dopaminergic fibres from the mesencephalic tegmentum in the marmoset causes severe torticollis with deviation of the head to the side of the lesion but lesions in the pontine tegmentum damaging ascending noradrenergic neurones induce contralateral torticollis. In animals with 6-hydroxydopamine lesions, amphetamine worsened the torticollis, low doses of apomorphine attenuated the condition and high doses of apomorphine reversed the direction of the deformity (Crossman and Sambrook, 1978). Carpenter (1956) showed that lesions restricted to the red nucleus of the monkey provoked tonic rotation and tilt of the head to the opposite side and that additional damage to the median longitudinal bundle was not essential for the effect to occur. Denny-Brown (1962) reported that a lesion between the red nucleus and interstitial nucleus of Cajal caused neck torsion in the monkey.

Eighth cranial nerve section and labyrinthectomy in lower animals produce striking ipsilateral inclination of the head but in the chimpanzee only minimal tilting occurs. Tarlov (1969) produced marked tonic neck postures in macaques with lesions in the vestibular nuclei but much slighter abnormalities occurred with similar lesions in baboons and chimpanzees.

Anticholinergic drugs and dopamine agonists had no effect on spasmodic torticollis induced by ventromedial mesencephalic tegmental lesions in the African green monkey, but dopamine antagonists, cholinergic and gabamimetic drugs all improved it (Battista et al, 1976).

PATHOLOGY

There are only a small number of necropsy reports of spasmodic torticollis and most of these are cases in which there was an underlying neurological disorder causing scattered lesions throughout the neuraxis. Grinker and Walker (1933) described a woman of 25 with torticollis who had evidence of encephalitis throughout the cerebral cortex, basal ganglia and cerebellum. Foerster (1933) reported a 23-year-old man with neck spasms and retrocollis who died after a cervical laminectomy and was found to have cavitations of the putamen and substantia innominata. Alpers and Drayer (1937) described a 90-year-old patient with bilateral choreo-athetosis and spasmodic torticollis who at post-mortem was found to have symmetrical bilateral caudate, putaminal and pallidal atrophy. Striatal damage has also been reported in two patients in which spasmodic torticollis was part of a more generalised dystonia (Cassirer, 1922; Wimmer, 1929). More recently Tarlov (1970) made a detailed pathological study of a 67-year-old woman who died of bronchopneumonia after a six-year history of spasmodic torticollis. Examination particularly of the interstitial nucleus of Cajal, basal ganglia and cerebellum, revealed no abnormalities. A further patient examined pathologically by Greenfield in 1936 and found to have no abnormality in the brain or spinal cord was re-examined by Tarlov who concurred with Greenfield's findings. It can be concluded that no distinctive histological abnormality has as yet been found in patients with spasmodic torticollis.

AETIOLOGY

A fruitless debate as to whether spasmodic torticollis is an organic or psychogenic condition continues to rage in many circles despite the substantial available evidence aligning the condition to the focal dystonias. The abnormal neck movements fulfil all the criteria for the diagnosis of dystonia and recognised associations exist with writer's cramp (Meares, 1971a), cranial dystonia (Tibbetts, 1971), segmental dystonia (Korein and Brudny, 1976) and generalised torsion dystonia (Marsden and Harrison, 1974). In most of the large series 5–10% of patients with spasmodic torticollis have also had mild dystonic movements in other parts of the body. In common with other idiopathic dystonias there is a strong link with essential tremor (Couch, 1975) and a less secure one with Parkinson's disease (Patterson and Little, 1943).

The first familial cluster of spasmodic torticollis was reported in 1896 by Thompson in which four siblings were affected. The onset was in childhood in one and in young adult life in the others. Three had tonic neck deviation to the left and the fourth had deviation to the right with some retrocollis. Van Bogaert (1941) reported a mother and two daughters with torticollis and noted tremor in other family members. One of Marsden's (1976a) 64 patients had a family history of the disorder and Tibbett (1971), in his series of 72 cases, quoted two family histories in which there was another affected member. Korein and Brudny (1976) reported a remarkably high figure of 15% of their patients with a positive family history. Gilbert (1977) has also reported familial cases which in view of the rarity of the disorder suggest a genetic factor in its aetiology.

Spasmodic torticollis has frequently been reported to follow rheumatic fever (Curling, 1860) and is also occasionally seen in a number of different diseases known to damage the central nervous system. For example, there are reports of torticollis in multiple sclerosis (Guillain and Bize, 1933), neurosyphilis (Schaeffer and Bize, 1934), malaria (Finney and Hughson, 1925), carbon monoxide poisoning (Solcher, 1957) and epidemic encephalitis lethargica (Martin, 1967) and a possible association with thyrotoxicosis has also been mooted (Gilbert, 1972). Spasmodic torticollis occurs as part of the clinical picture in diseases such as Wilson's disease and Hallervorden-Spatz syndrome which are known to affect the basal ganglia, and its occurrence following acute and occasionally long-term neuroleptic administration, indicates that a chemical derangement in extrapyramidal structures might underlie the spontaneously occurring condition.

It has been suggested that the dystonias may occur as a result of a primary abnormality of proprioceptive input. Meige commented as follows:

Some patients with mental torticollis seem to have lost the sense of position in their head, others evince a want of precision and assurance in the execution of different limb movements.

The ability to correct torticollis with a *geste antagonistique* and the reputed efficacy of biofeedback and behavioural therapy has been used as support for this notion. Cooper (1964) believes that torticollis is due to damage to the cerebello-thalamic pathways responsible for modulating the somatic motor pathways involved in the control of neck and head posture. Marsden (1976a), on the other hand, has emphasised the selective distortion of motor programmes in the basal ganglia as the possible cause.

It is a common experience in medicine that patients, on developing a disease, often attribute its appearance to some antecedent stressful life-event. Spasmodic torticollis is no exception and recent bereavements, marital dishar-mony, or business and financial worries are frequently blamed for its onset. However, the only possible triggering factor which consistently appears in the literature is mechanical trauma to the head and neck (David et al, 1952). Walsh (1974) reported significant preceding recent head trauma in five of his 46 cases, Shaw et al (1972) in six out of 18 patients and Korein and Brudny (1976) in nine of 48. Sixteen out of the 71 patients operated on by Sorensen and Hamby (1965) had experienced head and neck injuries at some stage. Sheehy and Marsden (1980) reviewed all the studies in the literature and found a history of recent neck trauma in 9% of 414 patients. These anecdotal reports suggest that a careful controlled study, with large numbers of patients, would be worth-while to pursue this point.

In view of the close relationship between the vestibular system and head and neck posture, a primary vestibular abnormality has also been suggested as the cause of spasmodic torticollis. Although minor degrees of labyrinthine preponderance and spontaneous nystagmus away from the direction of neck tilt and canal paresis and spontaneous nystagmus with the eyes closed are commonly reported, no uniform primary vestibular abnormality has ever been found.

In their monograph on tics Meige and Feindel wrote:

To establish the diagnosis of mental torticollis the existence of those psychical anomalies that are common to all who tic must first be substantiated and then must one essay the reconstruction of its mechanism. The enquiry may at first prove fruit-less, of course, but continuation of the search can scarcely fail to elicit the tokens of mental infantilism. In pursuance of this quest we shall find ourselves face to face with the 'big baby', the personification of childishness, obstinacy and caprice; we shall encounter the peevish, the sulky, the whining; we shall see how their impotence in the presence of their tic turns their nonchalance to profound despair, how their failure to adapt themselves to their malady convicts them remorselessly of volitional imperfection. The utter weakness of their will according to Déjerine [1914] justifies their being ranked as neurasthenics, but in the latter class of case obsessional ideas are both fugitive and fluctuating whereas mental torticollis is dependent on a fixed idea of peculiar tenacity.

Many subsequent authorities have affirmed the high incidence of neurotic traits in spasmodic torticollis. Paterson (1945) found 16 of her 21 patients to have a shy, anxious, immature disposition leading to difficulties in taking responsibility and in mixing socially. Tibbetts (1971) commented on the apparent frequency of vulnerable and obsessional personality traits in his patients and Meares (1971b) found a higher score for obsessional compulsive personality traits in his patients when compared with age-matched controls. None of these studies, however, provide any proof that spasmodic torticollis is due to some psychological illness and the behavioural abnormalities described might well have occurred as a reaction to the disorder.

Cockburn (1971) examined the hypothesis that spasmodic torticollis is either a psychiatric disease or that it occurs only in patients with abnormal pre-morbid personality traits. Fifty-five patients mainly referred from non-psychiatric sources were studied and 46 were seen and interviewed by the author. The pre-morbid personality was assessed by the length of the patient's longest job, the degree of marital stability, the number and type of psychiatric breakdowns, the incidence of alcoholism and the presence of neurotic traits. Patients were asked to fill out the Maudsley Personality Inventory N and E scores as they recalled their personalities before the onset of torticollis. Close relatives were also interviewed when possible and independent data obtained. Age-matched controls were selected from surgical patients admitted for operations in which psychological factors were believed to be unimportant. No significant differences could be found between the patients and controls except that the controls actually had a somewhat higher incidence of obsessional traits than the patients. The study by Matthews et al (1978) also failed to detect a characteristic pre-morbid personality in spasmodic torticollis.

Meares (1971b, 1973) believes that two subgroups of patients can be distinguished on the basis of their anxiety and neuroticism scores. The eight of his cases who spontaneously remitted had evidence of marked marital or sexual disturbance and higher anxiety scores. As a group they were also somewhat younger and their torticollis had begun with an aching or jerking presentation. Herz and Glaser (1949) also drew attention to the marital difficulties of many of their patients but attributed them to the effects of living with the disorder. They also noted about half their patients to be unstable, irritable, moody and sensitive, expressing dissatisfaction with life and having problems coping with their jobs. One of the female patients at University College Hospital frequently alluded to her unfaithful husband as 'the pain in her neck' and, following a spate of infidelities on his part, she finally killed him in his sleep. This, however, led to no permanent improvement in her neck deformity. Depression also occurs commonly in spasmodic torticollis and 14 of Tibbetts' (1971) 72 patients required specific psychiatric treatment.

Psycho-analytically-oriented physicians have postulated that the stiff neck may symbolically represent an erect phallus and result from Oedipal conflicts or castration anxiety (Abse, 1966). Cleveland (1959) found that his patients with spasmodic torticollis attached particular significance to the eyes and the act of looking providing support for the idea that torticollis was a symbolic rejection or turning away from the world (Whiles, 1940). Others elaborated on this idea pointing out that the movement of the neck in torticollis was not that of simple aversion and the only normal movement it resembled was breast searching in the neonate. These extraordinary notions now receive little credence and the view that torticollis is a form of conversion hysteria is equally untenable despite the occasional remarkable anecdote such as the ballerina from Balham whose neck started to twist away from her partner in the middle of a *pas de deux*.

CLINICAL DESCRIPTION

There is usually a gradual onset with an involuntary twisting or jerking of the head. In some patients there is a particularly leisurely onset with a mild turn or tilt of the chin usually first remarked upon by a friend or relative. A minority of cases appear to start with rheumatic pains in the posterior cervical muscles. No two patients have quite the same neck deformity but in most typically the head is pulled over one shoulder and the abnormal posture is accentuated by stress or walking and improved by lying down or supporting the head. The position of the head and neck in space is quite abnormal but by a marked effort of muscle contraction it is possible for normal individuals to imitate torticollis. Sometimes the head protrudes forwards (pro- or anterocollis) or backwards (retrocollis) and in some patients the head may actually turn in one direction

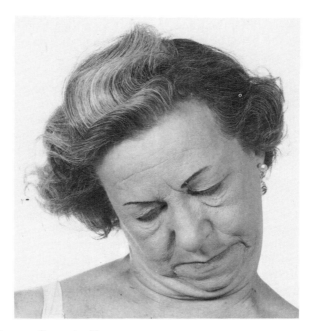

Figure 11.1. Spasmodic torticollis.

and rotate in the other. The established position of the neck is by no means immutable with some patients' torticollis changing strikingly in appearance over the years. A fixed deformity with marked nuchal muscle hypertrophy may finally develop but in many patients a limited degree of mobility is preserved and the tonic spasms may remain intermittent. Clonic tremulous head jerks and bobs are a frequent accompaniment and may be more evident than the underlying primary torsion. The direction of deviation of the chin to right or left is approximately equal and it has been suggested that in the individual patient there is a correlation between the predominant direction of postural functions and the direction of the rotatory component of the torticollis. This implies that the pathophysiology of spasmodic torticollis might involve the release of postural rotational laterality (Stejskal and Tomanek, 1981).

The muscle most commonly affected in spasmodic torticollis is the sternocleidomastoid which causes rotation to the opposite side with flexion of the neck to the side of the contracted muscle but this may be variably modified by contraction of both trapezii, the ipsilateral sternocleidomastoid, the splenii and the levatores scapulae (Figs 11.1 and 11.2). Flexion of the head to the side it is rotated is due to contraction of the sternocleidomastoid on one side and contraction of the splenius on the other side, whereas retrocollis is due to bilateral contraction of the splenii and trapezii. In fact electromyographic recording often confirms widespread prolonged contraction of several neck muscles sometimes with superimposed rhythmical discharges, even when the neck posture

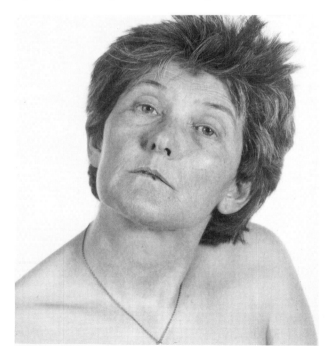

Figure 11.2. Spasmodic torticollis.

suggests relatively isolated contraction of one sternocleidomastoid muscle. Co-contraction of antagonists on both sides of the neck can also be demonstrated, an event which never occurs with normal movement.

The intensity, frequency and duration of the abnormal neck movements vary considerably but the early morning after sleep seems to be the time when symptoms are mildest. The tempo of the head movement also varies from rapid twitches to a slow, sinuous, graceful bending. If the patient attempts to correct his torticollis, an oscillatory component often becomes apparent and, as increasing force is applied with resulting emotional stress, worsening of the neck movement often occurs.

In contrast the *geste antagonistique efficace* sometimes corrects the deformity. This consists of a light touch to the side of the chin which may work by enhancing defective proprioceptive input or by reflex inhibition. The side of the chin which is touched or the particular hand used seems unimportant and indeed Kinnier Wilson described a patient who only had to make a gesture as if to touch the chin for realignment of the neck to occur. Korein reported a man who obtained partial relief of his torticollis by hanging a rubber band from his ear. Counter-pressure such as placing the hand on the back of the neck or wearing a high neck collar may also be beneficial.

Podivinsky (1968) made a careful study of the inhibitory and enhancing effects of different forms of movement and sensory stimulation. He observed, using electromyographic recordings, that a slight touch on the side of the neck towards which the chin is turned reduces the spasm whereas contralateral stimulation increased it. He also reported that supporting a weight in one or other hand markedly increased muscle discharge from the neck muscles. Other authors, however, have been unable to confirm the efficacy of the *geste antagonistique* (Matthews et al, 1978).

Additional neurological abnormalities are not uncommon in spasmodic torticollis. A spread of the dystonia to the shoulders, face and arms is commonest and a slight increase in muscle tone in the arm contralateral to the direction of chin deviation may be present. Postural tremor of the arms and head is often seen and there is a single unconfirmed report of a high incidence of blue irises.

Severe cervical spondylosis is a common late complication causing painful radiculopathies and spinal cord compression.

LABORATORY INVESTIGATIONS

A mildly elevated cerebrospinal fluid protein is occasionally found. Kjellin and Stibler (1974) found an extremely alkaline end fraction in the gamma globulin component of the spinal fluid in three patients similar to that seen in Huntington's disease and multiple sclerosis. Curzon (1973) found no changes in lumbar cerebrospinal fluid homovanillic acid or 5-hydroxyindoleacetic acid levels in nine patients. In a further study by Lal et al (1979) the concentration of homovanillic acid was low in the ventricular cerebrospinal fluid of three of four patients when compared with patients with a pain syndrome or obsessive-compulsive neurosis. In lumbar cerebrospinal fluid, basal concentrations of 5-hydroxyindoleacetic acid but not homovanillic acid were low in 15 patients compared with controls. Following probenecid pre-treatment, there was a marked increase in both acid catabolites even when basal values were low. Growth hormone response to apomorphine, however, did not differ from controls.

DIFFERENTIAL DIAGNOSIS

Congenital torticollis due either to fibrosis of one sternomastoid following a haematoma in the muscle or a congenital hemi-vertebra can be distinguished by the age of onset. Posterior fossa tumours in childhood, syringomyelia and colloid cysts of the third ventricle also cause neck tilt as does ocular muscle imbalance as from a trochlear nerve palsy. Fibrositis, inflammed lymph glands in the neck, cervical vertebral disease and cervical radiculopathy may all also cause a twisted neck. Hysterical torticollis is rare and often begins suddenly, sometimes giving the impression that the neck is resting on the shoulder. A primary gain must be sought and if the characteristic combination of tonic and clonic elements with recoil seen in spasmodic torticollis is present, or if there are motor abnormalities elsewhere, it should never be diagnosed.

COURSE

As a generalisation, spasmodic torticollis gets progressively worse over the first two to five years and then plateaus out or slightly improves. Pain, however, often increases steadily with the development of secondary cervical spondylosis. The disorder may stabilise at any stage and partial or even complete remissions are not uncommon in the first few years. In their follow-up study Patterson and Little (1943) found that 25% of cases had deteriorated, 12% were unchanged, 12% were slightly improved, 42% were definitely better and 7% of these cured. Ten significant remissions occurred in Meares' 41 patients (1971c) nine of which occurred in the first year. Five of these were only short-lived, however, but six more patients had remissions for more than one year between the second and fifth year and a single further patient had a remission between the sixth and 10th year. Good prognostic signs in this study included high anxiety and neuroticism scores. Similar encouraging remission rates were reported by Tibbetts (1971) 19 of whose patients remitted, and by Lang and Marsden (1982) 10 of whose 100 patients improved spontaneously. The findings of Matthews et al (1978) were less encouraging. Only one of 30 patients was cured at the time of review; six others had shown remissions but subsequently relapsed. These authors concurred with the general view that spontaneous amelioration tended to occur early if at all. Our own data from University College Hospital in which 26 patients were followed up for a median period of 10 years revealed a frequency of sustained remission of 23%, the median duration of remission was eight years and median duration of torticollis before remission was three years. Improvement when it occurred was usually gradual and in some appeared to have been accelerated by self-taught sensory reinforcement techniques (Jayne et al, 1984). Herz and Glaser (1949) studied a group of patients seen between 1930 and 1940 at the Neurological Institute of Columbia University with an overall disease duration of 6.4 years. At follow-up the course appeared to have been static in 34, six had improved, three were cured and three others had shown remissions.

TREATMENT

In common with the other adult onset focal dystonias, spasmodic torticollis is notoriously difficult to treat. Individual patients may idiosyncratically respond strikingly to one of a wide range of drugs but the available literature does not permit any definitive statement to be made about the clinical pharmacology of the disorder. Most physicians sequentially administer a range of drugs known to have disparate effects on central neurotransmitter function in the hope that one may provide benefit. Probably the best hope of lasting improvement, however, is a spontaneous remission which occurs in at least 10% of cases. Good results have been claimed for surgical treatment but morbidity is high and the results are unpredictable. Psychotherapy and more recently behavioural techniques including sensory biofeedback are occasionally useful. Measures such as the use of cervical collars, plaster casts and traction are quite useless and may injure the neck.

PSYCHOTHERAPY

The overall lack of success of psychiatric treatment was one of the factors precipitating the move away from psychogenic aetiological theories in spasmodic torticollis. Nevertheless, good results have been reported in individual patients. Paterson (1945) induced complete remission in five of her 21 patients using psychotherapy complemented by hypnotic suggestion. Tibbetts (1971) also considers that in suitably selected patients psychotherapeutic approaches may be beneficial. Fourteen of the 30 patients of Matthews et al (1978) were referred initially to psychiatrists and received a variety of treatments including electro-shock therapy without benefit.

BEHAVIOURAL THERAPY

Aversion therapy has been used to treat patients with spasmodic torticollis, electric shocks being applied on movement of the head (Brierly, 1967). Massed practice techniques have a long history (Poore, 1873) but the results have generally been disappointing (Agras and Marshall, 1965; Meares, 1973). Systemic desensitisation with reduction of coexisting anxiety by relaxation or hypnotherapy seems the most promising behavioural approach (Meares, 1973).

SENSORY FEEDBACK THERAPY

This technique, also referred to as operant conditioning, consists of detecting a signal from a physiological source and presenting it as a processed display to the patient. In the case of spasmodic torticollis the signal consists of the integrated surface electromyographic activity from the dystonic neck muscles. Korein and Brudny (1976) have used an EMA bioconditioner with a digital integrator to reflect, as a continuous trace, the intensity and duration of neck muscle activity on an oscilloscopic screen. Using this apparatus they have treated 48 cases with a mean duration of disease of five years, who were refractory to other forms of therapy. The patients were given a 12-week course of five weekly 45 minute sessions in a quiet, distraction-free environment. After the patient had learned voluntary control, various goals were set, such as minimising muscle activity when standing as well as in the sitting position. When this had been achieved the visual feedback would be withdrawn. Patients were instructed to reinforce these sessions at home with mirror drill and with the help of a simple portable biofeedback apparatus. Encouraging results were achieved. Most learned to control their head posture during therapy but only 26 maintained a substantial improvement once the treatment had stopped; 20 of these continued to improve for from three months to three years. Patients with a shorter disease duration fared better on the whole and the only complications occurring during the treatment were cervical root lesions in four patients and lumbar radiculopathies in two. Korein has suggested that this form of therapy may work by augmenting existing systems by resonating or matching activity with a defective servo system. By this means missing information may be supplied or new patterns formed which could then override a deficient feedback loop.

DRUG TREATMENT

Lal (1979) has reviewed the 42 drug treatment trials in 33 papers published between 1937–1978 which involved approximately 148 individuals. Most of these studies are difficult to evaluate because of small sample size, clinical heterogeneity, the design of the study not allowing for spontaneous remission and the short period of follow-up. Only two of the trials used double-blind crossover methods, and objective methods of assessment were rarely applied. A few studies used video-rating with horizontal grids and others mechanical devices for quantifying head tilt.

ANTICHOLINERGIC DRUGS

Of the 25 cases in the literature reviewed by Lal (1979) only three improved with anticholinergics. Lang et al (1983) gave acute intravenous challenges of atropine (0.6 mg), benztropine (2 mg), chlorpheniramine (10 mg) and saline control injections to eight patients without improvement and also reported disappointing overall results with oral therapy. Lal et al (1979) on the other hand reported sustained improvement in five of 10 patients [all of whom had improved with an acute benztropine challenge (2 mg)]. Four of the five therapeutic failures in this study had also failed to improve after a single injection of the drug. One of my own patients has also had an unequivocal excellent dose-dependent response to benzhexol (6 mg/d) making a trial and error approach reasonable despite the generally disappointing results.

DOPAMINERGIC ANTAGONISTS

Gilbert (1972) claimed excellent sustained benefit from a combination of high doses of haloperidol (4–14 mg/d) and amantadine (300 mg/d) in seven cases and these findings were generally supported by a further study by Couch (1976) using a mean dose of 7 mg haloperidol as sole treatment in 16 cases. It has been suggested, however, that good results only occur at the expense of iatrogenic Parkinson's syndrome and smaller doses of haloperidol are ineffective (Shaw et al, 1972). Korein and Brudny (1976) reported a few patients who improved with haloperidol and amantidine but others deteriorated. Lal et al (1979) reported benefit in 4 of 9 patients with pimozide but the responders all developed drug-induced Parkinson's syndrome and the same authors found acute challenges with dopaminergic antagonists unhelpful in predicting therapeutic response. Equally capricious results have been reported with the substituted benzamides tiapride and sulpiride (Trillet et al, 1977). The results with tetrabenazene are equally disappointing. At a mean dose of 150 mg/d none of the nine patients of Shaw et al improved and Swash et al (1972) noted improvement in only one of their three patients. Lang and Marsden (1982) treated 14 patients with a mean dose of 100 mg of tetrabenazene, one patient with a three-year history improving markedly. Another patient improved slightly, two were made worse and six were unable to tolerate the drug. The addition of alpha-methylparatyrosine did not improve the figures appreciably.

DOPAMINERGIC AGONISTS

A number of trials have reported negative results with high doses of L-dopa (3.0–7.0 g/d) (Barrett et al, 1970; Ansari et al, 1972). Shaw et al (1972) reported a single idiosyncratic therapeutic response to L-dopa in a patient with retrocollis, the other 16 patients being unresponsive. The patient who improved developed peak-dose chorea with sustained treatment. When bromocriptine became available a switch over to this drug (70 mg/d) was achieved without loss of control of the retrocollis and disappearance of drug-induced chorea. Of the other nine patients treated with bromocriptine in high dosage (15–80 mg/d), eight were unresponsive and one worsened (Lees et al, 1976). Lisuride, another dopamine receptor agonist has, however, been reported in a dose of 3 mg/d to be of benefit in three patients (Micheli et al, 1982). Two trials using amantadine alone have demonstrated no therapeutic effects (Shaw et al, 1972; West, 1977). In acute challenges with apomorphine six of 13 patients showed a clinical change, in four there was improvement and in two worsening. When the same patients were given L-dopa, two of the acute apomorphine responders improved and one of the patients who got worse on apomorphine also deteriorated with L-dopa (Lal et al, 1979).

Other drugs Benzodiazepines have been reported of benefit in a few patients but the improvement may result from non-specific sedative effects (Pernikoff, 1964). Good results have also occurred with lithium in some patients and quinine, L-tryptophan, alcohol, clonidine and propranolol have all been tried with occasional success.

SURGICAL TREATMENT

In a disorder in which the natural history is one of relatively unchanging non-life-threatening disability, effective therapy needs to abolish all symptoms without risk of serious complication. None of the present surgical methods can be said to achieve this aim in spasmodic torticollis. Nevertheless, in patients with severe long-standing painful disability unresponsive to drugs, cervical rhizotomy should be considered as a last resort, and cervical cord stimulation shows promise for the future.

PERIPHERAL SURGERY

CERVICAL RHIZOTOMY

Procedures aimed at reducing the excessive muscular contraction of the neck muscles in torticollis have a long history. Extraspinal division of the first three cranial nerves on one side was first performed in 1891 by Keen, and Taylor carried out the first intraspinal operation in 1915. Section of individual muscles was first attempted 300 years ago but despite a recent enthusiastic report (Chen, 1981) this technique is unlikely to be universally revived.

Finney and Hughson (1925) and Dandy (1930) were the first surgeons to report good results by peripheral surgery and Dandy's method of intradural section of the first three anterior cervical roots on both sides remains the basic approach today. Some contemporary surgeons also advocate section of the spinal accessory nerve which has an important contribution to the first cervical root and the fourth cervical root on the side showing greater posterior neck muscle contraction.

There are a number of large surgical series reporting benefit from these denervation procedures. Sorensen and Hamby (1965) obtained excellent initial improvement in 37 patients, moderate improvement in 22, minimal improvement in seven and no improvement in four, with one death. Seventeen required additional operations, however, and three had a total of three operations and one five separate procedures. Twenty-four of the patients were followed for up to one year, 20 for one to five years, and 26 for 6–10 or more years. At follow-up, 44 were without symptoms, 17 had minimal torticollis and nine had moderate residual torticollis. Late complications included weak necks in 34, limitation of head movement in 50, three of whom required neck braces, and eight collars or head supports. Atrophy of the sternomastoid and trapezius was present in 23, shoulder droop in 10, persistent dysphagia in 19 and sensory loss in four. Arseni and Maretsis (1971) reported 39% satisfactory results in 52 patients and Tasker (1976) noted an impressive immediate improvement in 29 of 47, six more having modest benefit. Fabinyi and Dutton (1980) claimed 18 good results out of 20. Unfortunately, none of these studies permits a comparison with unoperated cases and the indications for surgery are rarely stated. Some authors consider early surgery to be indicated to prevent fibrosis and cervical spondylosis whereas others reserve surgery for patients with fixed painful neck contracture. The methods of evaluating benefit are also variable and uncritical in most studies, the results being judged by the operator. Hernesniemi and Laitenen (1977), in a follow-up of 56 patients, noted that, although most patients considered the early results of peripheral surgery to be good, subsequently their opinions changed, some regretting the procedure. Meares (1971c) reported that the operation failed to abolish the involuntary movements in some patients and that some showed severe disability of a kind not seen in unoperated cases. Matthews et al, (1978) also found surgery to be generally ineffective. Other uncommon complications of rhizotomy included spinal cord or brain-stem ischaemia, subluxation of the cervical spine and permanent weakness of the upper limbs.

SUPPRESSION OF LABYRINTHINE ACTIVITY

This approach is based on the unproven premise that spasmodic torticollis is due to a small lesion in the reticular formation near the brachium conjunctivum which results in a release of the ipsilateral vestibular nuclei from normal inhibitory influences. Svien and Cody (1969) recommended the repeated iontophoresis of the middle ear with hyaluronidase and tolazoline and reported benefit in an 80-year-old woman with a six-month history of torticollis. Subsequent trials with this method led to a further excellent result in six other patients but as yet these results have not been duplicated.

STEREOTAXIC SURGERY

Although there is no longer any place for bilateral stereotactic thalamolysis in the management of torticollis, this operation was widely performed between 1960 and 1970. The demonstration that direction-specific turning movements of the head and neck can be induced in animals following stimulation of the internal segment of the globus pallidus or its thalamic connections provides the rationale for the procedure. Cooper, one of the main proponents of this approach, considered that torticollis was due to an abnormality of the motor-modulating sensory connections between the cerebellum and motor cortex. The frequent occurrence of tremor in association with torticollis was used as support for this view and he considered that interruption of these pathways at thalamic level might ameliorate torticollis.

Experience with 160 patients treated by stereotactic thalamolysis revealed that, although excellent results were sometimes obtained, overall the results were disappointing when compared to those obtained with segmental limb dystonia. Extensive procedures were required with bilateral lesions in the ventrolateral, ventropostero-medial, centromedianum nuclei and often the pulvinar. Even then lasting relief did not always occur and only about 60% of cases reported improvement (Cooper, 1977). Morbidity was considerable including dysarthria in about one-fifth of cases.

Hassler and Riechert (1958) believed the nucleus ventralis oralis internus to be the optimum target site because of its cephalic representation but their good early results were often not sustained. Rotatory movements of the head and neck occur in animals following stimulation of the interstitial nucleus of Cajal and its thalamic connections in the posterior part of the ventralis oralis internus while turning movements may be mediated by pallidothalamic fibres. Dieckmann (1976), by lesioning both these sites, abolished the abnormal neck movements in 47% of his patients and improved a further 29%. Andrew carried out thalamotomies on 22 cases and bilateral procedures to Vim, Vce-Vci and Cem were performed in 16 of them. Ten (62%) of those cases who had bilateral operations obtained good relief, three others initially improved but then relapsed. Over half, however, were left with dysarthria (Andrew et al, 1983). An interesting observation was that optimum therapeutic effects occasionally did not occur until several months after the operation. Subcortical neglect in the contralateral extremities appeared in 16% of cases.

Bertrand (1982), with 30 years of surgical experience in the management of spasmodic torticollis, initially performed cervical rhizotomies but then switched briefly in the 1960s to stereotactic lesioning in the posterior part of the nucleus of the ventralis oralis internus. Satisfactory results occurred in only 50%, however, and when bilateral lesions were performed dysarthria occurred in 25% of cases. He then employed a combined approach with unilateral thalamolysis supplemented by selective peripheral denervation if necessary, using local nerve blocks to isolate the residually affected muscles. With this combined approach good results were obtained in eight of nine cases. On the basis that it is the contralateral sternomastoid to the side to which the head turns and the ipsilateral posterior cervical group which are the main offenders, Bertrand's current policy consists of selective posterior cervical rhizotomy under light anaesthesia using stimulation. In rotational torticollis, he sections only the branches of the spinal accessory nerve to the sternocleidomastoid and in laterocollis he denervates those to the trapezius muscle. For spasmodic torticollis avulsion of the posterior rami of C2, C3, C4, C5 and C6 are also avulsed to eliminate all motor response from the posterior cervical group of muscles. In retrocollis, denervation to C4 on one side and C5 on the other is recommended. With this purely peripheral approach excellent results have been obtained in 90% of patients with torticollis, the results being slightly less good with retrocollis. Bertrand now recommends a unilateral thalamolysis only in failed cases or those with associated tremor.

CERVICAL CORD STIMULATION

Promising results have been reported in spasmodic torticollis following the percutaneous implantation of a two or four-electrode system into the epidural space between C2 and C4 (Waltz, 1982). The patient's response to stimulating specific electrode combinations is then studied and once the best electrode combination has been found the system is fixed in place with a subcutaneously placed receiver. The external system consists of a radio-frequency antenna and receiver and, when the antenna is placed over the receiver, radio-frequencies are converted to minute electrical impulses (100–1400 Hz) which in turn are conveyed to the cervical electrodes. Of 26 cases treated, a third have obtained marked improvement and approximately another third moderate benefit. Broken electrodes are the major complication and infections occasionally occur. This approach has also been used to treat cerebral palsy, generalised dystonia, intractable epilepsy and spasticity and may act either directly by neuromodulation of the reticular formation or indirectly via the release of neurotransmitters in this area.

MEIGE SYNDROME

Synonyms Cranial dystonia, Brueghel's syndrome, blepharospasm-oromandibular dystonia syndrome, idiopathic orofacial dystonia, orofacial cervical dystonia, mental trismus.

Definition An idiopathic focal dystonia symmetrically affecting the facial musculature and causing blepharospasm, grimacing and oromandibular torsion.

A possible example of bilateral facial spasm in a 62-year-old man was reported in 1870 (Talkow, 1870). In their monograph on tics, Meige and Feindel recorded the case of a 47-year-old metal polisher who presented to Brissaud's clinic at l'Hôtel Dieu with intermittent involuntary eyelid closure (Meige and

Feindel, 1902). In 1904 Gaussel described a 23-year-old soldier who developed torticollis, blepharospasm and bilateral tonic contractions of the face and a further two cases of blepharospasm and facial spasm were reported by De Spéville (1906). One year later at the Societé de Neurologie in Paris, Rochon-Duvigneaud and Weill presented an example of blepharospasm with synchronous facial contortions which was treated successfully by avulsion of both supraorbital nerves. In response to this paper Henry Meige concurred that tonic spasms of the midline facial muscles do sometimes occur with blepharospasm and affirmed that although related to tics, this condition was distinguished by the tonic nature of the involuntary movement and by its usual emergence in late adult life. In 1910 Meige reported 10 examples of 'spasme facial median' which he delineated from tics, hemifacial spasm and post-paralytic facial contracture. All his patients had presented in adult life with tonic involuntary movements affecting the orbicularis oculi most severely, but also causing wrinkling of the forehead, eyebrow raising, wincing of the chin, pulling up of the lips and twitching of the nostrils. The spasms fluctuated appreciably during the day but always disappeared in sleep. Triggering factors included looking upwards, walking and emotional stresses. Most of his patients were depressed and in one case there was a family member with spasmodic torticollis. Three improved with prolonged re-educative mirror drill but Meige opined that this disorder was much more resistant to this mode of treatment than tics. He was also of the view that the disorder should be looked upon as a neurosis caused by an irritative focus within the pons or midbrain. Sicard, who was also interested in the disorder, believed it to be closely related to spasmodic torticollis (Sicard and Hagueneau, 1925). In Kinnier Wilson's textbook the condition receives a few lines and is considered to be allied to hemifacial spasm. There is also a photograph of a young man who appears to have oromandibular dystonia attributed to epidemic encephalitis lethargica.

The syndrome was then virtually ignored in the medical literature until 1956 when Henderson reported 135 patients with essential blepharospasm seen at the Mayo Clinic. 21% of these cases had dystonia of other facial muscles. In 1972, Paulson reported three further cases and coined the eponym Meige syndrome, and Altrocchi described a further convincing case in which oromandibular dystonia was a prominent feature. Marsden then described the clinical features of an additional 29 cases and suggested that the syndrome should be renamed Brueghel's syndrome after the 16th century Dutch painter who, in his portrait 'De Gaper', appears to have captured the characteristic facial dystonia (Marsden, 1976b). Several other large representative series have now also been published (Gollomp et al, 1981; Tolosa, 1981; Jankovic and Ford, 1983).

EPIDEMIOLOGY

The peak age of onset is in the sixth decade of life but 10–20% of patients present before the age of 40 years. The youngest reported case in one recently published series was 10 years and the eldest 76 years (Jankovic and Ford, 1983).

There is a 3:2 female : male preponderance for both essential blepharospasm and the full-blown syndrome.

For most of this century the condition has been ignored and probably gone largely unrecognised. For example, Henderson in 1956 was only able to find 35 cases of essential blepharospasm in the literature. Nevertheless, the disorder has now been reported from Europe, the United States of America and Japan and occurs in the Negro and Indian races. I have seen 23 cases at the National Hospital for Nervous Diseases over the last five years and Marsden has examined over 50 cases at King's College Hospital over a similar period. Although precise incidence figures are unavailable, it seems probable that it is as common as spasmodic torticollis.

PATHOLOGY

There are now two published autopsy reports in which different histological findings have been reported. In the first case of a 62-year-old female with a seven-year history of Meige syndrome no histological abnormalities were found within the central nervous system (Garcia-Alba et al, 1981).

The second case, a Filipino male who died of aspiration pneumonia after a six-year history of involuntary jaw opening, facial grimacing, dysphagia and dysarthria, showed neuronal loss in a distinctive mosaic pattern in the dorsal halves of the caudate and putamen (Altrocchi and Forno, 1983). I have examined a further case of a 68-year-old man who committed suicide by self-poisoning after a 14-year history of blepharospasm and oromandibular dystonia. Shortly before his death his swallowing had become so severe that a gastrostomy had been performed. No histological abnormalities within the corpus striatum, zona reticularis of the substantia nigra, globus pallidus, nucleus of Darkeschwitsch, interstitial nucleus of Cajal or the cerebellum were found. Neurochemical studies and detailed cell counting within selected areas of the basal ganglia may prove more fruitful.

AETIOLOGY

The cause of Meige syndrome is yet to be established but there is some indirect evidence to suggest that altered basal ganglia function may be important. Blepharospasm and oromandibular dystonia occasionally occur in post-encephalitic Parkinson's syndrome, athetoid cerebral palsy, Wilson's disease and the Steele-Richardson-Olszewski syndrome and isolated blepharospasm is common in Parkinson's disease. Damage to the basal ganglia occurs in all these diseases and extrapyramidal symptoms, including loss of arm swing, rest tremor, chorea and mild rigidity can occur in Meige syndrome. A family history of Parkinson's disease has also been reported in about 10% of cases of Meige syndrome. Strokes or demyelination of the rostral brain-stem causes facial dystonia or blepharospasm (Fisher, 1963; Jankovic and Ford, 1983) and stimulation of the midbrain ventral to the superior colliculus causes abnormally rapid blinking (Nashold et al, 1979). One of my own cases with blepharospasm had an arterio-venous malformation on the dorsal surface of the pons with more involvement of pyramidal fibres than transverse pontine fibres. No characteristic radiological abnormalities have, however, been found in subcortical structures in Meige syndrome. Another interesting observation was that of Irvine et al (1968) who observed reflex blepharospasm in premature infants on tactile stimulation of the eyelids which disappeared as the infant matured and was not present in full term infants.

A link between Meige syndrome, the other focal dystonias and idiopathic torsion dystonia has recently been emphasised by Marsden (1976a). In support of this thesis is the similarity in the characteristics of the muscle spasms, their prolonged duration, repetitive and irregular timing and their provocation by action. A high incidence of essential tremor also occurs in all these conditions. Ten of Marsden's cases (1976a) developed dystonia outside the cranial musculature. In two of these patients the presenting complaint was actually writer's cramp and torticollis respectively; four more developed spasmodic torticollis after the onset of Meige syndrome, three others had respiratory dystonias, two flexion of the trunk and one of the patients with torticollis also had limb dystonia. These additional dystonic postures all appeared within three years of the onset of cranial dystonia. Seven of Tolosa's seventeen patients (1981) had tonic deviation of the neck and chin and in two of these there was mild limb dystonia. In the Houston study, 51% had torticollis, 25% arm dystonia, 11% leg dystonia, 11% truncal dystonia and 11% respiratory muscle dystonia. There also appeared to be a marked overlap with spasmodic dysphonia (Jankovic and Ford, 1983).

A genetic predisposition to Meige syndrome is supported by the occasional occurrence of the disorder in identical twins (Jankovic and Ford, 1983) and siblings (Nutt and Hammerstad, 1981). Three (18%) of Tolosa's cases and seven (7%) of Jankovic's patients gave a family history of cranial dystonia but this association was not observed in Marsden's series. Two of my own cases gave a family history of spasmodic torticollis, the son of one female patient and the brother of another male patient. Interestingly the son spontaneously remitted from his torticollis three years after its onset and has not relapsed again after a follow-up period of 12 years.

There is, however, very little to support the contention that Meige syndrome might be a forme fruste of idiopathic torsion dystonia. Severe stimulus-sensitive blepharospasm and oromandibular dystonia are unusual in the generalised disorder and there are only a few reports of Meige syndrome occurring in the relatives of patients with idiopathic torsion dystonia (Zeman et al, 1960).

A strong family history of essential tremor occurs in the relatives of patients with Meige syndrome. Four (24%) of Tolosa's patients, all of whom had hand tremor themselves, gave a family history of essential tremor and 12 (12%) of Jankovic's cases had at least one affected family member. In my own cases three (15%) gave a family history of essential tremor and four gave a definite family history of tics. I have also seen two patients who developed Meige syndrome in middle age who had suffered from tics during childhood and adolescence. Tolosa also reported a family history of tics in two of his cases.

Central dopaminergic abnormalities are suggested with the induction by L-dopa of end of dose cranial dystonia in Parkinson's disease (Lees et al, 1977; Weiner and Nausieda, 1982) and its occurrence with neuroleptics either as part of an acute dystonic reaction or as a potentially irreversible tardive dystonia (Weiner et al, 1981). However, the inconsistent pharmacological response of Meige syndrome to drugs known to modify central dopaminergic activity and the lack of post-mortem neurochemical data preclude the construction of a convincing theory implicating dopaminergic mechanisms at the present time.

The link between depressive illness and Meige syndrome is of great interest. Meige drew attention to the melancholic introspective personality of several of his patients but considered this to be a reaction to their appalling incapacities. Fourteen (35%) of Marsden's cases had depression at the onset of their illness and seven (41%) of Tolosa's series were also depressed. In five of Tolosa's patients the depression preceded the cranial dystonia by 1–35 years and in the other two it started two years after the onset. In three there was a family history of depression. No correlation was found, however, between the duration, severity or mode of therapy of the depression and the time of onset of Meige syndrome or its severity (Tolosa, 1981). One-quarter of Jankovic's patients also had marked depression and he also emphasised the high incidence of other psychological abnormalities such as mania, anxiety and obsessive-compulsive personality traits. Marsden (1976a) has pointed out that in order to prove conclusively that a physical complaint is psychogenically determined it is essential to show that a psychiatric illness is present at the beginning, that the physical disorder persists as long as the psychiatric condition remains and that it abates promptly once the mental ailment is cured. Clearly the above findings do not fulfil these rigorous criteria but in several of my own cases I have been struck by the close interplay between emerging psychopathology and the onset of Meige syndrome. One of my cases, a young woman in her 30s with a 15-year history of manic-depressive psychosis, developed Meige syndrome during her longest remission from mental illness. Treatment with anticholinergics rapidly alleviated her blepharospasm and facial dystonia but led to a severe recurrence of depression. Another patient in her 50s developed writer's cramp following a series of stressful life-events at home and work. This improved following their resolution. Several years later she presented with Meige syndrome, again coinciding with conflicts at work, but following her retirement several months later the facial spasms rapidly abated. It remains possible that there is some substance in the insistence of earlier neurologists such as Oppenheim and Meige that these disorders tended to occur in patients with a neuropathic disposition, in which a positive family history of disorders of neurological inferiority such as tremor, tics and depression occurs frequently. It is also conceivable that depression and Meige syndrome may share an underlying abnormality of central monoamines.

CLINICAL DESCRIPTION

Blepharospasm is the presenting symptom in at least two-thirds of cases. It usually starts as clonic involuntary contractions of the eyelids but frequently develops into persistent tonic spasms of eyelid closure. The onset is gradual with occasional painless involuntary blinking or winking of one or both eyes. The patient is not much inconvenienced at this stage and may brush off the symptom as merely a sensitivity to bright lights. Actual photophobia and eye irritation do occur early in a few cases when the patient may resort to the use of sun-glasses. A unilateral onset is unusual and the other eye is virtually always affected within a few weeks, after which the eye blinking is stereotyped and symmetrical. As the disorder progresses the patients find involuntary eyelid closure interfering with an increasing number of daily activities. For instance the eyelids may go into spasm on crossing the road making it difficult to avoid passing traffic, or occur so frequently in the course of a manual worker's job that it becomes difficult to complete deadlines. Most patients discover a selection of trick manoeuvres to combat the eyelid closure and some of the commoner ones together with the major provoking factors are listed in Table 11.1. Unfortunately these ploys become less reliable as the disease progresses and in the late stages the patient is often obliged to walk about prising his eyelids open with his fingers. Many patients become increasingly withdrawn and depressed as they find that any outside contact or pleasurable excitement

Table 11.1 EXTERNAL INFLUENCES ON MEIGE SYNDROME

Relieving tricks	Provoking factors
Forced jaw opening	Reading
Yawning	Watching television
Singing	Driving
Prising eyes open	Bright sunlight
Lightly touching side of upper eyelid	Embarrassment
Neck extension	Emotional stress
Gentle pressure on eyebrow	Fatigue
Drinking water or alcohol	Looking up
Pinching back of neck	Wind in the eyes
Humming	Crowded places
Combing hair	Walking
Closure of one eye	Depression
Pulling eyelid	
Walking	
Belching	
Whistling	
Blowing out cheeks	
Chewing on toothpick	

increases the spasms. Equally, however, solitary pastimes such as reading, watching television or doing needlework may induce eyelid closure so that the patient's daily activities become increasingly limited and he may eventually lose his job and social independence. Rest is the most effective relieving factor and, after a good night's sleep, blepharospasm often disappears for an hour or two in the early morning. Patients often attempt to compress all their daily chores into this brief pocket of freedom before their eyes begin to close again. Although there is a tendency for the frequency and severity of the eyelid spasms to increase with time, the disorder waxes and wanes *pari passu* with life's stresses and strains and temporary remissions for several hours or even days may occur. Henderson (1956), for example, relates the story of one of his patients, a 62-year-old woman who had a second myocardial infarction and was placed in an oxygen tent for four days. During this period her blepharospasm disappeared completely only to return subsequently. As with tics, blepharospasm may actually disappear during a medical consultation but may be brought out by getting the patient to read and write, tapping the bridge of the nose or observing the patient surreptitiously from afar.

In its most severe form the patient experiences virtually continuous irregular tonic contraction of the orbicularis oculi and surrounding muscles with only occasional respites lasting seconds at most. The patient has to be led around as if blind, and loss of normal eye to eye contact may cause considerable emotional problems with respect to the patient's loved ones. Profuse lachrymation is common and conversely dry eyes have occasionally been reported. Occasionally eyelid muscle hypertrophy occurs with entropion, but visual acuity, pupillary reactions and extraocular muscle motility are normal.

In some patients the disorder remains restricted to the eyelids when the term essential blepharospasm has been used. In the large ophthalmological series only 21% of cases in fact had more generalised orofacial dystonia at the time of examination. In Marsden's series (1976a), however, 58% had involvement of other facial muscles and an even higher figure of 77% was reported by Jankovic and Ford (1983). It seems likely, therefore, that if examined methodically and repeatedly over several years most patients with essential blepharospasm will be found to have some involvement of other midline facial muscles.

Surface electromyographic recordings have confirmed that, in most patients, each bout of dystonia begins with tonic, symmetrical, bilateral irregular contractions of variable duration in the eyelids and upper face and then spreads within seconds to involve other muscle groups which are affected with differing intensity. Sometimes it is the lower half of the face which is initially affected and less commonly all the affected cranial muscles fire off synchronously. Brief clonic contractions sometimes precede the dystonia especially in orbicularis oculi and frontalis muscles.

Meige emphasised the predilection for midline facial muscles:

> If one examines these patients with careful attention and for sufficient time, one can
> soon notice that the majority of the facial muscles participate in this spasmodic

phenomenon, always both sides simultaneously. The frontals muscle and especially the eyebrows contract along with the orbicularis oculi muscles. All the muscles of the nose (pyramidals, elevators, the triangular muscles the dilators of the nostrils) re-involved and the same goes for the labial muscles, especially the medial fascicles of the orbicularia oris and for the cheek and chin muscles. On the other hand the zygomatic muscles are much less affected and contract only exceptionally and weakly.

These facial convulsions closely resemble those occurring in hemifacial spasm. One may recognise the same partial palpitations, the same type of quivering contracture and the resultant small grimaces which do not correspond to any mimic expression. One sees sometimes for example, a mild folding between the eyebrows and at other times wrinkling of the nose or brief pulsations, beatings, contractions of its wings as well as a pulling of the lips and a wincing of the chin.

During a full-blown attack the expression of patients suggests the smelling of some acrid irritant such as ammonia with severe grimacing and eye closure (Fig. 11.3). Between attacks, however, provided the patient avoids any movements of the cranial muscles, facial expression usually returns to normal. Common facial movements during an episode include mouth retraction, frowning, eyebrow elevation, neck spasms, platysmal contractions, jaw opening, lip pursing, mouth clenching and nasal wrinkling. Slow tongue protrusions may also occur and pharyngeal and palatal dyskinesia may produce swallowing difficulties and dysarthria. Spasmodic dysphonia is also frequent in the late stages

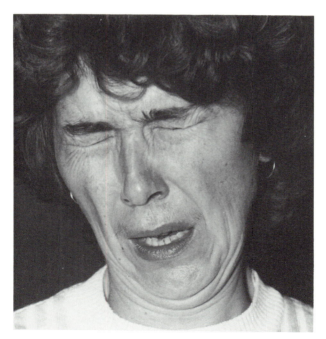

Figure 11.3. *Meige syndrome.*

(Marsden and Sheehy, 1982). Laboured breathing with inspiratory catching occurs in the late stages and death from aspiration pneumonia is a significant hazard. A few patients also develop abdominal and truncal spasm and clicking, throat clearing and choking noises may also occur during a dystonic attack.

Marsden drew attention to oromandibular dystonia as an important component of the disorder largely neglected by Meige. It is occasionally the presenting feature but the dystonia rarely remains restricted to the jaw. Presenting complaints include facial stiffness or swelling, jaw pain or bruxism. The jaw may be held open with associated lip retraction and platysmal contractions or be forcibly closed with lip pursing. Sometimes patients may alternate rapidly between these two positions but all complain of a lack of control over smooth jaw movement. For jaw dystonia stress, talking and chewing are potent triggers. Facial and jaw movements are of normal strength but repetitive opening and closing of the mouth is impossible because of the induction of dystonia. Marsden (1976a) described a patient who was able to sing but not talk without provoking spasms.

DIFFERENTIAL DIAGNOSIS

Meige syndrome must be distinguished from idiopathic orofacial dyskinesia (senile chorea) and the bucco-linguo-masticatory syndrome due to chronic neuroleptic treatment. In these disorders the movements are more rapid, choreic in nature and not induced by voluntary movement of the affected muscles. Meige syndrome, at least in the early stages, is also more spasmodic with long symptom-free intervals between each dystonic burst. Tardive dystonia can be excluded by taking a careful drug history.

Occasionally, blepharospasm or the related apraxia of lid opening may be the presenting feature of multisystem degeneration or the Steele-Richardson-Olszewski syndrome and it may occur rarely with tumours, strokes or multiple sclerosis involving the midbrain. Although blepharospasm commonly occurs in Parkinson's disease, it is never the presenting feature. An acquired cranial dystonia may occasionally follow viral encephalitis.

Tics of the eyelids and face are more abrupt and unpredictable and rarely so symmetrical. Furthermore, Meige syndrome is a rarity in childhood whereas tics uncommonly present for the first time in adult life. Use of the affected muscles rarely exacerbates tics. The distinction between clonic hemifacial spasm is also usually straightforward. Here the contractions are not stimulus sensitive, are almost invariably confined to one side of the face, and the involuntary spasms are strictly localised to muscles innervated by the facial nerve. Hemifacial spasm also may continue during sleep. Post-paralytic facial contracture or facial spasm from an intrinsic pontine tumour are rarely bilateral and blepharospasm does not occur.

Ocular myotonia in which there is a delayed relaxation of orbicularis oculi following forceful eyelid closure leads to delay in eye opening and lid lag and is seen in hyperkalaemic periodic paralysis, mytonia congenita, dystrophia myotonica and hypothyroidism. Myasthenia gravis is another common misdiagnosis.

Psychogenic spasm of eyelid closure exists but is rare. It occurs usually in young women of neurotic disposition who complain of photophobia and blindness and may have associated eyelid drooping of a non-organic type.

COURSE

An up-and-down course with sometimes dramatic and seemingly inexplicable relapses and remissions is characteristic. The detrimental effect of inner tensions and grief on the disorder has also been recognised since the earliest accounts. Tolosa (1981) re-emphasised the vicissitudes of the illness but most of his patients steadily deteriorated over the first five years and then remained static or only marginally worsened. However, the time from onset to maximal severity varied from two months to 18 years (mean 10 years). The duration of the illness in Marsden's cases (1976a) ranged from 1–28 years and, in some, oromandibular dystonia appeared several years after the onset of blepharospasm. Gollomp et al (1981) reported no spontaneous remissions over a mean five-year follow-up but I have seen one spontaneous complete recovery and there are a number of other reasonably well-documented complete or partial remissions in the literature, most of which were attributed to the eradication of underlying psychopathology. Nevertheless, as a rule, the disorder gets imperceptibly worse as time goes by. Depression tends to increase and the last few years of many patients' lives are spent in virtual total darkness with severe articulation, swallowing and breathing disabilities. Aspiration pneumonia and suicide are the two commonest disease-related causes of death but most patients succumb to intercurrent illnesses.

TREATMENT

There is no consistently effective remedy for Meige syndrome. Occasional patients remit spontaneously early in the course of the illness and others appear to respond convincingly to psychotherapy. Anticholinergic drugs, dopaminergic antagonists, lithium and benzodiazepines seem to be the most promising medications but less than a quarter of cases derive lasting benefit from drugs. Surgical approaches for intractable blepharospasm have met with considerable success but post-operative complications are common and there are recurrences.

PSYCHOTHERAPY

Marsden (1976b) reported that many of his patients had received behavioural therapy, hypnosis, aversion therapy, psychological counselling and acupuncture without benefit and Bird and McDonald (1975) were equally gloomy about the value of psychotherapy. Cole (1973) drew a distinction between essential blepharospasm in which psychiatric conditions often accompany the disorder but in which a cause and effect has not been proven, and psychogenic blepharospasm occurring in younger people which he believed to be a form of conversion hysteria and amenable to psychotherapy.

Meige (1910) reported three patients who were cured following prolonged psychomotor drill exercises. Langworthy (1952) described four individuals with blepharospasm who had previously derived temporary benefit from hypnosis and who responded well to psychotherapy. All the patients were middle-aged with no evidence of overt psychopathology and three fully recovered with intensive treatment. Similarly spectacular results have been claimed for behavioural therapy in individual cases (Reckless, 1972; Sharpe, 1974). Cavenar et al (1978) described four cases of essential blepharospasm, all of whom had concurrent significant psychological illness. One had severe depression and the other three were described as having neurotic or conversion behaviour patterns. Psychotherapy led to improvement in some cases but with the unmasking of a cryptic psychosis. Pursuing this aetiological line, Volow et al (1980) proposed a joint therapeutic approach using drug treatment and psychotherapy together.

DRUG TREATMENT

There is no one medication which reliably ameliorates the symptoms of Meige syndrome. However, therapeutic effects have been demonstrated with a number of drugs which differ markedly in their pharmacological properties. Although acute intravenous drug challenges may be of some limited benefit in predicting the likely response to oral administration, the physician has no alternative at present than to try a list of promising treatments one after the other in the hope that a gratifying response will occur to at least one.

ANTICHOLINERGIC DRUGS

Anecdotal reports of modest benefit from anticholinergic drugs are common in the literature (Henderson, 1956; Altrocchi, 1972; Paulson, 1972). Tanner et al (1982a) improved all six patients in an acute study with scopolamine (0.8 mg i.m.), an effect which was consistently reversed by physostigmine (2.4 mg i.m.). Twelve of 13 patients treated with long-term anticholinergics (benztropine 1–3 mg/d, trihexiphenidyl 2–8 mg/d) also improved. Tolosa and Lai (1979) also reported improvement in acute studies using intravenous methylscopolamine bromide and deterioration following physostigmine. Duvoisin (1983) described a marked response in a single patient to 12–16 mg/d of benztropine, the unwanted peripheral side-effects being controlled by ambenonium, 15 mg/d. Jankovic and Ford (1983) noted marked lasting improvement in 37% of their cases treated with trihexiphenidyl and Gollomp et al (1983) reported that four out of nine of their patients treated with high doses of anticholinergics (trihexiphenidyl 30 mg/d or ethopropazine 800 mg/d) benefited.

Others have been less enthusiastic. Casey (1980) actually noted worsening in one of his two cases on 3 mg/d of benztropine, and Nutt et al (1983), after encouraging open studies, failed to demonstrate benefit to 12 mg/d of trihexiphenidyl in a controlled study in five patients. Lang et al (1982) carried out acute studies using three different anticholinergics, benztropine, atropine and chlorpheniramine and noted only mild improvement which they attributed to sedation. Furthermore, in a retrospective note survey only four of 25 patients who had received anticholinergics had responded and they concluded that cholinergic mechanisms were not of primary importance in the pathogenesis of Meige syndrome. Side-effects are common at high doses including confusion, memory loss, blurred vision, dry mouth and sedation.

DOPAMINERGIC ANTAGONISTS

Tolosa and Lai (1979) noted improvement in four of their five patients treated with haloperidol in a dose of 1.5–12 mg/d, whereas four patients of Tanner et al (1982) derived no response, one improved and one worsened. Jankovic and Ford (1983) obtained a lasting benefit in 26% of their cases with tetrabenazene and Gollomp et al (1983) improved 37% of their patients with haloperidol or tetrabenazene. Similar figures were obtained by Lang and Marsden who treated 10 patients with tetrabenazene. One case derived marked benefit and a further four mild to moderate improvement. Alphamethyltyrosine improved only two of nine cases (Lang and Marsden, 1982).

DOPAMINERGIC AGONISTS

L-dopa exerts no effect on the majority of patients but occasional idiosyncratic therapeutic responses occur (Jankovic and Ford, 1983). Some patients are made worse (Tanner et al, 1982) and in one of my own patients L-dopa in combination with a peripheral dopa decarboxylase inhibitor (Sinemet 125, 8-hourly) aggravated the facial dystonia and at the same time induced reversible dose-related chorea in a rigid right arm (Hardie et al, 1983).

Beneficial effects have been noted with apomorphine (1–2 mg) in acute studies (Tolosa and Lai, 1979), and lisuride (0.6–1.2 mg) and apomorphine, but not bromocriptine (20 mg), produced marked improvement in two cases (Micheli et al, 1982).

Other drugs Benzodiazepines are widely prescribed for blepharospasm and clonazepam has been claimed to be particularly effective. Jankovic and Ford (1983), however, obtained improvement in only one of 10 patients. A number of reports of benefit from lithium carbonate have recently appeared and 26%

of the Houston patients responded (Jankovic and Ford, 1983). Gollomp et al (1982) obtained improvement in five of 11 patients with baclofen (60–120 mg/d) and other drugs which have been said to help include sodium valproate, tricyclic and tetracyclic antidepressants, monoamine oxidase inhibitors and amantadine.

SURGICAL TREATMENT

The surgical attempts to reduce severe blepharospasm over the last century have been reviewed by Henderson (1956). Early, generally unsuccessful, procedures included attempts to weaken the orbicularis oculi by direct interference with the muscle, section of the facial nerve branches as they entered the lateral side of the muscle and more recently the use of frontalis slings using non-absorbable materials. During the early part of this century alcohol injection into the facial nerve at differing sites was the treatment of choice. The results were often initially good but always short lived.

The most successful results of facial denervation have been achieved by selectively dividing the upper branches of the nerve within the parotid gland. Electrical stimulation of the nerve branches to identify their precise innervation before section has proved a useful refinement of this technique. The facial nerve branches are first identified at the anterior border of the parotid gland and the temporal, zygomatic and buccal branches are avulsed bilaterally. The function of the mandibular branch is then assessed by electrical stimulation and, if it innervates the orbicularis oculi or surrounding muscles it is also sectioned. In one recently published series from Moorfields Eye Hospital the 22 patients operated upon using this method all had immediate relief of symptoms provided denervation was adequate (Talbot et al, 1982). Twelve patients, however, required secondary surgery and there was an impressive list of minor post-operative complications. Ectropion occurred in 12, epiphora in four, difficulty in eating in four, difficulty with dentures in three, dribbling in three, blepharochalasis in two, ectopic parotid secretion in two, brow droop in one, ptosis in one, lid swelling in one, trichiasis in one, corneal exposure in one and facial pain in one. Secondary surgery comprised ectropion correction in five, blepharoplasty in two, brow elevation in one, tarsorrhaphy in one, ptosis correction in one, face lift in one and clot evacuation in one. The most striking cosmetic changes were symmetrical brow droop due to loss of action of the frontalis muscle and weakness of the elevators of the corner of the mouth giving rise to a most remarkable flat, expressionless facial appearance. This sometimes improved over the few months after surgery. All the patients were routinely prescribed artificial tear preparations and antibiotic ointment at night and provided with spectacles with side-shields. Four patients were re-operated on for recurrence after a mean interval of 14 months from the first operation. Despite these drawbacks every patient bar one was satisfied with the result and often for the first time in years they were able to see again and return to full employment.

Less radical approaches are being used by others in order to minimise long-term cosmetic complications (Battista, 1982). One procedure involves thermolytic coagulation of the nerve and is carried out using local anaesthesia and intravenous analgesics. Then, using a percutaneous needle probe, the nerve branches to the upper face are identified by electrical stimulation. With the patient's cooperation thermolytic lesions are then applied until spontaneous spasms are relieved. This usually requires 8–38 lesions on each side. Although the recurrence rate is high the procedure has several advantages; general anaesthesia is avoided, post-operative complications such as facial paresis are less, and because scarring is minimal the procedure may be repeated in stages. Similar promising results are being obtained with the local administration of botulinus toxin into the orbicularis oculi muscle.

Cricopharyngeal myotomy has occasionally been tried for dysphagia in Meige syndrome but without lasting improvement, and stereotactic thalamolysis is of little use because of the high morbidity associated with bilateral lesions.

SPASMODIC DYSPHONIA

This uncommon disorder was first described by Traube in 1871 and subsequently referred to by Schnitzler (1875) as spastic dysphonia. Until relatively recently it was regarded as a psycho-neurosis and terms such as stammering of the vocal cords, laryngeal neurosis and psychophonasthenia were used by laryngologists. Heaver (1959) even looked on it as a form of conversion hysteria somatised to the larynx. Two forms were distinguished, an occupational mogiphonia affecting teachers, barristers and the clergy and a much commoner traumatic form due to chronic stress (Arnold, 1959). Schnitzler described two patients with this disturbance who had associated wrinkling of the forehead, tics and limb dyskinesias and Meige (1914) reported a 4-year-old child with athetoid birth damage who developed strained speech and stereotyped gestures. Critchley (1939) coined the term inspiratory speech and described three patients with 'constrained, forced and barely intelligible voice', two of whom had additional tic-like contractions of the neck and face and one of whom had a tremor. In a study by Robe et al (1960) on 10 patients, nine were said to have minor non-specific electroencephalographic abnormalities and a total of 84 'soft neurological signs' were elicited with a high incidence of basal ganglia abnormalities. Aronson et al (1968), in a comprehensive study from the Mayo Clinic on 27 cases, reported facial and tongue twitches in eight, tremulous voice in 14 and a hand tremor in six patients. One additional patient had spasmodic torticollis. These authors introduced the term spasmodic dysphonia and considered an organic cause possible with a close link with benign essential tremor. They also commented, however, that their patients as a group tended to be rigid and over-conscientious. Lang and Marsden (1983) have reported a patient with both spasmodic dysphonia and Gilles de la Tourette syndrome.

In most of the published series the sex incidence is equal, which is in sharp contrast to psychogenic voice disorders such as mutism which have a strong female preponderance. In Aminoff's paper (1978), however, 10 of the 12 cases were female. The peak age of onset for spasmodic dysphonia is in the fourth and fifth decades and the onset is usually insidious, increasing in severity over several months; abrupt onsets, however, have been reported. In typical cases the voice sounds strained, tight and hoarse and is of low pitch and volume. There is a loss of melody (chanson de parler) and it often sounds as if the patient is attempting to vocalise whilst being choked. Phonation may be staccato or tremulous and individual patients may have difficulties with particular groups of consonants. Irregular stoppages and pitch breaks with grunts are common. There may be an explosive harsh accentuation of certain vowels. In the full-blown condition most patients prefer to talk in whispers and in attempting to vocalise often develop tic-like contractions of the neck and face, throat clearing noises, facial flushing and cyanosis with occasional contractions of the abdominal musculature. In the early stages the speech disturbance may be intermittent and triggered only by stressful events. The voice may be stronger shortly after waking and may be improved by alcohol or relaxation. The singing of familiar songs or shouting may be easier than normal speech and laughing, coughing and crying are usually unaffected. Talking normally in sleep has also been observed. Trick movements like pinching the nose may be helpful and associated complaints include nasal congestion, dysphagia, choking sensations and chest tightness.

Indirect laryngoscopy usually reveals no abnormalities, but this procedure only permits the vocal folds to be visualised during sustained falsetto phonation which many patients are able to perform normally. General neurological examination is also usually unremarkable although a proportion of patients have a postural tremor of the limbs and a few have cranial dystonia, torticollis or focal limb dystonia. Aronson (1973) described two types, the commonest being due to excessive adduction of the vocal cords when the speech sounds strained and harsh and occurs often in inspiration with associated facial grimacing. Much less common is excessive abduction of the cords leading to intermittent aphonia, sudden drops in pitch and a certain breathiness to the voice (Merson and Ginsberg, 1979).

The cause is completely unknown. The speech has some similarities to that found in some forms of extrapyramidal disease and the association with essential tremor and focal dystonias and its capricious variability in response to specific triggers also provides circumstantial evidence for dysfunction of the basal ganglia. McCall et al (1971) used videofluoroscopy to demonstrate tonic laryngeal and pharyngeal spasm occurring during speech and in quiet respiration. Subsequent studies also revealed irregular tonic avocal contractions of the extrinsic laryngeal muscles which would be compatible with a dystonic aetiology.

Spontaneous remissions are exceptional and there is a tendency for the disorder to progress steadily over a number of years ultimately leaving the patient aphonic. Medical treatment with anticholinergic drugs, benzodiazepines and dopaminergic medications has been generally ineffective. Symptomatic relief, however, has been reported following the section of one recurrent laryngeal nerve in selected cases. The procedure is carried out only if phonation improves significantly following topical infiltration of local anaesthetic around one recurrent laryngeal nerve. Clarity of tone, improvement in control of pitch and elimination of associated movements occurred in all operated patients, but mild residual hoarseness and breathy voices were complications in a few. Interestingly, structural abnormalities were reported in 30% of the recurrent laryngeal nerve specimens which were removed (Dedo, 1976; Dedo et al, 1977).

WRITER'S DYSTONIA

Synonyms Writer's cramp, scrivener's palsy, writer's angina, graphospasmus, mogigraphia, anapeiratic paralysis, cheirospasmus, graphic dyskinesia, schreibkrampf, crampe des écrivains, fingerkrampf.

Definition A focal dystonia of the hand primarily affecting the act of writing but often spreading to involve other dextrous manual activities.

The brush writers of ancient China are reported to have suffered occasionally from disabling hand cramps and Da Grado may have reported the condition as early as 1470 in the West (Murphy, 1955). Ramazzini in his account of the diseases of scribes and notaries in 1713 also provides an early description of the disorder. Bruck (1831) in Germany and later Sir Charles Bell in England (1833) were both aware of the disorder, attributing it to the advent of the steel nib. Solly (1864) considered it to be due to a granular disintegration of the cervical cord brought about by excessive writing.

Its incidence may indeed have increased in England in Victorian times with the movement for mass education and the increasing number of people employed as copper plate clerks and scriveners. A typical example of the arduous toil inflicted on city copying clerks at that time is the case of the wretched employee of Jarndyce and Jarndyce in Charles Dickens' *Bleak House* who was required to reproduce tens of thousands of Chancery folio pages frequently writing without respite for hours on end. It has been suggested that Woodrow Wilson, the brilliant but controversial President of the United States, may have had the disorder and, at times of stress in his work, he was also noted to have facial tics. At the age of 28 he wrote to his fiancée:

I have been writing all day long and my hand begins to rebel against its hard usage

Subsequently he was forced to use his left hand to write and received a variety of treatments ranging from rest of the hand to electrical therapy (Marmor, 1982). Duchenne de Boulogne (1883) reported cramps in writers and similar affections occurring in other professions, considering them all to be caused by repetitive volitional stimulation and due to a disorder of the spinal cord. Erb (1887) believed writer's cramp to be a disorder of nutrition of the central nervous system which caused damage either at spinal cord, brain-stem or cerebral cortical level. Two physicians at University College Hospital, London, Poore (1878) and Gowers (1877), wrote extensively on the subject of writer's cramp. Poore (1897) who saw at least 300 patients with writing difficulties over a 20-year period drew attention to the problem that many sufferers of writer's cramp had with other manual activities such as winding a watch or holding a salt spoon and postulated that the affliction was due to 'abuse of the proper rhythm of volition, muscles becoming repugnant to the will'. Gowers distinguished simple and dystonic forms and initially believed that faulty penmanship led to a derangement of the centre for writing in the cerebral cortex. In his later writings, however, he stressed the importance of anxiety as a pathogenetic factor. Osler (1892) considered a dysfunction of the brain's writing centre as the likely cause and Jelliffe (1910) also subscribed to the view that disordered cortical control was responsible. Collier and Adie (1922) writing in Price's *Textbook of Medicine* believed writer's cramp to be a disorder of the basal ganglia, probably arising from a dysfunction of the thalamus. Barré (1952) also considered it to be an organic condition related to torticollis and maladie des tics. At around this time behavioural treatments based on the premise that writer's cramp arose out of a faulty learning experience (Janet, 1925) were increasingly in vogue and slowly psychological explanations superseded the original organic hypotheses. By the 1940s most authorities considered writer's cramp to be a psycho-neurosis occurring most commonly in obsessional, anxious or hysterical individuals (Culpin, 1931). Pai (1947), for example, grouped the disorder into tremulous, spastic, genuine or ataxic forms and attempted to correlate each subgroup with a different psychological disorder. In recent years neurologists such as Critchley, Liversedge and Marsden have reasserted the original view that the condition is due to a primary dysfunction of motor control.

EPIDEMIOLOGY

The commonest age of presentation is between 20 and 50 years with a peak incidence in the third and fourth decades of life. This is in contrast to spasmodic torticollis where the peak incidence is in the fourth and fifth decades and Meige syndrome where the onset is usually in the fifth and sixth decades. Writer's dystonia may also be the first symptom of idiopathic generalised torsion dystonia in childhood and cases of isolated writer's dystonia in the elderly have also been reported. Possibly as a result of the predominance of men employed in clerical office duties at the turn of the century, early series reported male to female incidence ratios as high as 10:1. More recent studies have failed to confirm these figures. Sheehy and Marsden (1982), for example, reported the disorder to occur equally in the two sexes. Writer's dystonia has been reported in all races although its relative frequency in different ethnic groups is quite unknown. I have seen a number of recent examples in African postgraduate students preventing them from completing their studies or examinations. Sarkari (1976) reported an estimated incidence of 5.4 per 1000 office workers and Pai (1947) isolated 171 cases of primary writing disturbance among 1880 neuropsychiatric cases admitted to hospital between 1941 and 1946. Gowers believed laywers' clerks to be at particular risk because of their cramped writing style and drew attention to the fact that shorthand writers were in his view never affected. In fact I have seen two patients in whom shorthand writing became quite impossible. Subsequent studies have generally confirmed that those involved in writing for long periods every day, particularly under the pressure of deadlines, seem to be particularly at risk (Liversedge, 1961). Twelve of Sheehy and Marsden's (1982) patients were clerks, five accountants and four were students who were involved in considerable amounts of writing. Left-handers do not appear to have a higher incidence of the disorder and there is no association with stuttering. It seems likely that the advent of dictaphones and typewriters has reduced the overall frequency of this disorder to a considerable degree.

ANIMAL MODELS

There is, of course, no paradigm for writer's dystonia within the animal kingdom but an analogy has recently been drawn with the male canary's song (Lancet, 1982). Every year the male canary learns its love song by improvisation and listening to its rivals. Recently it has been demonstrated that the more elaborate the bird's song the larger become the brain nuclei, perhaps as a result of neurones extending their dendrites over a wider field. In late summer the canary falls silent and shrinkage of these nuclei occurs. Retracting dendrites and the canary losing his song might therefore offer a mechanism for loss of a dextrous skill such as writing. This suggestion would, of course, be more plausible if particularly amorous canaries occasionally lost their song in midsummer as a result of over-use of their vocal cords.

PATHOLOGY

Gowers (1893) reports a single case of writer's dystonia coming to post-mortem in which no histological abnormality was found. No neurochemical studies on the brains of patients dying from writer's cramp have as yet been carried out.

AETIOLOGY

Most recent authors have adopted a dualistic view with respect to writer's cramp believing those cases with isolated writing difficulties to be predominantly psychogenically determined, while at the same time accepting that there may be a subgroup of patients with dystonic hand deformities. The progression of simple writer's cramp to involve in some cases other activities such as shaving, holding a fork and using a screwdriver suggests that no clear distinction can be drawn between these two types. In Marsden's material 21 of 49 segmental dystonics presented with writer's cramp and 13 patients out of 60 with generalised idiopathic torsion dystonia also had writing problems as their first symptom. Spread of the dystonia up the arm may also occur in adult onset writer's cramp and spasmodic torticollis may coexist. In common with the other dystonias an associated tremor is common and often most evident when the patient attempts to write.

Handwriting is a highly individual skill usually acquired in childhood over a number of years as a result of maturation and training. When the child starts to write all attention is directed towards the mere mechanics of writing, but eventually he is able to write almost automatically, attention then shifting to the formulation of content. This ability must involve the establishment of neural circuits of combined sensory and motor function which, when needed, operate smoothly and promptly without the close surveillance of those areas of the cerebral cortex normally involved in conscious voluntary action. It is not clear, however, whether particular subcortical centres are primarily responsible for this sort of learned programme or whether there is a much more fluid adaptable interplay between cortex and subcortex.

Gowers considered that deranged action within the part of the cerebral cortex concerned with writing was the underlying cause of writer's cramp, and faulty penmanship acted as the trigger. Eighty years later Liversedge (1961) would go no further than to implicate a disorganised servo-mechanism due to an electromechanical abnormality of structural neural mechanisms. Marsden believes a breakdown of central motor engrams arising in subcortical centres to be important and points out that one's signature remains instantly recognisable whether it is written on paper, with chalk on a blackboard, whether it is written upside down or with the eyes shut, and even in the absence of gravity or with an anaesthetised hand.

A few familial cases have been described in the literature and there are also reports of other focal dystonias occurring in close relatives. One of Gower's female patients had an affected father and in Sheehy and Marsden's series a similar example is quoted. Vance quoted by Wilson alludes to a man who developed writer's cramp and on seeking rest for his hand visited his brother who lived in a remote part of the country and was amazed to find that he too had become affected with the condition. One of my own patients has both a father and brother who are mildly affected. Dystonic writer's cramp has also been reported in families containing a case of generalised torsion dystonia (Eldridge, 1970).

Peripheral trauma to the affected hand has been implicated occasionally. Gowers, in his textbook, describes a naval officer who sprained his thumb and was then required to do an inordinate amount of writing for a survey report before he had time to recover. Kinnier Wilson also considered that a wrist sprain might sometimes be the provoking factor for the onset of writer's cramp. It is now known that peripheral limb injuries may cause central pain so it is not inconceivable that local injury might lead to dysfunction of subcortical structures. Simmons (1982) has even suggested that ischaemia of the affected muscles may be involved in the pathogenesis of the condition.

Gowers considered that patients with writer's cramp were irritable and sensitive and bore overwork and anxiety badly. Many of his cases were under chronic stress from deadlines and arduous schedules. Others were noted to have domestic difficulties or business worries at the time of onset. Culpin (1931) believed writer's cramp to be a form of conversion hysteria and Cameron (1947) that it arose out of the 'would-be writer's ambivalent attitude towards his endeavour'. Oppenheim stated that it occurred only in neurasthenics and de Ajuriaguerra (1956) that it arose out of emotional conflict in individuals of psychomotor personality type. Bindman and Tibbetts (1977) regarded their 10 patients to have obsessional personalities and Crisp and Moldofsky (1965) described their cases as tense, striving, over-conscientious and controlled with a need to help others and a tendency to become over-dependent in their interpersonal relationships. Despite all these anecdotal observations, as Critchley has put it, 'to look upon the craft palsies as problems in psychopathology has not proved satisfying even to psychiatrists'. Sheehy and Marsden (1982) in a controlled study using the Present State Examination found no higher incidence of psychiatric disturbance in their patients.

CLINICAL DESCRIPTION

The slight tongue protrusion of many adults or the curling of a child's leg round his chair at school testifies to the delicate motor skills involved in writing. When writer's dystonia appears, a steady regression occurs back along the path upon which the skill was initially learned and there is an increasing application of inappropriate muscles with the adoption of abnormal postures. The onset is usually gradual with early complaints of cramping, drawing or tightness after prolonged periods of writing. There may also be some mild deterioration in the legibility of the script and occasional unprovoked involuntary jerks or tremors of the writing hand. Rarely the disorder begins acutely particularly if the individual is under time pressure to complete large amounts of paper work. After writing for some time he begins to notice that his pen is not moving quite as intended and that the down strokes may be becoming too thick. A painful fatigue develops in the muscles of the hand and a dull ache over the metacarpal bones. Tenderness may in fact be present in front of the wrist, below the elbow and even as high as the shoulder muscles. The alacrity of writing is affected and this is accentuated if the patient is under surveillance. Sometimes the fingers repeatedly slip off the pen and on other occasions the writing implement may be held too tightly and driven through the paper. The grip often steadily tightens so that to the affected individual it feels as if a weight is attached to his hand. Frequently the thumb and first finger flex at the proximal metacarpophalangeal joint and there may be hyperextension of the distal interphalangeal joints (Fig. 11.4). The pen is usually held tightly with a semiflexed posture of the index finger. Less commonly the fingers are extended or the

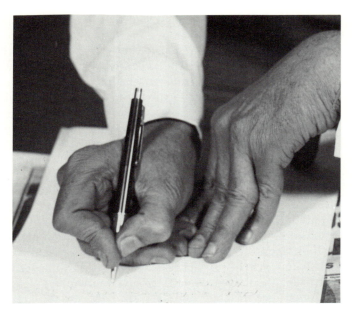

Figure 11.4. Writer's cramp.

middle and right finger are held in spasm. The wrist may be flexed, extended or supinated and finally the whole arm may contort. As the disorder progresses many patients find it impossible to even pick up the pen or start to write and for others painful fatigue appears after only a few letters have been written. Many patients attempt to counteract the spasms by holding the pen between the extended middle and index fingers, supporting the writing hand with the other hand or even the top of the pen with their chins. Some find a more bulbous writing instrument beneficial and felt-tipped pens and pencils are easier to use than a fountain pen. In some individuals the major incapacity appears to be a tremor on writing and a few patients have striking intermittent clonic jerks of the hand. Although there are no characteristic features enabling the script of a patient with writer's dystonia to be confidently recognised, when compared with the patient's former writing it tends to be smaller, more cramped and jerky and less legible and it may also appear somewhat tremulous (Fig. 11.5). Some patients find that a slight change of body position may improve their capacity to write, standing for example may be beneficial and free writing movements in mid-air are often unaffected so that, for example, writing on a blackboard where the hand does not touch the writing surface may be carried out normally. Slight loss of arm swing and increase in tone in the affected limb is quite common and occasionally mild dystonic features are detected in other parts of the body.

Gowers considered there to be two main components involved in writing: the way in which the pen is held and the way in which the movements are accomplished, the latter being the most important. He considered writer's

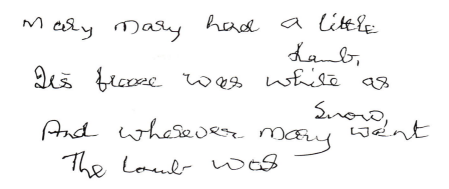

Figure 11.5. *Script of a patient with writer's cramp.*

cramp to occur particularly in those who write with the little finger at a fixed point of support, the pen being moved up and down by the thumb and first two fingers and lateral movements being carried out by slight supination. Using this style, only a few letters can be written without movement of the little finger. The other common method of writing which also carried risks was that in which the wrist is used as a fixed point with vertical strokes being made by flexion and extension of the fingers and thumb and lateral movements by ulnar abduction of the wrist. Gowers advocated learning to write from the middle of the forearm or upper arm, the forearm, wrist and fingers resting on the table. In this way the pen is held lightly and can be moved freely across the page without pen and paper breaking contact.

DIFFERENTIAL DIAGNOSIS

Tenosynovitis, carpal tunnel syndrome, ulnar nerve lesions, cervical radiculopathy and brachial plexus palsies may all cause pain on writing and must clearly be distinguished from writer's cramp. Parkinson's disease occasionally presents with pain and spasm on writing. Focal dystonia of the hand may follow a hemiparesis due to a stroke or occasionally occur as a direct result of thrombosis of a lenticulostriate artery causing striatal and capsular damage. Midbrain trauma and tumours of the basal ganglia are other uncommon causes. Tardive dystonia due to chronic neuroleptic administration may also produce a focal dystonia of the hand but the disability always involves all dextrous activities and is not restricted to writing.

COURSE

Most commonly writer's dystonia slowly increases in severity over several weeks and then tends to remain static and disabling as long as the patient continues his attempts to write. In many cases the disorder progresses to involve other manual activities. Occasionally it is intermittent at the onset of the illness, and spontaneous partial remissions have been reported especially after a period of complete rest from writing. Although fluctuations in severity are characteristic, the disorder is usually chronic: arrest of progression may occur at any stage. Four of Sheehy and Marsden's patients developed a similar problem in the contralateral limb on learning to write with the other hand and Gowers reported a 50% chance of the other hand becoming affected.

TREATMENT

Early attempts to treat writer's dystonia by tenotomy or immobilisation were soon abandoned. Charcot advised complete rest of the hand whereas Gowers stressed prevention by the teaching of improved writing styles in the classroom. Both Poore and Gowers also considered early abstinence from writing to be important and recommended patients to learn to write with their left hand or use a typewriter. Tonics containing strychnine, Indian hemp, subcutaneous morphine, inunctions of belladonna, and glycerine and aconite ointments were also recommended. Gowers was unimpressed by electrical treatments such as faradism but recommended flexion- extension movements of the fingers. Galvanic stimulation, however, had many influential adherents, the anode being placed over the nape of the neck and a cathode attached to the affected muscles. Fifteen-minute treatment sessions three times a week were recommended. At the turn of the century a peculiar combination of massage and exercise advocated by Wolff, a teacher of penmanship in Frankfurt, came to have an unwarranted reputation for success and some of the more affluent European sufferers of the time made pilgrimages to his consulting rooms for treatment. Mechanical devices designed to make an alternative set of muscles work were also popular in the early part of this century. These ranged from simple, sensible ploys such as a large soft, cork pen holder and an easy nib to elaborate contraptions such as the Nussbaum bracelet which consisted of a thin oval band of hard rubber slipped over the fingers and thumb with the pen held on the dorsum of the hand by a clamp attached to the rubber band.

PSYCHOTHERAPY

Hypno-analysis, insulin coma therapy, psychodrama and relaxation techniques have all been reported to lead to improvement in individual cases, but no satisfactory controlled studies have been carried out. Psycho-analysis has also been said to be useful (Brun, 1964). In a recent report postural correction under hypnosis led to marked improvement in two patients. On the basis of this the authors suggest that writer's dystonia may be a reversible learned response to posture-induced neuromuscular dysfunction and fatigue (Besson and Walker, 1983). Crisp and Moldofsky (1965) used relaxation techniques together with formal psychotherapy and reported beneficial results in six of seven cases. Bindman and Tibbetts (1977), however, found this approach unhelpful in their 10 patients.

BEHAVIOURAL THERAPY

Janet (1925) believed that writer's dystonia occurred as a bad habit arising out of a faulty learning process and used the re-educational techniques devised by Kouindjy with apparent success. These included formal exercises to strengthen hand extensors, the patient then being taught to write with his hand supinated to encourage extensor muscular activity and discourage excessive digit flexion. A series of devices were used to develop accurate finger movements including keyboards, pigeon holes and triangular prisms. De Ajuriaguerra (1956) treated 19 patients with relaxation techniques, 10 showing improvement for up to six years. Liversedge (1961) used an avoidance conditioning paradigm consisting of a pen constructed to administer a mild electric shock if the finger pressure became excessive. This was used in conjunction with a specially designed metal board with holes, trenches and tapes of different sizes, the patient being asked to trace round these obstacles with the pen. If the stylo left the side of the obstacle a shock was applied. Once this tremor board had been mastered graded self-administered writing exercises were used. Thirty-eight patients were treated in this manner, 28 of whom were improved appreciably three to six weeks after the treatment period had finished. Following a longer follow-up period of four months to four years, most maintained some improvement but five subsequently relapsed. An associated tremor and a long history were poor prognostic signs. Beech (1960) advised negative practice therapy, the patient exercising with a dynamometer to reduce the overactive grip. Bindman and Tibbetts (1977) have also reported some success with electromyographic biofeedback techniques used over four or five sessions. Cottraux et al (1983) used a combination of relaxation techniques, systemic desensitisation and assertive training through role playing, combined with EMG biofeedback technique with some benefit in some patients. They concluded that writer's dystonia was a response to stress related to working conditions.

DRUG TREATMENT

Over 100 years ago Vance recommended 1/60th grain of atropine three times a week and since that time there have been repeated reports that medication with central anticholinergic properties might be beneficial. Liversedge (1961) reported improvement in four of his cases with benzhexol and six of Sheehy and Marsden's (1982) patients were helped by benzhexol in doses of 6–24 mg/d. Acute pharmacological challenges, however, with 0.6 mg of atropine, 2 mg of benztropine or 10 mg of chlorpheniramine led to no improvement in five patients (Lang et al, 1983).

SURGICAL TREATMENT

Rouquier (1951) performed a bilateral prefrontal lobectomy in a patient with anxiety, writer's cramp and Parkinsonian features with apparent benefit. Siegfried et al (1969) reported a successful result in a 60-year-old man with a severe tremulous writer's cramp following stereotactic surgery to the ventro-lateral nucleus of the thalamus, writing being normal after three months' follow-up. There can, however, be no indication for the general application of these procedures.

OCCUPATIONAL DYSTONIAS

Synonyms Occupational cramps, craft palsies, occupational palsies, occupational neuroses.

The occupational dystonias are a group of conditions characterised by the break-down of a particular learned motor skill, essential for the normal execution of the affected individual's trade. Those people in occupations in which repetitive, intricate, finely co-ordinated hand and finger movements are demanded are particularly at risk but dystonias of the feet in ballerinas and of the lips in wind brass players have been described. In the occupational dystonias there is a dilapidation of a single skilled act which has often been acquired by tedious practice and is capable of being carried out virtually automatically with great speed and economy, often for long periods without fatigue. Once dysfunction has set in, however, attempts to overcome the incapacity by concentration or will power or by downgrading the motor skill to a more voluntary action are ineffective. Disorganisation of the range and rate of prime movers, synergists and antagonists is characteristic and local pain and spasm often occurs, a point distinguishing this group of disorders from the dyspraxias which are painless and generally involve unskilled movements. In many instances a tremor compounds the dystonic spasm.

In fact many of the large number of occupational cramps described in the literature at the turn of this century occurred as a result of peripheral nerve injuries, radiculopathies, spinal cord claudication and musculoskeletal injuries such as tenosynovitis. Occasionally idiopathic Parkinson's disease also presents as an occupational cramp. Nevertheless, spontaneously occurring dystonias undoubtedly occur and a list of the most convincing are given in Table 11.2

Parliament, at the turn of the century, recognised that certain trades were particularly liable to induce these disorders and legislation requiring employers to pay compensation to the victims was passed. Personal idiosyncrasies, however, are undoubtedly of prime importance in their causation with fatigue from chronic ill-health or stress playing an additional background role. It has

Table 11.2. LIST OF PROFESSIONS IN WHICH OCCUPATIONAL DYSTONIAS OCCUR

Writers	Barbers
Telegraphists	Watch-makers
Typists	Artificial flower-makers
Professional musicians	Ballerinas
Professional sportsmen	Sewing-machine workers
Cotton-twisters	Enamellers
Tailors	Money-counters
Sailmakers	Locksmiths
Seamstresses	Knitters
Cobblers	Tinsmiths
Cigar-rollers	Diamond cutters
Gold-beaters	Letter sorters
Knife-grinders	Engravers
Saddlers	Cabinet-makers

also been suggested that afflicted individuals are as a group more neurotic than their workmates. One interesting point appears to be the fact that loss of one learned motor skill may ultimately lead to the disruption of other related skills suggesting that the primary learning mechanism for motor proficiency may become damaged in some ill-understood way. Collier and Adie (1922) described a telegraphist who developed dystonia and could not continue his job whereupon he was relegated to counter duties, only to be struck down with writer's cramp. He was then demoted further to sealing envelopes only to develop cramp again so that he finally finished his post office career as a messenger. Critchley (1977) also reports a lady of 55 with pianist's palsy whose affliction spread to involve her ability to play both the organ and the oboe.

Technological advances, increasing automation and shorter working hours have helped to eradicate many occupational dystonias, but typists and telegraphists remain at risk and classical musicians and some groups of professional sportsmen may also be affected.

DYSTONIAS IN MUSICIANS

Most of the disorders which devastate a professional musician's career are due either to local orthopaedic problems or psychogenically-determined phobias of one sort or another. Essential tremor is a further incapacitating and not uncommon symptom which often prematurely curtails a violinist's career. Dystonias do occur, however, particularly in concert pianists and once established are virtually untreatable in view of the virtuosity required to play this instrument at the highest level. James Paget once heard Janotha play a presto by Mendelssohn and recorded that she played 5595 notes in four minutes three seconds, each one involving two movements of one finger and 72 movements per second for the piece. Hochberg et al (1983) interviewed 100 musicians with hand difficulties. Virtually all were professional musicians who spent several hours every day practising and more than three-quarters were pianists, the rest included violinists, guitarists, cellists and harpists. Most of the pianists began to experience hand difficulties in mid-career at an average age of 31 years and complained of pain, tightening or weakness, most commonly starting in the fourth or fifth fingers. Loss of control, diminished facility and reduced endurance or speed were also mentioned. In fact the commonest cause was found to be tendinitis or tenosynovitis of the finger extensors which occurred in approximately half of the musicians. 15% of hand difficulties were caused by entrapment neuropathies and only one-quarter were considered to be due to idiopathic loss of motor control. 50% of the 49 patients examined had weakness and wasting, 40% had an abnormal posture, about 20% had tendon contractures and 8% had sensory loss.

Pianist's dystonia is probably somewhat commoner in females than males and may affect either or both hands. It usually comprises a tonic spasm of the finger extensors which prevents rapid finger movements and at times a single finger may remain extended for a few seconds instead of striking the correct note appropriately. It is usual for two or three fingers to become affected simultaneously and aching pain in the forearm extensors often radiating up the arm to the shoulder is a frequent accompaniment. There is a tendency for all the fingers to run together in staccato passages; some pianists complain of the left forefinger constantly touching the keyboard.

Technical deterioration seems to set in far earlier with professional violinists than pianists and this may be related to the fact that the whole act of violin playing is by its very nature excessively tiring as a result of the asymmetrical hand techniques and the twisted posture. The left hand is more often affected than the right leading to exaggerated finger pressure, torsion of the upper arm against the chest wall, rolling of the arm to the left or right or flatness of finger application. If the right hand is affected this is even more troublesome as the defect cannot be concealed. Prolongation of the bow movements may disrupt the whole timing of the orchestra leading to the so-called violinist's cancer. In fact spasm of the extensor muscles may actually ultimately draw the bow right off the strings and in severe cases the musician may be unable even to pick up his instrument.

Much less commonly dystonias have been reported in cellists, drummers, harpists, zither players and flautists, and there is a recent report of horn player's palsy being improved with bromocriptine (James and Cook, 1983).

DYSTONIA IN PROFESSIONAL SPORTSMEN

Such are the physical rigors of modern professional sport at the highest level and so prodigious the financial rewards that it is scarcely surprising that those sportsmen involved in games which demand delicate and sustained manual skills occasionally develop dystonias. The game of golf demands that a player drives a hard $1\frac{1}{2}$ inch ball 200 yards or so straight up the course with the aid of an elegantly-shaped club. The golfer must then make the green with further shots and is then required to hole out putting the ball into a $4\frac{1}{4}$ inch hole submerged in the ground. It is this last aspect of the game in which the master golfer excels and which may win or lose him vast sums of money depending on his ability to gauge the tilt or borrow of the green. Most illustrious professionals can recall at least one disastrous miss, frequently in a pressurised situation, which occured as a result of an edgy jerky shot, but there are a few whose careers are threatened or even ruined by what is known in the game as the 'yips'. Foster (1977) described the rise and fall of Ben Hogan who, after being generally acknowledged as the greatest golfer of his generation, in 1953 suddenly began to freeze at short puts finding he was unable to take the putter away from the ball because of spasm in the forearm and hands. The elegant stylist Sam Snead also became a victim of these jerks. In order to continue in the game he had to learn to put facing the hole with the ball between his legs. When this revolutionary technique was declared illegal he perfected a side-winding technique in which he would crouch, feet together, with the club held at the top with a reverse left-hand grip and the right hand, index finger extended, pushed down the grip of the putter, 18 inches or so separating the hands. The ball was then hit outside the line of his right foot with a fluent swing.

I have also observed a case of a professional snooker player who developed loss of cue skill only when using the rest or spider so that he was quite unable to make contact with the ball at all when using these particular pieces of equipment. Shots without the rest were completed as usual with consummate skill. Olympic marksmen and fencers are also occasionally afflicted with dystonia. Another case I have seen involved a 36-year-old keen amateur darts player who developed pain and spasm when throwing, leading to embarrassing excursions in his shots and rarely to an incapacity to let go of the dart at all. Before the onset of his disabilities this man would spend about four hours a night practising at his club or in the pub and would also practise at home on Saturdays. Initially he noted difficulty in releasing the darts in tournaments, following which he began to use jerky forearm movements and to stand on his tip-toes to overcome the handicap but his symptoms steadily got worse. Curiously after three months he had a brief remission for a week but the symptoms then recurred and have remained ever since. At the time of examination he found it quite impossible to release the dart from his right hand and went through a curious ritual of repetitive flexion and extension movements of the arm and abduction of the shoulder. If he threw the dart underarm there was no problem and he had a normal throwing action on the left. If the dartboard was put on the floor then he could accurately throw the dart with his right hand. He was able to play snooker, throw a ball and carry out intricate hand movements in his job as a welder without difficulty. There had been some intermittent pain around the right shoulder since the onset of the disorder and as a result of his difficulties he had been forced to give up playing team darts altogether. He did not suffer from writer's cramp and there was no family history of focal dystonia or tics and nothing else of relevance in the past medical history, in particular no history of psychiatric illness. On general examination there were no abnormalities and the neurological examination, apart from some slight difficulty with fine finger movements and a tendency for his head to twist to the left, was quite normal. He was able to pick up his darts quite normally and adopted a normal throwing position but he then became stuck despite trying to rock himself into releasing the dart. He had tried drinking alcohol, getting in a rage and all manner of other tricks to no avail. Holding a pencil as if it were a dart was equally difficult.

TELEGRAPHIST'S DYSTONIA

In 1844, as a result of the discovery of electromagnetic induction, Morse sent a telegraph by wire from Baltimore to Washington and thereby started a revolution in long-distance communication. Within a few years the Morse machine was in wide use throughout the post offices of the world and literally thousands of people were employed in telecommunication. The Morse machine is a clumsy brass instrument which requires the movement of a key by the operator's hand and wrist extensors against a spring resistance of 2–4 oz. Up to 515 muscular contractions may occur per minute in order to produce the up and down movements required for rapid transmission of messages. It is not surprising, therefore, that dystonia affected a considerable percentage of operators at some stage in their careers. Particular difficulty would occur with letters involving a series of dots especially at the end of a word, often because of difficulty in getting the key up again quickly enough. Operators would become acutely aware of problems with particular types of word sequences and on occasions developed secondary phobic reactions. The disorder was at one time so common that Thompson and Sinclair (1912) in their governmental report were able to identify 230 cases, 42 of whom developed the disorder in their first five years of service. Collier and Adie (1929) reported that in 1911 4% of operators in the Post Office were affected and that many of these had additional writer's cramp and difficulty with dextrous acts such as shaving. Most, however, appeared able to supervene their difficulties and continued to work until retirement, although tell-tale signs were always evident when watching these affected individuals at work. Smith et al (1927) considered 31 of their 41 subjects with the disorder to be psycho-neurotic and emphasised the importance of chronic stress in its pathogenesis. A recent study in Australia by Ferguson (1971) confirmed a union claim that 14% of 516 telegraphists with seven or more years' service had experienced dystonia and a further 5% myalgic pains in the hand and wrist. 74% had had specific difficulties with Morse, 65% with the new keyboard instruments and 50% with writing. 13% had developed the affliction in the first year of work and a third of the men had endured symptoms for 10 years. When using Morse instruments the thumb, index and middle fingers were most commonly involved whereas the ring and little finger tended to be affected more in keyboard operators. The affected individuals were more likely to be ambidextrous and work overload was considered a potent trigger. About three-quarters of the sufferers were considered to be psycho-neurotic, 25% had stammers, 5% had had tics, 14% were nail biters and 8% had obsessional neuroses. This study clearly shows that the disappearance of Morse instruments has not entirely eradicated this disturbance in telegraphists.

TYPIST'S DYSTONIA

Loss of speed, pain in the fingers and an involuntary flexing or extending of the little or ring fingers are characteristic premonitory signs of typist's cramp. The disorder may begin in one hand and spread to the other or affect both simultaneously and may increase in severity to such an extent that it is impossible to type at all. Macé de Lepinay (1909) described a patient with both writer's and typist's cramp. Meige reported a patient with writer's cramp in the right hand, typist's cramp in the left and a bilateral pianist's cramp. Sheehy and Marsden (1982) reported four patients with typist's cramp; in one the disorder spread over several months to involve difficulty in picking up objects such as a pencil because of stiffness of the fingers and wrist.

12

The Drug-induced Dyskinesias

The unexpected occurrence of abnormal involuntary movements in patients receiving antipsychotic drugs provided the initial stimulus for the current wave of interest in the neuropharmacology of extrapyramidal diseases. The appearance of dyskinesias in Parkinsonian patients on long term L-dopa therapy and the development of stereotypies, chorea and tics in chronic amphetamine addicts were equally tantalising and use of these drugs as investigational tools has helped to formulate many of our current notions on the pathophysiology of abnormal movement disorders. Although tics are one of the least common of the iatrogenic dyskinesias, the mere fact that they occur at all and may be seen in association with chorea and athetosis implies that they could be triggered by a central biochemical disturbance.

Neuroleptics, L-dopa and amphetamines have quite different pharmacological actions, but all three classes of drug share the ability to influence dopamine metabolism profoundly. The distinctive regional distribution of dopamine in the brain led Blaschko in 1957 (Blaschko, 1957) to suggest that it might have an important function of its own and not simply be an intermediate by-product in the biosynthesis of noradrenaline. It occurs in very high concentrations in the substantia nigra (80% of total brain dopamine) and elegant histochemical methods have now characterised four well-defined dopamine-containing neuronal pathways. Confirmation of a substance as a neurotransmitter requires it to possess post-synaptic actions identical to those of the transmitter normally released at the synapse and it must also be possible to collect the substance from the synaptic cleft after firing of the pre-synaptic neurone. The absence of clear-cut synapses and the relative inaccessibility of the central nervous system has presented major obstacles to the absolute confirmation of dopamine as a neurotransmitter. Furthermore, it has proved extremely difficult to detect the release of a chemical substance in the brain without destroying the neurone's functional and structural integrity. Nevertheless, compelling evidence has accrued to suggest that dopamine is a chemical messenger in the central nervous system and it is now thought that the nigrostriatal dopaminergic bundle is involved in the integration of normal motor function. The tubero-infundibular hypothalamic tract regulates prolactin and possibly gonadotrophin release and the mesolimbic and mesocortical dopamine pathways may be concerned with mood, motivation and attention.

Dopamine receptors occur on pre-synaptic cell bodies and terminals as well as the post-synaptic membrane. These autoreceptors control transmitter synthesis and release and may also occur on small interneurones in the substantia nigra where they respond to dopamine from neighbouring dendrites. Anatomical, pharmacological and physiological evidence is now available to support the existence of at least two and probably more discrete, dopaminergic receptor systems. One set of receptors are adenyl-cyclase linked (D1) whereas another group, the D2 receptors, are not. It is probable that greater understanding of the specific function of these different receptors, their neuronal connections and interaction with other neurotransmitters, will help to explain many of the paradoxical drug-induced phenomena now to be described. The chapter has been sub-divided as follows:

1. Neuroleptic-induced dyskinesias
   (a) Acute dyskinesias
   (b) Akathisia
   (c) Tardive dyskinesias.
2. Psychomotor stimulant-induced dyskinesias
   (a) Pundning
   (b) Chorea
   (c) Tics.
3. L-dopa-induced dyskinesias
   (a) Chorea-athetosis
   (b) Dystonia
   (c) Myoclonus
   (d) Tics.

1. NEUROLEPTIC-INDUCED DYSKINESIAS

GENERAL INTRODUCTION

The healing powers of the snake-root plant (Rauwolfia serpentina) have long been acknowledged in the Indian sub-continent where it has been used for centuries by the lower castes of the northern plains and foothills as a sedative. It is mentioned in Sanskrit incunabula and the early Ayurvedic commentaries, and its Bengali name *Chandra*, meaning moon, suggests a link with lunacy. The late Mohandas Gandhi took Rauwolfia infusions for years to control his hypertension and it seems possible that his serene and bland disposition in later life may have owed something to the plant's ataractic properties.

Phenothiazines were synthesised in Europe in the late 19th century as part of the development of aniline dyes and Ehrlich in one of his many prophetic statements suggested that some of these, including methylene blue, might be useful in treating mental illness. These early pointers were unfortunately ignored and it was not until chlorpromazine was synthesised by Charpentier in

1949 and Woodward extracted and purified the alkaloid reserpine from Rauwolfia that psychopharmacological properties of these compounds really began to be appreciated in the West. In spite of their widely different chemical structures, reserpine and chlorpromazine possess similar pharmacological characteristics. Their injection into laboratory animals induces a curious, rigid immobility called catalepsy which closely resembles the flexibilitas cerea seen occasionally in catatonic schizophrenia. In man a state of affective indifference appears with loss of drive and a reduction of aggression and impulsiveness. Mild sedation is usual but normal subjects always respond appropriately to questions and intelligence; memory and conceptual reasoning are not significantly impaired.

Early clinical studies by Kline using Rauwolfia extracts and later reserpine showed both these preparations to possess useful but modest antipsychotic properties. Unfortunately a large number of unwanted effects including sialorrhoea, diarrhoea, postural hypotension and sedation frequently spoiled the therapeutic response. The results were much more encouraging with the phenothiazine chlorpromazine. After early reports of benefit to paranoia by Sigwald, and to mania by Colonel Paraire and other psychiatrists at the military hospital Val de Grace, Delay and Deniker published their research which had led them in 1952 to the conclusion that chlorpromazine possessed inherent antipsychotic properties which were quite separate from its anxiolytic qualities. By the mid 1950s chlorpromazine was commercially available and its value in the management of psychotic conditions began to be generally appreciated. Many other structurally related phenothiazines and thioxanthenes were soon marketed and by 1958 Janssen had developed the first butyrophenone (phenylbutylpiperidine), haloperidol. In the last few years other classes of compounds including dibenzodiazepines, benzamides and diphenylbutylpiperidines, all with similar pharmacological profiles and antipsychotic effects, have been developed.

To emphasise their similarities and to distinguish them from general anaesthetics, hypnotics and opiates, Delay and Deniker introduced the term neuroleptic. In Europe this is generally used synonymously with anti-psychotic although there has been a recent tendency to restrict it more to the unwanted neurological effects.

The impact of neuroleptics on psychiatric practice has been considerable. Hundreds of millions of patients have taken these drugs in the short time since their introduction, and partly as a result of their beneficial effects the number of long-stay psychiatric in-patients has begun to fall. Acute psychotic relapses can now often be managed in the community with the help of antipsychotic drugs and some chronic schizophrenics, after years in asylums, have returned home to live happy and rewarding lives. Neuroleptics are also useful in the symptomatic control of toxic confusional states and in the containment of acutely disturbed patients. They are also widely dispensed as antiemetics, for the treatment of vertigo and intractable hiccoughs and for mania and severe refractory anxiety neuroses.

As with most momentous therapeutic advances, initial euphoria was almost immediately tempered by concern about the frequent occurrence of a number of different distressing neurological side-effects. Abnormal involuntary movements were the most alarming, most occurring in the first few weeks of treatment. These were reversible on stopping the offending drug and improved with anticholinergic medication (Table 12.1). However, after chronic therapy a more disturbing tardive dyskinetic syndrome appeared in some patients which sometimes persisted for many years after drug withdrawal. These extrapyramidal side-effects, undesirable as they were in the clinical context, provided a fruitful stimulus to basic research in biological psychiatry.

Already by the late 1950s it was known that reserpine depleted brain monoamines and while initial attention was focused on 5-hydroxytryptamine and noradrenaline it was not long before Carlsson showed dopamine deficiency to be primarily responsible for the cataleptic state (Carlsson et al, 1957). This together with the revelation that reserpine could cause Parkinsonism in man paved the way for the ultimate confirmation of idiopathic Parkinson's disease as a dopamine deficiency state. Subsequent work has confirmed that both reserpine and tetrabenazene act by blocking monoamine storage mechanisms in pre-synaptic terminals.

In contrast, blockade of dopamine receptors is almost certainly responsible for the neuroleptic effects of the butyrophenones and phenothiazines. Although many of these drugs also possess alpha-adrenergic receptor blocking actions these are more likely to mediate their sedative properties.

One of the most hotly debated issues in the first 10 years after the introduction of neuroleptics was the relationship between their antipsychotic properties and the extrapyramidal side-effects. Many authorities considered mild extrapyramidal symptoms such as subtle bradykinesia to be an essential prerequisite for therapeutic effects whilst recognising that severe Parkinsonism need not be present and could be possibly detrimental (Haase and Janssen, 1965). It is now evident that these two effects are quite independent and can be clearly separated from one another.

Histochemical methods have distinguished several discrete dopamine pathways in the brains of animals. The nigrostriatal bundle originates in the zona compacta of the substantia nigra and ascends in the dorsal hypothalamic area through the internal capsule to terminate mainly in the putamen and caudate nucleus. Another group of dopaminergic neurones known as the mesolimbic tract originates in the midbrain dorsal to the interpeduncular nucleus and terminates in the nucleus accumbens, olfactory tubercle and amygdaloid nuclei. Mesocortical pathways also exist terminating in the medial frontal and cingulate areas. There is an important tubero-infundibular system which arises from the arcuate and periventricular nuclei of the hypothalamus and ends in the median eminence close to the hypophyseal-portal system and is known to control prolactin release. Scattered dopaminergic neurones are also found in the retina, globus pallidus and area postrema of the medulla oblongata (the vomiting centre).

Several observations suggest that the antipsychotic and extrapyramidal actions of neuroleptics are mediated through different structures. For instance,

Table 12.1. NEUROLEPTIC-INDUCED EXTRAPYRAMIDAL SIDE-EFFECTS

Side-effects	Symptoms	Usual time of onset	Approximate incidence in routine practice	Age predisposition
Early reversible				
Acute dyskinesia	Painful dystonia, choreo-athetosis, Pisa syndrome	1–4 d	3–10%	Children and young adults
Akathisia	Dysphoria and motor restlessness	10–90 d	10–20%	None
Parkinson's syndrome	Rigidity, bradykinesia Rest tremor	14–90 d	10–20%	Middle-aged and elderly
Rabbit syndrome	Perioral nibbling movements 5 cycles/s	14–90 d	3–5%	Middle-aged and elderly
Late Potentially irreversible				
Tardive dyskinesia	Bucco-linguo masticatory dyskinesias Limb choreo-athetosis, dystonia	$\frac{1}{2}$–5 y	10–20%	Elderly

anticholinergic agents efficiently abolish acute dyskinesias and Parkinsonism while the antipsychotic effects are left more or less unaffected. There are also a few novel antipsychotic drugs such as clozapine which do not appear to induce extrapyramidal side-effects at all. Finally sustained antipsychotic effects occur in many patients without any overt evidence of extrapyramidal disability.

The antipsychotic drugs can be divided into classes that differ fundamentally in their actions at a molecular level as well as in their structures. All, however, reduce the activity of dopamine receptors and it seems safe to conclude that inhibition of dopaminergic function is central to their action. The exact brain site through which their therapeutic effects occur is not known but what evidence there is points to the mesolimbic or possibly mesocortical dopaminergic pathways. The primary disturbance in schizophrenia, however, may not lie within the dopaminergic synapse at all but in some other system in intimate relationship with it.

With respect to the neuroleptic-induced dyskinesias, the dopaminergic-cholinergic balance hypothesis is most popular. This states that the balance between the inhibitory dopaminergic and excitatory cholinergic neuronal activity in the corpus striatum is disturbed and the early reversible dyskinesias are due to a shift towards cholinergic excess whereas tardive dyskinesia is due to dopaminergic predominance. This simplistic view, however, will almost certainly prove to be incomplete.

Only the hyperkinetic abnormal movements (acute dyskinesias, akathisia and tardive dyskinesia) are covered in this section (see Table 12.1). Neuroleptic-induced Parkinsonism, the neuroleptic malignant syndrome and the related rabbit syndrome (Jus et al, 1972; Villeneuve, 1972) are excluded.

ACUTE DYSKINESIAS

Synonyms Hyperkinetic transitory syndrome, Excitomotor crisis, acute dystonic reaction, early dyskinesias, initial hyperkinesias.

Definition Reversible, predominantly dystonic movements which occur within the first few days of starting neuroleptic treatment or following an increase in dosage and are rapidly improved by the parenteral administration of anticholinergic drugs.

EPIDEMIOLOGY

Data is still scanty on the incidence of acute dyskinesias and recent studies are to some extent in conflict with the earlier literature. Ayd (1961) reported an overall incidence of 2.3% in 3775 patients (3.1% of 1833 males and 1.5% of 1942 females) treated with phenothiazines, almost half of whom had received chlorpromazine. In another comprehensive survey, fluphenazine and trifluoperazine provoked acute dyskinesias in 3% of patients, other phenothiazines were less hazardous (1–1.5%) and reserpine (0.5%) least of all (Goldman, 1961). Indeed there is some debate as to whether reserpine can induce acute dyskinesias at all despite one or two other case reports (Priori and Schettini, 1958; Wolf, 1973).

The Boston Collaborative Drug Surveillance Programme followed 1152 patients receiving neuroleptics and recorded acute dyskinesias in 116 (10.1%). Torticollis occurred in 35, a swollen dystonic tongue in 20, trismus in 17, oculogyric crises in 7, opisthotonus in 4 and a variety of other dystonic syndromes developed in the rest. The disparity between this high figure and those previously reported has been explained by the much greater incidence of acute dystonic reactions with haloperidol (16% of 200 patients) and 11.7% of 137 patients treated with the depôt phenothiazine fluphenazine. In fact the figure of 3.5% in the 679 patients who took chlorpromazine is quite similar to that previously reported by both Ayd and Goldman (Swett, 1975). Freyhan (1959) noted acute dyskinesias in 19.2% of 104 in-patients treated with 3–30 mg/d of trifluoperazine. Garver et al (1976a,b) observed acute dyskinesias in 8 of 13 schizophrenics given a single 40 mg oral dose of the piperazine phenothiazine butaperazine. Abuse of trifluorperazine by eight youths in the mistaken belief that they were taking amphetamines led to dystonia in seven within 24 hours after 60 mg oral doses. Autosuggestion may have played some role in the high incidence in this report (Fitzgerald and Fitzgerald, 1969). Finally Binder and Levy (1981) observed dyskinesias within the first 14 days of haloperidol therapy (5–70 mg/d) in 10 of 20 orientals, nine of 20 American blacks, and 11 of 40 whites of North European stock.

Acute dystonia is much commoner in young adults and children (Gupta and Lovejoy, 1967) and some papers have reported a male preponderance (Ayd, 1961). However, above the age of 50 the sex incidence is approximately equal (Swett, 1975).

Very few predisposing factors to acute dyskinesia have as yet been found. There is a single account of a number of patients with untreated hypoparathyroidism experiencing dystonia a few hours after small doses of prochlorperazine (Schaaf and Payne, 1966), increased nervous excitability due to hypocalcaemia or associated basal ganglia calcification being possible aetiological factors. Dehydration and impaired hepatic function may also increase susceptibility, probably as a consequence of altered drug metabolism (Mowat, 1973). It has also been claimed that there is a high incidence of acute neuroleptic-induced dystonia in the relatives of patients with idiopathic torsion dystonia (Eldridge, 1970) and that patients who are taste-sensitive to quinine develop a reaction more frequently than those who are not (Knopp et al, 1966). Finally a few families have been reported who appear especially vulnerable (Ayd, 1960).

ANIMAL MODELS

Research into the underlying pathophysiology of acute dyskinesias was hampered for some time by the apparent absence of comparable phenomena in neuroleptic-treated laboratory animals. However, reversible dyskinesias have now been induced in a number of different non-human primates (Paulson, 1972b; Liebman and Neale, 1980) although the repeated administration of neuroleptic drugs has often been necessary. Weiss et al (1977), using Cebus monkeys, were obliged to give haloperidol 0.5–1.0 mg/kg orally five days a week for several months before dyskinesias emerged but these then recurred consistently one to six hours after a daily injection of 0.5–0.1 mg/kg of haloperidol. Further challenges, even with very small doses, then continued to induce dyskinesias one year after drug withdrawal suggesting persistent sensitisation.

Meldrum et al (1977) gave haloperidol (0.6–1.2 mg/kg i.m.) to a colony of 25 adolescent Senegalese baboons (Papio papio) and observed jaw opening, tongue protrusion, twisting of the neck and trunk, grimacing and licking in two susceptible animals within 5–10 minutes of administration. Several other antipsychotic drugs including pimozide (0.5–2.5 mg/kg), chlorpromazine (5–26 mg/kg), metoclopramide (1.5–1.7 mg/kg) and oxiperomide (0.25–1.0 mg/kg) induced a similar reaction but interestingly thioridazine (3–7 mg/kg), which posesses inherent anticholinergic properties, did not. The anticholinergic drugs scopolamine (0.02 mg/kg i.v.) and benztropine (0.2 mg/kg i.v.) abolished the dystonic movements whereas the anti-cholinesterase physostigmine (0.1 mg/kg i.v.) predictably exacerbated them. Pre-treatment of the baboons with reserpine (2 mg/kg i.p., 24 hours before) to deplete dopamine stores and alphamethylparatyrosine (200 mg/kg i.p. four to six hours before) to inhibit dopamine synthesis, strikingly attenuated the dystonic response to haloperidol in the susceptible animals, although administration of either drug alone did not produce comparable effects.

PATHOPHYSIOLOGY

The observation that acute dyskinesias occur as often with relatively selective dopaminergic antagonists such as haloperidol and pimozide as with chlorpromazine which possesses noradrenergic blocking properties suggests that dopamine is probably the important mediating catecholamine. Meldrum's studies (1977) in the baboon strongly suggest that pre-synaptic dopaminergic mechanisms may constitute one important aetiological factor.

Following the acute administration of an antipsychotic drug, a compensatory increase in dopamine turnover occurs as a consequence of increased synthesis (Nyback et al, 1967), increased release (Bartholini, 1976) and increased firing of dopamine-rich neurones in the substantia nigra (Bunney et al, 1973). These changes occur in an effort to override the simultaneous blockade of the post-synaptic dopamine receptors. The controlling feedback systems are still inadequately understood but almost certainly involve antagonism of pre-synaptic dopaminergic autoreceptors (Kehr et al, 1972) and a number of striato-nigral loops. After repeated neuroleptic administration, this increased release of dopamine attenuates and eventually disappears (Scatton et al, 1975).

A further point in favour of the relevance of increased dopamine release in the causation of acute dyskinesias is the fact that similar dystonias may occur after L-dopa, the natural precursor of dopamine, is given in large doses to healthy monkeys (Mones, 1973; Sassin, 1975). Sustained L-dopa therapy can also induce dystonic phenomena in Parkinsonian patients several hours after each dose as a withdrawal phenomenon (Lees et al, 1977). Furthermore, anti-cholinergic drugs which abolish acute dyskinesias in man are known to reduce neuroleptic-induced dopamine release (O'Keefe et al, 1970; Anden, 1972).

However, at the time of increased dopamine release the post-synaptic receptors are blocked and theoretically should be totally unresponsive. It is now known that there are at least two subtypes of striatal dopamine receptor (Kebabian and Calne, 1979) and as Stevens and Matthyse (Matthyse, 1973) have suggested it is conceivable that a subpopulation of dopamine receptors remains responsive to the increased dopamine release. Indeed Skirboll and Bunney (1979) have now detected two subpopulations of receptors, the effects of dopamine on one of which cannot be blocked by haloperidol.

Neuroleptics also cause delayed compensatory changes in post-synaptic receptor sensitivity. Twenty-four hours after acute butyrophenone administration rodents exhibit increased stereotypies or climbing behaviour when challenged with dopaminergic agonists (Christensen and Moller-Nielsen, 1974; Martres et al, 1977).

Marsden and his group (Kolbe et al, 1981) have recently devised a study to investigate these complicated interactions. They gave butaperazine (40 mg/kg orally) to rats and then followed the changes in apomorphine-induced stereotypy (0.5 mg/kg subcutaneously given 15 minutes beforehand), striatal dopamine, homovanillic acid (HVA) and dihydroxyphenylacetic acid (DOPAC) serially over the next three days. Apomorphine-induced stereotypy was abolished for the first eight hours and markedly reduced for 12 hours, whereas over the same period of time striatal HVA and DOPAC were greatly increased with no change in dopamine suggesting an increased striatal dopamine turnover. Twenty-four hours later, however, apomorphine provoked a normal or slightly exaggerated stereotypic response at a time when striatal HVA and DOPAC were falling but still increased compared with controls. After 72 hours no difference could be found in either the behavioural or biochemical parameters between the butaperazine and control animals.

In the careful clinical study by Garver et al (1976a, 1977) using oral butaperazine, all but one of the acute dystonic reactions occurred in the first 24 hours and Marsden's studies show that it is during this crucial period that animals given the same drug have an increased striatal dopamine turnover at a time when the post-synaptic receptor sensitivity is normal or increased, as gauged by apomorphine-induced stereotypy.

On the basis of this study Marsden and Jenner (1980) have suggested that acute neuroleptic-induced dyskinesias might occur as a result of enhanced dopamine release at a time when decreasing brain neuroleptic concentrations have left a population of normal or even supersensitive post-synaptic dopamine receptors exposed. Possible explanations for the low incidence of acute dyskinesias in clinical practice might be that it is dose-related and would occur in everyone if the initial dose were large enough, or alternatively that the response may be related to some genetically-determined idiosyncrasy (Eldridge and Gottlieb, 1976).

CLINICAL DESCRIPTION

Although probably first reported by Labhardt (1953) in Switzerland and Kulenkampff and Tarnow (1956) in Germany, the most complete and comprehensive early descriptions can be found in the writings of the French psychiatrists, Delay and Deniker (1959, 1969), and Sigwald et al (1959b). For the purpose of clinical description the syndrome may be broadly subdivided into three groups — the acute dystonic reaction, buccolingual dyskinesias with limb choreo-athetosis reminiscent of tardive dyskinesia and, finally, the isolated occurrence of severe tonic flexion of the spine (the Pisa syndrome).

THE ACUTE DYSTONIC REACTION

This is by far the commonest of the three presentations beginning either abruptly or in a more stuttering step-wise fashion over several hours. Generalised torsion is more likely to result in children whereas local or segmental varieties are usually seen in adults. The syndrome is painful and distressing. Curiously, suggestion can trigger an attack and countersuggestion may be helpful in treatment, observations which no doubt contribute to the frequent misdiagnosis of hysteria.

Involvement of the ocular muscles is particularly characteristic and clinical presentations include blepharospasm, periocular twitches ('winking spasms') and protracted staring episodes. Oculogyric crises, once regarded as pathognomonic of post-encephalitic Parkinsonism, are quite common. These commence with a feeling of malaise or restlessness followed by a sustained, upward, adversive rotation of the eyes so severe that often during an attack only the white of the eye is visible. The patient may be momentarily able to correct the tonic spasm to command but almost immediately the eyes resume their upturned posture. Occasionally clonic movements occur and sometimes the eyes are downturned or much more rarely converged or laterally deviated. Not uncommonly the head may be simultaneously hyperextended, the mouth opened wide and the tongue protruded. Autonomic storms can occur and the patient may be anxious or even delirious. An attack may last anything from a few minutes to 72 hours and is followed by severe exhaustion. Very occasionally an acute dystonic reaction may be followed by severe hyperpyrexia, electrolyte disturbances with hyponatraemia, akinesia, stupor, pulmonary congestion and even death (the neuroleptic malignant syndrome).

Intermittent or sustained trismus, forced mouth opening, sensations of tongue swelling, facial grimacing, tongue protrusion, and abnormal lip movements are other common manifestations. Platysmal contraction and severe torticollis are even more frequent and the tonic muscular contraction may fluctuate from muscle group to muscle group over short periods of time. Characteristically all these disturbances are acutely painful and are often associated with an inner restlessness, a reduced pain threshold, a fine postural tremor of the tongue and hands and facial immobility.

Reported complications include dislocation of the temporo-mandibular joint, severe tongue injuries and chipped teeth. Laryngeal dystonia and glossopharyngeal spasms may cause a jerky voice or even aphonia, dysphagia, foaming at the mouth and occasionally stridor and life-threatening dyspnoea requiring emergency tracheostomy and bronchial lavage. More generalised spasms are also seen including opisthotonus, tortipelvis, scoliosis, malleable dystonic limb spasms and tetanic contractures. Slow bowing trunk movements (chorée salutante), mobile bladder spasms, and episodes of abdominal distension (gros ventre pseudocyesis) due to diaphragmatic contractions are also sometimes seen.

EARLY OROFACIAL DYSKINESIAS AND GENERALISED CHOREO-ATHETOSIS

Acute choreiform dyskinesias unaccompanied by severe muscle spasm may also occur. These tend to be somewhat more stereotyped and rhythmical than those seen after prolonged neuroleptic treatment and may occur in conjunction with drug-induced Parkinsonism or akathisia. Grimacing, tongue twisting and protrusion, pouting of the lips, lip smacking, shoulder shrugging and jerky or writhing movements of the limbs are some of the most commonly observed phenomena. These may occur after a few weeks of treatment as well as in the first few days.

THE PISA SYNDROME

Ekbom et al (1972) described this characteristic postural disturbance occurring 3–10 days after the administration of the butyrophenones, methylperone and haloperidol in three patients suffering from dementia. In all three the trunk was tonically flexed to one side and slightly rotated backwards and, in one patient, the head and neck were also bent towards the same side. On walking, the trunk and body twisted obliquely backwards towards the side of the curvature so the patient tended to rotate in the opposite direction to the path of walking. The patients had less difficulty in turning to the side of the flexion; turning to the opposite side was conducted in stages through a relatively wide arc. One patient walked alternately forwards or backwards or round her own axis. None of the patients showed dystonia of the eyes, face or mouth. The symptoms disappeared on drug withdrawal and were also improved by anticholinergics.

COURSE

Most acute dystonic reactions occur within the first few days of drug treatment. In Ayd's study (1961) 90% occurred within the first four days and a similar figure was reported by Swett (1975). In Garver's study (1976a,b, 1977) using oral challenges of 40 mg butaperazine, the dystonia began between 23 and 28 hours in seven and one late response was seen at 54 hours. Peak plasma and red cell butaperazine levels occurred as early as 2–8 hours and by the time the extrapyramidal side-effects appeared the levels had fallen to 3–33% of the initial maximum value. No difference was found between the plasma levels of the drug in those with dystonia and the unaffected group. However, red cell butaperazine values were six times higher in the dystonic group, red cell half-life was greatly prolonged and the area under the absorption curve was also increased in the dystonic patients. Part of the red cell butaperazine is membrane bound and this parameter might therefore be a better indicator of brain concentration than plasma. This data could be used to support the notion that acute dyskinesias are dose-determined and raises the possibility that the reaction might be minimised by the use of smaller initial doses.

Acute dyskinesias subside usually within a few hours or at most two or three days after drug withdrawal. What is much less clear is what happens if neuroleptics are continued once they have appeared. It is generally believed that the higher the initial dose the more likely are dyskinesias to occur but, apart from Garver's study, there is no evidence to support this at present. Furthermore, the notion of side-effect breakthrough has been mooted on the basis of one intriguing but as yet unconfirmed report in which very large doses of neuroleptics in young patients reduced the incidence of dyskinesias and Parkinsonism (Rifkin et al, 1971).

A few patients, particularly those receiving depôt tranquilliser preparations, have recurrent acute dyskinesias a few hours after each injection. They reappear in others on switching to approximately comparable doses of a new neuroleptic or following sudden large increases in dosage. Another reason for the apparent repeated recurrence during presumed sustained therapy is poor compliance, the patient restarting treatment after a period of self-prescribed abstinence.

DIFFERENTIAL DIAGNOSIS

Hysteria is still the commonest error in diagnosis; the contortions are often so bizarre and grotesque that, if never previously observed, it is easy to understand how this phenomenon might be construed as psychogenic (Angus and Simpson, 1970).*Habitués* of accident and emergency rooms are not infrequently turned away when they return with painful dystonia a day or so after prescription of a tranquilliser. The matter is further complicated by the fact that suggestion can frequently induce the reaction in susceptible individuals and the symptoms can fluctuate spontaneously over hours. There is even a report of *folie à deux* in which a serviceman, on taking his schizophrenic wife's haloperidol to help him sleep, developed severe dystonia and was followed shortly afterwards to the casualty department by his wife who had developed identical dystonic conversion symptoms (Cavenar and Harris, 1980). Enquiry into recent antipsychotic drug ingestion is an essential step in arriving at the correct diagnosis. Phenytoin intoxication, tricyclic antidepressants, antihistamines, antimalarials and central nervous system stimulants such as amphetamine and fenfluramine may also occasionally provoke acute dyskinesias and the antiemetic metoclopramide is another common cause of acute dystonia.

Tetanus (Gleckman et al, 1969), rabies, strychnine poisoning, encephalitis and meningitis, tetany, status epilepticus, strokes and catatonia are other frequent diagnostic errors. The absence of meningism, the presence of hypertonicity between spasms and the frequency of ocular spasms in the drug-induced syndrome are helpful distinguishing features. If doubt remains, however, the slow intravenous injection of an anticholinergic agent should be carried out as a diagnostic test.

TREATMENT

Discontinuation of the offending antipsychotic drug and the simultaneous parenteral administration of an anticholinergic drug is probably still the treatment of choice for all three subtypes of acute dyskinesias. Atropine was the first anticholinergic to be used (Priori and Schettini, 1958) but it is now more customary to use procyclidine (5–10 mg), biperiden (1–5 mg), benztropine (1–2 mg) or the antihistamine diphenhydramine (10–50 mg) given intramuscularly or by slow intravenous injection. If improvement does not occur, a repeat dose may be given after 30 minutes. Normally, however, amelioration begins within 10 minutes and may continue for three to four hours. Cover for 48 hours with the equivalent oral anticholinergic preparation is probably wise in order to avoid immediate recurrence. Acute dystonia is so distressing that a case can be made for the use of prophylactic anticholinergic medication for three to seven days after starting neuroleptics as it has been shown that this can strikingly reduce the incidence (Stern and Anderson, 1979). However, breakthrough dystonia on withdrawing the anticholinergic may still occur. An alternative approach might be always to use an antipsychotic which possesses inherent anticholinergic properties such as thioridazine.

The slow intravenous injection of the benzodiazepines, diazepam (10 mg) and clonazepam (1 mg) is also very effective in controlling acute dystonic reactions (Korczyn and Goldberg, 1972; Gagrat et al, 1978). In patients with glaucoma, a history of confusional episodes or acute prostatism, this is probably the treatment of choice and it has been claimed that, if the dose is carefully titrated by slow injection, relief of symptoms with pleasant relaxation can occur without significant respiratory depression or induction of sleep.

Smaller starting doses of neuroleptics are said to be less likely to cause acute dyskinesias. Swett (1975) has reported that the incidence of chlorpromazine-induced reactions is higher when doses above 300 mg/d are used and Crane (1967) considers doses of haloperidol above 15 mg/d to be more hazardous. Large incremental increases should also probably be avoided with the butyrophenones and depôt phenothiazines.

A wide range of other drugs with different pharmacological effects have been reported to alleviate acute dyskinesias including the parenteral administration of caffeine (Kulenkampff and Tarnow, 1956; Freyhan, 1959), pethidine (Perez, 1961), diphenhydramine and promethazine (Sigwald et al, 1959) and sodium amylobarbitone (Gailitis et al, 1960). The use of intravenous calcium has been advocated on theoretical grounds (Lichtigfeld, 1964).

It is of considerable interest that drugs which enhance dopaminergic activity have been reported to attenuate acute dystonia. Methylphenidate, which increases dopamine release and blocks its re-uptake, produced prompt relief in two patients when given intravenously (20–50 mg) (Fann, 1966). Gessa et al (1972) conducted a controlled study using apomorphine, a dopamine agonist, in 13 schizophrenics with haloperidol-induced dyskinesias. Within 15 minutes of their onset 5 mg apomorphine or 1 ml distilled water were administered intramuscularly. In the six saline-treated controls dystonia continued for at least three hours whereas, in the seven treated with apomorphine, suppression occurred in all of them within 15 minutes. Three of the apomorphine-treated patients experienced relaxation and drowsiness.

AKATHISIA

Synonyms Paradoxical behavioural reactions, turbulent reactions, tasikinesia.

Definition A state of mental and motor restlessness in which there is a total inability to remain seated and an irresistible compulsion to incessantly move about.

EPIDEMIOLOGY

The difficulty in delineating mild akathisia from hypomania and acute anxiety, severe akathisia from chorea, and the absence of any hard diagnostic criteria pose major problems in obtaining accurate data. Nevertheless, there is agreement that in contrast to neuroleptic-induced dyskinesias, akathisia occurs with approximately equal frequency throughout adulthood (Ayd, 1961) and that the early reports of a striking female preponderance (Ayd, 1961) were probably artefactual. Children may be affected and depôt phenothiazines seem particularly hazardous.

In a double-blind multi-centre study designed to assess the comparative efficacy of three drugs with antipsychotic properties in 400 newly admitted young schizophrenics, akathisia occurred in 6% of the patients treated with chlorpromazine (mean dose 650 mg/d), 12% of fluphenazine-treated patients (mean dose 6 mg/d) and in 5% of those who received thioridazine (mean dose 700 mg/d). The comparable figures for drug-induced Parkinsonism and acute dyskinesias respectively were: chlorpromazine (15% and 4%), fluphenazine (24% and 7%) and thioridazine (4% and 1%). A chastening aspect of this study was a 4% incidence of akathisia reported by experienced psychiatrists in the placebo-treated group (National Institute of Mental Health, 1964). A comparably low incidence was also reported by Goldman in his extensive survey of 5000 patients. Figures of 7% were recorded for trifluoperazine and prochlorperazine, 5% for haloperidol, 4% for thioridazine and 3% for chlorpromazine. Only three of 651 (0.5%) patients given reserpine experienced akathisia but, of four patients receiving the related shorter-acting drug tetrabenazene, one developed akathisia (Goldman, 1961). In fact the incidence of akathisia with tetrabenazene probably approaches that reported with the commonly used antipsychotic drugs. Freyhan (1957) also observed that coexistent akathisia was more common with reserpine-induced Parkinsonism than with the chlorpromazine-induced state. In a further study Freyhan (1959) reported a figure for akathisia of 12.5% in 104 psychiatric in-patients treated with trifluoperazine (3–30 mg/d) and excluded the milder syndromes where diagnostic doubt may have existed.

Ayd (1961) found akathisia present in 21.2% of 3775 psychiatric patients treated with phenothiazines. Braude et al reported a similar figure of 25% in an acute psychiatric admission ward and Kennedy et al (1971) reported an even higher figure of 39% in 63 residential schizophrenics who had been receiving anti-psychotic drugs mainly in the form of trifluoperazine (mean dose 17 mg/d) for 4–13 years. However, in 10 of the 24 affected individuals, the symptoms were mild. Finally, in a recent study in which motor restlessness was only considered to be drug-induced if it improved after intramuscular biperiden (5 mg) and not after a placebo saline-injection, 45 of 110 patients (49%) receiving butyrophenones or phenothiazines without anticholinergic prophylaxis experienced akathisia (Van Putten, 1975). There are very few studies designed to elucidate whether akathisia is dose-dependent but Gardos et al (1974) have reported that thioxanthene is more likely to cause akathisia at 40 mg/d than at 10 mg/d. Braude et al (1983) also observed an increased frequency after a large initial dose or after a relatively rapid dosage increase.

PATHOPHYSIOLOGY

Akathisia remains a paradoxical enigma and is one of the least understood of the neuroleptic-induced side-effects. It has been regarded as a basal ganglia mediated disturbance on the tenuous grounds that it occurs in idiopathic and post-encephalitic Parkinsonism (Delay et al, 1957), but related phenomena such as Ekbom's restless legs are usually considered to be of peripheral origin and Sovner and Dimascio (1978) consider it to be a primary sensory phenomenon.

One currently fashionable notion is that selective blockade of nigral pre-synaptic dopaminergic autoreceptors may be involved. Under normal circumstances dopamine released from the pre-synaptic terminals stimulates these autoreceptors and leads to a feedback inhibitory control on dopamine synthesis and release (Carlsson et al, 1972). A preferential effect on these receptors by a neuroleptic would enhance dopamine synthesis and its release on to unblocked post-synaptic receptors. In fact low doses of haloperidol can increase motor activity in rodents which is reversed with higher doses (Costall et al, 1972) and paradoxical inhibition of locomotion can occur with small doses of the dopaminergic agonist apomorphine (Strombon, 1977). However, a number of clinical observations militate against this hypothesis. The fact that the dopamine depletors, reserpine and tetrabenazine, can cause akathisia and that it occurs in Parkinson's disease where loss of nigral neurones leads to impaired dopaminergic transmission suggests that enhanced pre-synaptic dopamine release is not important. Furthermore the simultaneous occurrence of akathisia and drug-induced Parkinsonism argues against preferential blockade. Finally, there is no evidence as yet that akathisia is more likely to occur when small doses of antipsychotics are used, in fact the reverse seems more likely.

Marsden and Jenner (1980) have recently postulated an alternative hypothesis implicating blockade of the mesocortical post-synaptic dopamine receptors. In laboratory animals, destruction of this pathway caused increased locomotor activity (Tassin et al, 1978) with an increase in activity in subcortical dopamine systems (Carter and Pycock, 1980). The mental accompaniments of akathisia make a hypothesis which involves the cerebral cortex particularly appealing, but further work is necessary to establish its validity. Alternatively, effects on dopamine receptors in the spinal cord might provide an attractive link with Ekbom's restless legs.

Psychodynamic theories have also been propounded. Winkelman (1961), for example, suggested that intact mental functioning depends on the constant outlet of psychic energy. In some way this overriding need is impeded by neuroleptics resulting in akathisia as a means of expression of emotional conflict. Van Putten (1975) also considered the condition to be primarily emotional and a wide range of behavioural syndromes have been reported as presenting features. These, however, may not be symptoms of akathisia but reflect the difficulties in distinguishing the condition from symptoms of mental illness.

CLINICAL DESCRIPTION

Sigwald was probably the first to recognise drug-induced akathisia whilst using promethazine in 1947; Steck (1954) reported its occurrence with reserpine and Lehmann (1955) and Delay et al (1957) provided two of the early reports incriminating phenothiazines. Complaints of mounting inner tension and unease ('the jitters') usually herald motor restlessness and occasionally intense feelings of fear, rage and sexual craving may appear early. An unbearable, irresistible compulsion to move then often ensues with shuffling and tapping of the feet and constant shifting of body weight from one leg to the other (*le balancement lent du corps*). Formication, pins and needles, sensations of warmth or vibration, pulling, drawing feelings in the legs, and muscular cramps add to the discomfort especially when lying down and finally the patient is forced to his feet. He then begins to pace up and down sometimes breaking into a trot, is quite incapable of any form of mental concentration and may continue to parade up and down for hours on end. Stereotyped marching on the spot ('marking time') is also common and compulsive dancing, climbing or rocking may be seen. Rocking from foot to foot may occur very occasionally with tremors or myoclonic jerks of the feet. Inactivity immediately provokes profound mental and physical torment and restlessness may be so intense as to prohibit sleep. If forced to sit down the patient immediately rises again and starts aimlessly circling round and round like a caged beast. An exacerbation of the underlying psychosis may occasionally occur *pari passu* with the hyperactivity and there is always a distressing feeling of inner tension and malaise (Van Putten, 1975).

Denham and Carrick (1961) have provided an excellent vignette:

> From a state of complete inertia there rises one in which there is a desire of incessant activity. Although the muscle hypertonia is if anything more pronounced than that seen in the second state, thus making movement very difficult, the patient is compelled to move. He cannot sit or stand inactive. He must walk about constantly but will not be satisfied with one part of the ward, ever seeking a change of action and locality. It is at this stage that he may endeavour to work, but as with all his other activities any attempt at one particular task is soon superseded by the desire to try something different. Questioned as to his behaviour the patient may say that only by constant walking can he allay his restless feelings or that 'something pushes him on'. The predominating mood is depression, but there may be mood-swings, short periods of euphoria interrupting the former, particularly in the evening. When this akathisic condition is marked, insomnia may be present but is not a common cause for complaint.

The American patient's description reproduced by Van Putten (1975) is also instructive:

> Mentally I feel like I am going at 90 miles per hour . . . my nerves are just jumping. I feel like I'm wired to the ceiling. I just feel impatient and nasty. I can't concentrate, it's like I got ants in my pants; my nerves are raw I just feel on edge. I feel just nasty. I feel like jumping out of my skin if this feeling continues. I would rather be dead. I can't describe the feeling. I'm quivery from the waist up, I want to climb the walls. I feel all revved up, it's like I got a diaper rash inside.

It can be seen from these accounts that an agonising dysphoria and the compelling urge to move are the two cardinal features of akathisia. Of all the neuroleptic-induced side-effects it is the one which is the most distressing to patients and the one most likely to lead to poor drug compliance. It has been suggested that the excessive motor restlessness is particularly likely to occur in the legs (Braude et al, 1983) but I have observed severe akathisia in the trunk, head and arms in a paraplegic on sulpiride.

COURSE

Although akathisia usually begins at least one week after starting treatment there are well-documented instances of its onset within a few hours (Crane and Naranjo, 1971; Kendler, 1976). A steadily increasing prevalence occurs in the six months after starting therapy, Ayd (1961) reporting only 50% of the total reactions occurring in the first month. It usually appears a few days before Parkinsonism in patients who experience both side-effects and spontaneous remissions, and relapses on fixed dosage are not uncommon (Borenstein et al, 1962). Some patients lose their motor restlessness altogether after the first few months of treatment whereas others may continue to have distressing hyperactivity for several years. Forrest and Fahn (1979) have drawn attention to the frequent coexistence of tardive dyskinesias and akathisia and the subjective anguish commonly present with the latter.

Discontinuation of the offending drug generally leads to a slow resolution of symptoms but this is by no means invariable. Kruse (1960) described three patients aged over 50 years who experienced persistent motor restlessness for from 3–18 months after withdrawal of medication. Hershon et al (1972) gave placebo for 16 weeks to 32 institutionalised schizophrenics continuing an age- and treatment-matched control group on phenothiazines. They found a significant increase in akathisia in the placebo-treated group which could not be explained by a reduction in Parkinsonian disabilities. Furthermore, five of the patients on placebo developed withdrawal akathisia.

DIFFERENTIAL DIAGNOSIS

The term akathisia was originally used by Haskovec (1901, 1903) to describe a curious mental state in which there was a total inability to remain seated. He considered it to be psychologically determined and compared it to the hysterical form of astasia-abasia. His description was based around two male patients in whom motor restlessness identical to that now commonly seen with anti-psychotic drugs occurred. The first, a man of 40, also had paroxysmal laryngeal spasms and diaphragmatic tics and was thought to be hysterical, whereas the second, a 54-year-old, had a long history of neurasthenia and improved with treatment. A similar case had already been written up by Joffroy, and Raymond and Janet added a fourth (Raymond and Janet, 1902). Bing considered it to be a psychosis resulting from a morbid fear of sitting down, while Oppenheim suggested phobic anxiety as the aetiology and Kinnier Wilson believed it to be hysterical in origin. Further spontaneously occurring cases have not been recorded, however, and it seems likely that alternative diagnoses such as the restless legs syndrome or anxiety neurosis may subsequently have been given. Mild akathisia can undoubtedly occur in normal individuals particularly after a gruelling day. Catatonic excitement can lead to over-activity but this often has a clownish appearance and is usually distinguishable from the drug-induced reaction. For instance the schizophrenic patient will jump up and down, somersault and rush about dramatically, laughing or singing (Fish, 1976).

Drug-induced reactions may easily be mistaken for an exacerbation of the original mental illness, particularly in schizophrenics who have difficulty articulating their feelings. Anxiety in psychiatrically ill patients about taking drugs which affect their minds can also lead to understandable feelings of severe apprehension and fidgetiness (Sorwer-Foner, 1960; Raskin, 1972). Braude et al (1983) suggest that symptoms related to the legs associated with tasikinesia (inability to sit still) are the characteristic features whereas hand wringing and general restlessness are more likely to be due to the underlying psychiatric illness.

Akathisia occurs in idiopathic and post-encephalitic Parkinson's disease (Sicard, 1923) and distinction between these conditions and the drug-induced Parkinsonism-akathisia syndrome can only be made by taking a careful history. The relation of conditions like Ekbom's restless legs (1960) and molimimia crurum nocturna (Brenning, 1971) to akathisia is not clear. The restless legs syndrome first described by Thomas Willis in the 17th century gives rise to an unpleasant discomfort in the leg muscles when sitting and is particularly troublesome when the patient retires to bed. Mounting discomfort in the calves with formication, paraesthesiae and cramps occurs and after a period of agitated shuffling the patient is forced to get up and pace the floor to obtain relief. On lying down again similar symptoms may return and, as a consequence of chronic insomnia, depression may ensue. Examination of the nervous system and muscles has so far revealed no abnormality in these cases and a number of quite different secondary causes are now recognised including chronic poliomyelitis, uraemia, exposure to severe cold, diabetes mellitus, chronic obstructive airways disease and chronic venous insufficiency due to varicose veins.

TREATMENT

No clear guide-lines on management have as yet been formulated. Most authorities would recommend the use of parenteral anticholinergic drugs to control severe symptoms (Freyhan, 1959; Ayd, 1961) but the response is much more unpredictable than that seen with acute dyskinesias. Furthermore, the lack of response of two patients to physostigmine raises questions as to the importance of cholinergic mechanisms in the pathogenesis (Ambani et al, 1973). Braude et al (1983) noted improvement in all 10 of their cases in which the dosage of antipsychotic medication was reduced but, out of 20 patients treated with anticholinergic agents, only six improved. All the responders had additional Parkinsonian signs and they have suggested that two distinct pharmacological subtypes might exist. Benzodiazepines were ineffective in this study. There is a single unconfirmed report of drug-induced akathisia responding to the dopaminergic drug methylphenidate in a dose of 10–20 mg/d (Carman, 1972). There are anecdotal reports of akathisia burning itself out during the first few months of treatment and it may be possible to bide time by the concurrent prescription of a benzodiazepine such as diazepam. If all else fails, a switch to another antipsychotic drug should be tried.

TARDIVE DYSKINESIAS

Synonyms Terminal extrapyramidal insufficiency, persistent extrapyramidal hyperkinesia, complex or persistent dyskinesias.

Definition Tardive dyskinesia is a term used to describe a complex of persistent and occasionally irreversible abnormal involuntary movements appearing after sustained treatment with antipsychotic drugs. The movements are heterogeneous and include orofacial chorea (the bucco-linguo-masticatory syndrome), limb chorea, dystonia tics, stereotypies myoclonus and hemiballismus.

EPIDEMIOLOGY

Much of the evidence incriminating antipsychotic drugs in the production of tardive dyskinesias stems from epidemiological data. A number of studies have compared the relative prevalence of these abnormal movements in drug-treated and unmedicated patients within the same institutions (Faurbye et al, 1964; Pryce and Edwards, 1966) and in hospitals where neuroleptics are widely used compared with those where they have been used very little (Degkwitz and Wenzel, 1967; Crane, 1968a,b, 1971; Ogita, et al, 1975). With very few exceptions (Demars, 1966; Owens et al, 1982) all have shown a higher frequency of abnormal movements in the drug-treated groups.

Prevalence figures of between 0.5% and 40% have been quoted in chronic institutionalised psychiatric patients. This wide range reflects methodological differences and variable diagnostic thresholds. Probably at least 5–10% of patients treated for one year will develop the disorder (Gardos and Cole, 1980) and the frequency may be even higher in the elderly (US Task Force, 1980). However, it should be stressed that the incidence of severe and disabling forms of tardive dyskinesia is very low. Chronic institutionalisation was at one time considered a predisposing factor but Asnis et al (1977) have reported a prevalence of 43.4% in 69 (53 female, 16 male) randomly selected psychiatric out-patients treated for at least three months.

In some susceptible individuals very small doses of antipsychotic drugs can provoke tardive dyskinesia (Simpson, 1973; Thornton and Thornton, 1973) and as yet there is no wholly convincing data to indicate that large doses of neuro-leptics or prolonged treatment are especially hazardous (Smith and Baldes-sarini, 1980; Task Force, 1980). Because most patients receive a number of different major tranquillisers reliable information is also hard to come by with respect to the relative dangers of particular compounds. Phenothiazines are possibly more likely to induce the syndrome than butyrophenones, and tardive dyskinesia has only been occasionally reported with chronic reserpine therapy (Uhrbrand and Faurbye, 1960; Degkwitz, 1969; Wolf, 1973). The piperazine phenothiazines, which have a high incidence of acute extrapyramidal side-effects, have been claimed to be particularly likely to cause tardive dyski-nesias (Uhrbrand and Faurbye, 1960). Thioridazine, a piperidine phenothiazine with potent anticholinergic properties and a low incidence of reversible early dyskinesias, can also provoke tardive dyskinesias. Clozapine, on the other hand, which has a piperazine side-chain has a very low incidence of reported extrapyramidal reactions, but has been temporarily withdrawn from clinical practice in most countries because of the possible risks of agranulocytosis. Metoclopramide, which is used as an antiemetic, may also cause tardive dyski-nesias (Lavy et al, 1978) in non-psychotic patients but the incidence of tardive dyskinesia with this drug and the related substituted benzamides sulpiride and tiapride seems very low.

There is a suggestion that patients who develop a Parkinsonian syndrome early in the course of treatment are more likely to go on to get tardive dys-kinesias (Crane, 1972a). It is not yet known whether any correlation exists between the incidence of acute dystonic reactions and the subsequent occur-rence of tardive dyskinesia.

Smith and Baldessarini (1980) have recently reviewed the available data concerning the relationship between prevalence and severity of tardive dys-kinesia and age. On the basis of nine available studies in the literature they concluded that a strong linear correlation existed between the prevalence of tardive dyskinesia and age in the range of 40–70 years. Using their own data from two previous studies they also found that the severity of abnormal move-ments increased with age and that the duration of treatment or dosage were not sufficient to explain these findings. Kane et al (1982a) have conducted a prospective study in young, psychiatrically ill patients (mean 28 years) and reported an incidence of 14% at the end of four years' cumulative neuroleptic exposure with a uniform incidence rate of 3–4% per year.

There is also a suggestion that the female sex may be slightly more predis-posed to the disorder (Bell and Smith, 1978; Smith et al, 1978), although many of the early studies, which showed a higher frequency in females, probably only reflected their preponderance in the elderly populations studied (Hunter et al, 1964: Kennedy et al, 1971). The available data suggesting brain damage (Faurbye et al, 1964), previous leucotomy (Hunter et al, 1964), electro-shock therapy (Uhrbrand and Faurbye, 1960) and blue eyes in men (Brandon et al, 1971) as causative factors are unconvincing. A number of papers have commented on the higher incidence of tardive dyskinesias in the edentulous (Pryce and Edwards, 1966; Brandon et al, 1971: Asnis et al, 1977) but the spontaneous occurrence of dyskinesias in individuals with dental prostheses makes evaluation of these claims difficult. There is also no correlation between the occurrence of tardive dyskinesias and the diagnosis for which the medication was prescribed. Numerous examples of tardive dyskinesia occurring in non-psychotic patients have now been reported (Faurbye et al, 1964; Klawans et al, 1974).

While the epidemiological data implicating antipsychotic drugs is quite convincing, analysis is hampered to some extent by a relative lack of information on the prevalence of similar dyskinesias in the untreated elderly, brain-damaged and schizophrenic populations. However, in a survey by Mettler and Crandell in 1955 just before neuroleptics were introduced, choreo-athetoid movements and other dyskinesias were extremely rare, occurring only in a fraction of 1% of the total psychiatric hospital population. Greenblatt et al (1968) reported a prevalence of 2% in geriatric patients not on neuroleptics compared with 40% in those on drugs and Klawans and Barr (1982) documented a 0.8% prevalence of orofacial dyskinesias in individuals aged between 50 and 59 years, 6% between 60 and 69 and 8% between 70 and 79. Kane et al (1982b) have found similar low figures with a prevalence of 1.2% in the healthy elderly compared with 66.4% in neuroleptic-treated, psychiatrically ill, old people. However, Delwaide and Desseiles (1977) noted that 29% of 55 untreated old people in a nursing home had bucco-lingual dyskinesias and recorded an even higher figure of 39% in 185 psychogeriatric patients who had never received neuroleptics.

It is difficult to determine whether chorea or athetosis occurs in untreated chronic schizophrenia uncomplicated by neurological disease. Kraepelin (1919) reported choreiform movements of the face and fingers and Kleist (1960) noted continuous grimacing jerking and fragmentation of speech. Bleuler (1950, 1951), on the other hand, commented that he had never seen chorea in schizophrenia and it is probable that many of the choreic syndromes described in the earlier literature were due to organic neurological disease. Most of the recent surveys have concluded that choreo-athetosis is extremely rare in psychiatric populations and the 'chronic psychotic choreo-athetosis' described by Dincman (1966) was probably drug-induced. Yarden and Discipio (1971), however, were able to collect a number of untreated acute schizophrenics who manifested choreiform movements.

ANIMAL DATA

Early attempts to induce persistent dyskinesias with phenothiazines in non-human primates were unsuccessful. Paulson (1972b) gave chlorpromazine 30 mg/kg to 15 monkeys for three to nine months but could only provoke transient reversible oral dyskinesias. Carlson and Eibergen (1976), however, treated eight rhesus monkeys with the narcotic dopamine-receptor blocker methadone for 10–22 months and at intervals of 2–11 months after drug withdrawal, challenges with normally ineffective doses of methamphetamine consistently caused oral hyperkinesias. These abnormal movements were selectively blocked by dopaminergic antagonists, chlorpromazine and spiroperidol. Carlson (1977) had also reported that stress alone can produce dyskinesias in the same animal model. Gunne and Barany (1976, 1980) have now managed to produce a convincing paradigm for tardive dyskinesias in Cebus apella monkeys. The prolonged administration of haloperidol or flupenthixol to 19 animals produced oral dyskinesias in nine which persisted after drug withdrawal for varying periods up to six years. All the animals passed through a cataleptic state and also exhibited acute dyskinesias early in treatment. The monkeys with dyskinesias were found to have a 57% reduction of glutamic acid dehydrogenase in the nigra and a 20–30% reduction in the globus pallidus and the subthalamic nucleus with a concomitant fall in GABA levels which was not present in the neuroleptic-treated animals without movements. A regional decrease of dopamine catabolites (HVA and DOPAC) also occurred in the dyskinetic monkeys. On the basis of these findings the authors have suggested that strionigral degeneration of GABA neurones may be the primary abnormality in tardive dyskinesia. Casey has also reported that spontaneous orofacial dyskinesias can occur in old Cebus apella monkeys, five of his 27 animals being affected. Acute challenges with a range of dopaminergic agonists and haloperidol to these previously untreated animals revealed a wide range of individual sensitivity but all the trial drugs were capable of inducing short-lived orofacial dyskinesias in varying numbers of animals.

Research using a number of rodent species has confirmed that chronic neuroleptic treatment can lead to dopamine receptor hypersensitivity (Rubovitz and Klawans, 1972) and that anticholinergics will accentuate stereotyped behaviour induced by dopaminergic stimulation (Scheel-Kruger, 1970). Neuroleptics have also been shown to increase dopamine synthesis and turnover in the brain after acute administration (Carlsson and Lindqvist, 1963) probably by the blockade of pre- and post-synaptic dopamine receptors (Bunney and Aghajanian, 1976). With chronic administration, dopamine turnover diminishes slowly (Scatton, 1977) and after discontinuation the synthesis and turnover fall temporarily below the baseline level (Hyttel, 1977a,b).

Neuropathological studies in neuroleptic-treated animals have so far been as unrevealing as the scattered information available in man. Gerlach (1975) found no significant difference in cell counts in the substantia nigra between rats treated with perphenazine enanthate 3.4 mg/kg/14 days for 12 months or 40 mg/kg/14 days for six months and saline-treated controls. Fog et al (1976) also administered perphenazine 40 mg/kg/14 days to rats for six months and found no changes in the cell counts in the corpus striatum or cerebral cortex compared with controls. However, a 10% reduction (p < 0.05) in cells in the ventrolateral part of the striatum in rats after treatment with fluphenazine decanoate 4 mg/kg/wk was found by Nielsen and Lyon (1978) and it is possible that further morphological and biochemical studies using a non-human primate model might prove fruitful. Electron microscopic studies in rabbits with extrapyramidal syndromes after prolonged application of chlorpromazine and haloperidol have shown synaptic changes in the pallidum and hypothalamus that were considered to be caused by partial blockage of glycolysis and/or axonal transport. Changes in post-synaptic dendrites with deposition of granular and fibrillar material, shrunken boutons embraced by astroglia and vacuolation of pre-synaptic axon terminals also occur; changes reminiscent of those occurring in the striatal boutons after destruction of the nigrostriatal bundle (Koizumi and Shiraishi, 1973a,b).

PATHOPHYSIOLOGY

The mechanisms underlying the development of tardive dyskinesias are poorly understood. An important and relatively selective effect of the anti-psychotic drugs is to block the action of dopamine in the brain. It is also known that prolonged exposure to neuroleptics causes a number of compensatory physiological and biochemical changes in the dopaminergic neurones on which they act. The clinical pharmacology of tardive dyskinesias suggests that over-stimulation of central dopaminergic systems may be important. For example they closely resemble the dyskinesias which occur during sustained L-dopa treatment for Parkinson's disease and they may be enhanced by high doses of dopamine receptor agonists (Gerlach et al, 1974). They commonly occur for the first time on reduction or discontinuation of the offending neuroleptic and may be suppressed by dopamine depleting drugs such as reserpine and dopamine synthesis inhibitors such as alpha paramethyltyrosine. Paradoxically they are often temporarily improved by increasing the dose of the neuroleptic, an effect which occurs too rapidly to be ascribed to superimposed bradykinesia.

To overcome the problem of how a neuroleptic drug with dopamine receptor blocking properties can induce dopaminergic over-activity, Klawans (1973a) invoked the concept of drug-induced supersensitivity. Pharmacological inactivation or denervation of pre-synaptic neurones in the autonomic nervous system has been known for some years to produce post-synaptic receptor supersensitivity to the applied neurotransmitter. It is reasonable therefore to suppose that blockade of dopamine receptors might produce similar effects by depriving the post-synaptic apparatus of any access to its transmitter. Considerable support for this hypothesis is now available from animal studies. Chronic administration of phenothiazines to rodents for several weeks leads to dopaminergic supersensitivity as judged by an exaggerated response to dopamine receptor agonists days or weeks after drug withdrawal (Tarsy and Baldessarini, 1974). After one week of phenothiazine administration the number of dopamine receptors in vitro has also been shown to be increased using tritiated neuroleptic binding techniques (Burt et al, 1977).

However, these findings do not adequately explain the emergence of tardive dyskinesias in many patients in the course of sustained antipsychotic therapy where presumably the bulk of dopamine receptors are blocked. A recent series of experiments on rats in which trifluoperazine and cis-flupenthixol were given for up to a year throw some light on this apparent contradiction. After one month's neuroleptic administration all indices of brain dopamine activity were antagonised, i.e. apomorphine responsiveness, a reduction in dopamine-stimulated adenylcyclase activity in vitro, and dopamine receptor binding affinity which after a transient increase returned to normal. Between one and six months, despite regular drug intake, stereotypy with apomorphine reappeared, dopamine-stimulated adenylcyclase activity returned towards normal and the receptor binding levels remained unchanged. Between six months and one year this re-emergence of dopamine receptor responsiveness gradually transformed to a state of dopaminergic over-activity, apomorphine provoked greater stereotypy than in the controls, there was increased dopamine-stimulated adenyl cyclase activity and the number of tritiated spiperone bound receptors increased. The striatal dopamine receptor supersensitivity is also of functional significance as it is accompanied by changes in striatal acetyl choline and 3 glutamate release. The increase in the number of dopamine receptors and unexplained alterations in affinity persist for up to six months after drug withdrawal (Clow et al, 1978, 1979a,b; Murugaiah et al, 1982). No such effects have been observed following the chronic administration of sulpiride and clozapine. Marsden and Jenner (1980) have pointed out that administration of a drug for a year to a rat represents exposure for approximately one-third of its life-span and persistence of supersensitivity for six months may represent a change lasting 10 years or so in a human being. Crow and his colleagues, however, have failed to find any difference between the degree of dopamine receptor supersensitivity found in schizophrenics with or without tardive dyskinesias in post-mortem brain studies.

A primary reduction in dopaminergic neurotransmission may also be a crucial factor in the causation of tardive dyskinesias. The analogous but reversible L-dopa-induced dyskinesias only occur in Parkinsonian patients where there is a marked reduction in dopamine activity and the dyskinesias tend to be most intense in those parts of the body most severely involved by the disease process. There is also possibly a greater tendency for tardive dyskinesia to develop in patients who had drug-induced Parkinsonian features early in the course of therapy.

Secondary changes such as disuse or denervation post-synaptic dopaminergic hypersensitivity might cause the emergence and temporary persistence of tardive dyskinesias but these pharmacological changes are unlikely to be responsible for persistence of abnormal movements years after drug withdrawal. More profound changes might occur such as damage to the post-synaptic cell membrane and cellular respiration mechanisms. Neuronal destruction may also occur as a result of precipitation of neuromelanin particularly in dopaminergic nigral neurones (Forrest, 1974) or as a result of localised cerebral hypoxia. The fact that the elderly are much more prone to develop irreversible tardive dyskinesias could indicate that they have a reduced capacity to respond with compensatory changes to the long-term effects of neuroleptics and age and neuroleptic-related reductions in central dopaminergic and cholinergic activity might be important. At the present time there is no evidence that chronic neuroleptic therapy induces neurotoxic changes and it is possible that those cases of apparently irreversible tardive dyskinesias seen in the elderly are simply patients in whom the drug has unmasked an underlying spontaneously occurring dyskinesia.

At least two types of dopamine receptor are now known to exist in the corpus striatum of animals. Selective effects on these different subpopulations might offer an explanation for the well-recognised clinical observation of co-existing Parkinsonism and tardive dyskinesias. It is possible that the dopamine released as a result of neuroleptic administration may act on both a subgroup of blocked dopamine receptors and also a further group of receptors not affected by neuroleptics (Skirboll and Bunney, 1979).

Increased dopamine transmission in the striatum also invariably leads to a disturbance of the balance between the excitatory striatal neurotransmitter, acetyl choline and dopamine. A relative cholinergic under-activity occurs and it is known that anticholinergic drugs may uncover or aggravate tardive dyskinesias (Gerlach and Thorsen, 1976). Prolonged neuroleptic treatment also causes reduced acetyl choline turnover in animals (Sethy, 1976) and reduces acetyl choline receptor sensitivity (Dunstan and Jackson, 1977). There is no data, however, to suggest that concurrent therapy with anticholinergic drugs increase the risk of tardive dyskinesia (Gerlach and Simmelsgaard, 1978), and it is probable that cholinergic under-activity occurs essentially as a secondary effect consequent upon dopaminergic hypersensitivity.

PATHOLOGICAL DATA

The fact that tardive dyskinesias may be irreversible suggests that permanent structural changes might occur in the brain as a result of chronic neuroleptic therapy. Alternatively, neuroleptics might unmask an incipient pathological process. The few post-mortem light microscopy studies so far carried out have failed to show any consistent abnormalities. Scattered foci of neuronal degeneration with gliosis have been described following long-term phenothiazine administration (Roizin et al, 1959; Forrest et al, 1963) and individual case studies from patients dying with either neuroleptic-induced Parkinsonism and/or tardive dyskinesia have implicated the globus pallidus and putamen (Poursines et al, 1959), the caudate nucleus and substantia nigra (Gross and Kaltenbach, 1968), the medulla oblongata (Mackiewicz and Gershon, 1964) and the inferior olive (Grunthal and Walter-Buel, 1960). Degenerative changes in the substantia nigra were present in two of the three patients reported by Hunter but these were judged to be compatible with the patient's advanced age (Hunter et al, 1968). Christensen et al (1970) studied the brains of 28 patients with oral dyskinesias, in 21 of which the movements were thought to be drug-induced. Twenty-seven of them were found to have neuronal degeneration and gliosis of the substantia nigra. In contrast only seven of 28 age- and disease-matched controls showed similar changes. The average age in the dyskinesia material, however, was 74 years. Gliosis in the midbrain and brain-stem was also much more common in the patients with tardive dyskinesia. In 13 of 28 patients who had received long-term neuroleptics,

Jellinger (1977) found swelling of the large caudate nucleus neurones, increased glial satellitosis and occasional neuronaphagia with relative preservation of small neurones. Gliosis was most prominent in the anterior two-thirds of the caudate nucleus. Eight of the 14 patients with tardive dyskinesia (57%) showed these changes compared with five of the dyskinesia-free group (37.5%). No correlation was found, however, between the intensity of the morphological changes and the severity of the clinical syndrome. Infarctions in the anterior part of the corpus striatum and the frontal lobe have been described in a further study (Kameyama et al, 1975).

All these studies have methodological failings in the sense that the findings might be non-specific and age-related and that detailed cell counts in the basal ganglia were not attempted.

It is probable that the application of newer histochemical methods will in the next few years shed more light on the underlying pathology of irreversible tardive dyskinesia. The predilection of tardive dyskinesias for the tongue, lips and mouth suggests that the defect underlying the condition may be localised to a particular area of the basal nuclei. By means of autoradiographic techniques it is now possible via the somatotopically organised motor cortex to locate corresponding functional areas in the corpus striatum. The ventrolateral part of the corpus striatum has been implicated in the control of tongue and jaw movements in experimental animals (Nielsen and Lyon, 1978).

LABORATORY INVESTIGATIONS

The diagnosis of tardive dyskinesia is based on clinical observation and a positive history of sustained neuroleptic ingestion and no confirmatory laboratory test exists at present. Nevertheless, considerable research data has now accumulated and, although much of this is at present conflicting, some help to shed light on the central effects of prolonged neuroleptic treatment. There have been relatively few studies of cerebrospinal fluid monoamine metabolites in tardive dyskinesia. In one study after probenecid loading (3 g for two days) to block egress of metabolites from the lumbar sac, cerebrospinal fluid homovanillic acid (HVA) levels were normal (Pind and Faurbye, 1970). Chase (1976), however, obtained results in keeping with a diminished dopamine turnover and a reduced cerebrospinal HVA response to haloperidol.

In the course of long-term antipsychotic drug treatment, a fall in cerebrospinal fluid homovanillic acid begins after three to four weeks following an initial rise (Bowers, 1975; Post and Goodwin, 1975) and may approach normal. The effects on 5-hydroxytryptamine and noradrenaline metabolites vary depending on the particular neuroleptic given. Chase and Tamminga (1979) have reported a significant reduction in cerebrospinal glutamic acid dehydrodgenase (GAD), the synthesising enzyme of gamma-aminobutyric acid, but this seems to be a non-specific finding.

At present no evidence exists for post-synaptic hypersensitivity in the

hypothalamo-pituitary dopaminergic system. Challenge studies using the dopamine receptor agonist apomorphine revealed lower serum growth hormone
(GH) levels in the tardive dyskinesia patients compared with controls and the
baseline GH levels were also subnormal. These results suggest that the receptors might actually be hyposensitive in tardive dyskinesia (Ettigi et al, 1976).
Two other endocrinological studies also failed to show any hypersensitivity as
judged by serum prolactin and growth hormone levels after dopamine agonist
challenge (Smith et al, 1977; Tamminga et al, 1977). It is possible that the
hypothalamo-pituitary dopaminergic pathway reacts differently to chronic
neuroleptics from the other central dopaminergic systems and does not exclude
the possibility of striatal receptor hypersensitivity.

No distinctive radiological abnormalities have been found in tardive dyskinesia, although ventricular dilatation and cortical atrophy is a non-specific
finding on air encephalography and computerised axial tomography in some
patients (Gelenberg, 1976b). Owens et al (1984) have recently claimed that
schizophrenia with associated ventricular enlargement may represent a major
predisposing factor to the development of involuntary movements.

CLINICAL DESCRIPTION

Age considerably influences the type and pattern of abnormal movements.
In those over 50 years marked orofacial dyskinesias are most common, either
as an isolated phenomenon or together with chorea and athetosis of the limbs
and trunk. On the other hand isolated involvement of the mouth, lips and
tongue is rare in children who present more commonly with reversible choreic,
athetotic, myoclonic and hemiballistic syndromes of the limbs, head and trunk,

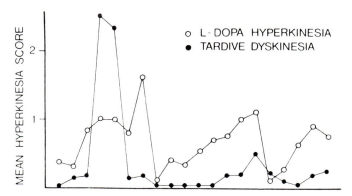

Figure 12.1. The relative distributions of L-dopa-induced dyskinesia and
tardive dyskinesia in different body regions. (By kind permission of Dr
Gerlach, 1977. In: Psychopharmacology, vol. 51. Springer, pp. 259–263.)

often with associated ataxia. In young adults a mixed picture of orofacial dyskinesias and limb chorea is found. Generalised or focal dystonia is relatively uncommon and neuroleptic-induced Gilles de la Tourette syndrome extremely rare. In comparison with L-dopa-induced dyskinesias, tardive dyskinesias have a predilection for the lips, tongue and jaw (Gerlach, 1977; Karson et al, 1983) (Fig. 12.1).

THE OROFACIAL DYSKINESIAS (BUCCO-LINGUO-MASTICATORY SYNDROME)

The original observations implicating neuroleptics in the aetiology of this disorder were made by Schoneker (1957) in Germany and Sigwald (1959 a,b) in France. Restricted vermicular movements of the tongue within the mouth have been claimed to be a premonitory sign (Crane and Naranjo, 1971) but the disorder is not generally recognised until the tongue starts to protrude out of the mouth. At first these lingual movements may only occur when the individual is under stress or engaged in some demanding manual activity. Eventually, however, they become more continuous. The tongue may assume a relatively fixed posture protruding from one side of the mouth or it may twist and writhe around the surface of the lips (Fig. 12.2). Pouting, described by Sigwald et al (1947) as *baillement de carpe*, slight sucking movements and lip pursing are common. The tongue may be driven rhythmically against the inner aspect of each cheek, as if the individual were chewing the cud, or alternatively roam sinuously over the ridges of the teeth. Teeth grinding, puffing out of the cheeks and lateral jaw movements are other frequent accompaniments. Initially the individual is quite unaware of their presence and, if the movements are drawn to his attention, he is able to suppress them totally. As the disorder intensifies, however, the dyskinesias become more complex and organised; a stereotyped regularity appears and a variety of superimposed mannerisms are occasionally devised in an attempt to conceal the grotesque contortions. The individual may now complain that his tongue is forcing itself out of his mouth against his will or that it is swelling up and being driven down his throat. Lightning reptilian flicks of the tongue ('the fly catcher's tongue') or slower, thrusting, rolling and curling movements begin often with incessant jaw opening, lip smacking, munching and champing. Atavistic facial expressions such as snarling, sneering and gnashing of the teeth may be prominent and coarse head and neck movements are sometimes troublesome. Repetitive retching movements with eye closure, tongue protrusion, gagging, eye bulging, suffusion of the face and intermittent cyanosis have been reported (Hunter et al, 1964). Blowing, flaring of the nostrils, chewing movements and intermittent prognathism are other components of the syndrome.

When severe, the movements may lead to intense social embarrassment and reactive depression with patients occasionally taking their own lives. Speech becomes nasal, slurred and fragmented, and oral ulceration, laceration of the tongue, broken teeth and continual protrusion of dentures make chewing

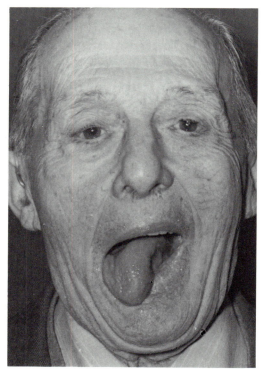

Figure 12.2. *Metoclopromide-induced tardive orofacial dyskinesias.*

difficult. Extrication of fillings and bruxism causing severe temporo-mandibular jaw pain are other problems and, in chronic severe cases, a general coarsening of features may appear. In some patients more serious and potentially life-threatening complications are seen (Casey and Rabins, 1978). Respiratory dyskinesias including inspiratory sighs and grunts, hyperventilation and irregular disorganised breathing patterns are not uncommon. These sometimes cause dyspnoea, choking episodes with cyanosis and are so disabling as to warrant a tracheostomy (Hunter et al, 1964). Dysphagia with marked weight loss, and recurrent aspiration pneumonitis can also occur; a number of factors including tongue hypertrophy, irregular palatal movements, aerophagy, asynchronous oesophageal contractions and paroxysmal abdominal distension may be responsible. Pharyngeal and laryngeal dyskinesias may compound the speech disturbance leading to an unintelligible dysarthria. Cricopharyngeal myotomy or gastrostomy is needed in severe cases.

Eventually each individual acquires a unique pattern of movements with fixed frequency (usually 0.5–2.0 cycles/second) and roughly constant amplitude. The movements are repetitive and usually lack the darting playfulness of chorea. They are frequently attenuated when the individual uses his mouth and may temporarily be suppressed by will power. Emotional stress and fatigue on the other hand make them worse. The movements are generally easy to imitate and are in fact inappropriate sham movements, reminiscent for example of those occurring normally during a hearty meal.

OCULOFACIAL DYSKINESIAS

Involvement of the upper half of the face is uncommon. Usually the forehead and eyes possess an impassive frozen appearance. Coexisting Parkinsonism (Degkwitz and Wenzel, 1967) is probably the cause for this and infrequent blinking, seborrhoea and a positive glabellar tap sign may be found on examination. Dyskinesias do occur occasionally, however, the commonest being brief vertical rotations of the eyes, eyelid blinking, blepharospasm, eyebrow raising and facial contortions (Crane and Naranjo, 1971; Ayd, 1974).

LIMB AND TRUNK DYSKINESIAS

These are mainly choreic or athetotic and are indistinguishable from those occurring following sustained L-dopa therapy in Parkinson's disease. They occur more commonly below the age of 50 but most elderly individuals with severe orofacial dyskinesia have some. The steady pressure of a dorsiflexed great toe has been reported to produce the unusual complication of a hole in the top of the shoe (Degkwitz, 1969). Pelvic thrusting movements and rocking of the trunk forwards and backwards are fairly common. The gait may be abnormal (Hunter et al, 1964); broad-based, walking on heels, stamping, excessive arm swing and dragging are some of the descriptions used (Simpson and Shrivastava, 1978) and an exaggerated lordosis of the trunk can also be seen (Fig. 12.3). Twisting, spreading flexion-extension movements of the fingers, tapping of the feet, hyperextension and abduction of arms and ballistic and myoclonic movements of the limbs are other features.

TARDIVE DYSTONIA

This is an uncommon sequela and has been most commonly reported in children and young adults. Torticollis, retrocollis and increased scoliosis of the spine have been described (Chateav et al, 1966; Harenko, 1967; Angle and McIntyre, 1968; Crane, 1973; Keegan and Rajput, 1973) either alone or combined with choreo-athetosis. The syndrome is frequently irreversible and unresponsive to anticholinergics or L-dopa. It has been suggested that generalised tardive dystonia is only seen in children or young adults whereas the focal forms are more usual in the middle-aged, thus bearing a striking resemblance to the age-related pattern of idiopathic dystonias. Burke et al (1982) have reviewed 42 patients with ages of onset ranging from 13–60 years and symptoms appearing after three days to 11 years of antipsychotic therapy. Irreversibility

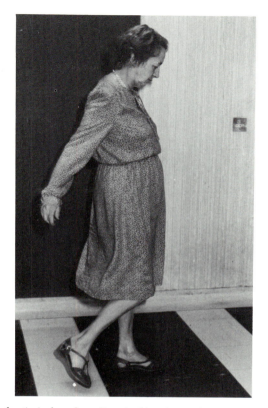

Figure 12.3. Neuroleptic-induced tardive dyskinesia to show abnormal gait and 'le gros ventre'.

despite neuroleptic withdrawal was much commoner than with tardive chorea and therapy was rarely totally successful, although tetrabenazene and anticholinergics were sometimes of use.

NEUROLEPTIC-INDUCED GILLES DE LA TOURETTE SYNDROME

It is now well established that sustained haloperidol therapy for idiopathic Gilles de la Tourette syndrome may occasionally lead to superimposed tardive dyskinesias. Conversely several instances of presumed drug-induced Gilles de la Tourette syndrome have now been reported after long-term antipsychotic medication (see Table 12.2). Most of these cases occurred following neuroleptic withdrawal, and the vocal and bodily tics abated in some on reinstitution of drug treatment. The case reported by De Veaugh-Geiss (1980) of a 65-year-old man treated with phenothiazines for six years is of particular interest. This patient developed drug-induced Parkinsonism early in the course of therapy which slowly worsened on continuing therapy. After four years he then developed

Table 12.2. THE CLINICAL FEATURES OF THE REPORTED CASES OF NEUROLEPTIC-INDUCED GILLES DE LA TOURETTE SYNDROME

Author	Age of patient at onset (yrs)	Sex	Diagnosis	Neuroleptic	Duration of therapy (yrs)	Dose	Clinical features
Klawans et al (1978)	24	F	Schizophrenia Epilepsy	Chlorpromazine Haloperidol	6	Not given	Facial tics, shoulder and arm tics, barking and clicking noises, teeth grinding, dystonic arm postures*
DeVeaugh-Geiss (1980)	65	M	Not specified	Thioridazine Perphenazine	6	100 mg/d–4yrs 4–12 mg/d–2yrs	Grunting, barking, tic-like movements in orofacial region*
Stahl (1980)	26	M	Autism	Not specified	9	Not given	Facial tics, sniffing, grunting, barking, tics of neck, trunk, diaphragm coprolalia*
Fog et al (1981)	22	M	Schizophrenia	Haloperidol	2	4–10 mg/d	Tics of head and body, grunts*
	54	M	Schizophrenia	Phenothiazines Haloperidol	14	5–15 mg/d	Arm tics, shouting, echolalia, door slamming
Mueller and Aminoff (1982)	50	M	Schizophrenia	Chlorpromazine + other phenothiazines	13	400–600 mg/d	Echopraxia/echolalia, howling, orofacial dyskinesia
	27	M	Autism	Thioridazine + chlorpromazine	19	2000 mg/d 2000 mg/d	Head jerks to right, tongue clucking, hand flapping, barking, orofacial dyskinesia*

* Onset on drug withdrawal.

choreiform movements of the head, neck, mouth and limbs typical of tardive dyskinesias. On gradual withdrawal of the drug over 10 months there was an initial increase of tardive dyskinesias but two months after total discontinuation the movements disappeared only to be replaced by grunting, barking and orofacial tics. These symptoms, characteristic of Gilles de la Tourette syndrome, continued for four months then ceased spontaneously. One of the patients reported by Fog et al (1981) had no bodily tics but presented with involuntary vocalisations and orofacial dyskinesias identical to those seen in tardive dyskinesias.

DIFFERENTIAL DIAGNOSIS

The diagnosis of tardive dyskinesias should always be considered in any patient on long-term neuroleptics who develops chorea, athetosis or orofacial dyskinesias. Particularly suggestive is their appearance following discontinuation or reduction in dosage. Acute neuroleptic-induced dyskinesias, while sometimes very similar to tardive dyskinesias, generally occur within the first few weeks of therapy and are improved by anticholinergics. However, occasionally patients receiving depôt preparations of phenothiazines may experience acute dyskinesias after each injection. In practice the main diagnostic stumbling-block is Huntington's disease.

Because this condition commonly presents with psychiatric and behavioural disturbances, which may require antipsychotic medication, and the positive family history may be concealed, the disorder may be mistaken for tardive dyskinesia until progressive dementia ensues. In Huntington's disease, however, there is usually less extreme involvement of oral structures, less stereotypy and a more fleeting, darting playfulness to the abnormal movements. Generalised tardive dystonia in children and young adults differs from the idiopathic form in that there is a positive drug history and it tends to be static or to resolve slowly on drug withdrawal. Copper studies should always be performed to exclude Wilson's disease and a wet blood film to eliminate neuroacanthocytosis. As discussed already, indistinguishable dyskinesias may occur in the unmedicated elderly, edentulous (Sutcher et al, 1971), demented and psychotic.

COURSE

Although a minimum treatment period of one year was traditionally considered necessary for the production of tardive dyskinesias, there are now a number of well-documented cases of the disorder beginning within the first three to six months (Crane, 1973). There is very little information regarding the long-term course of tardive dyskinesias in patients in whom no specific therapeutic interventions are performed. In one study 40% of patients became symptom-free after 15 months without drug modification (Heinrich et al, 1968). Chien and Cole (1973) reported no change in the severity of abnormal movements in 24

patients after 18 months. Finally, Degkwitz et al (1976) re-examined 70 neuroleptic-treated psychiatric patients again after two years and found that 26% had
increased symptoms of tardive dyskinesia, in 23% there was no change and in
10% the abnormal movements had improved. 15% of the patients revealed
tardive dyskinesia for the first time at the second assessment. From the paltry
data available it can be concluded that in the majority of patients tardive
dyskinesia does not appear to be a progressive condition.

Patients are usually still taking antipsychotic medication when the condition
appears but Crane (1973) has estimated that up to 40% of chronically treated
patients may develop dyskinesias on drug withdrawal. The majority of these
probably represent transient withdrawal dyskinesias which appear within the
first 10 days of stopping medication and resolve spontaneously within six weeks
(Jacobson et al, 1974; Gardos et al, 1978). For example in a group of 141
psychotic children, neuroleptic discontinuation led to withdrawal dyskinesias
in 48 (32%). Choreo-athetosis of the limbs, trunk and head were commonest
but mild orofacial dyskinesias and tics occurred in 16%. Rapid disappearance
of these movements resulted in 38% and in the others no opportunity to
observe spontaneous resolution was possible because the children's mental state
demanded the reintroduction of antipsychotic medication within seven days of
withdrawal (Polizos et al, 1973; Ayd, 1974). Dyskinesias which continue for
longer than six weeks after drug withdrawal have been termed covert dyskinesias (Gardos et al, 1978) and the likelihood is that they were being
suppressed by the drug treatment.

On reviewing the literature, Smith and Baldessarini (1980) concluded that
remissions after drug withdrawal were three times commoner in patients under
60 years than those over this age. Patients remitting within one month of
neuroleptic discontinuation were excluded from the analysis. The United States
Task Force on Late Neurological Effects of Antipsychotic drugs concluded that
as many as 50% of patients may improve markedly within a year and improvement may sometimes continue for several years after drug discontinuation (US
Task Force, 1980). The risk of irreversible tardive dyskinesias based on what
paltry data exists is about 10–20% but longer follow-up studies are required.
Prolonged pharmacotherapy may be more likely to lead to irreversibility
(Quitkin et al, 1977; Jeste et al, 1979), but this remains unsubstantiated. To
date complete recovery has been the rule in children and permanent irreversible choreo-athetotic dyskinesias are found almost exclusively in individuals
over 50 years of age. However, irreversible tardive dystonia may occur in young
adults. It is possible that a reduced biological buffer capacity in the elderly is
the explanation for this age difference (Gerlach, 1979).

TREATMENT

In the absence of a safe and effective therapy, prevention becomes of great
importance. In fact the indications for phenothiazines are few and their long-

term use for chronic anxiety states, manic-depressive illness, personality disorders, dyspepsia and persistent vertigo should be discouraged. Only in chronic schizophrenia is the use of maintenance therapy supported by hard data although it is also probably warranted in some cases of Gilles de la Tourette syndrome and chronic pain syndromes. In about 30 controlled studies an average of 56% (range 17–100%) of nearly 3500 schizophrenic patients who received placebo for from 3–12 months deteriorated symptomatically whereas only 17% (range 0–49%) of the patients receiving neuroleptics relapsed (Davis, 1975). While this difference is highly significant it should be noted that almost half the schizophrenics did not deteriorate on placebo.

The use of vigorous diagnostic criteria for schizophrenia is an essential prerequisite for long-term therapy and evidence of drug responsiveness, continuing psychosis or frequent relapses should also be forthcoming. Good medical practice demands a full explanation of the purpose and implications of medical treatment to the patient and his family. For medico-legal purposes a full written note in the patients records documenting the indications for therapy and the fact that the risks have been fully discussed is recommended. The need for continuing therapy must also be regularly reviewed and follow-up notes on this point should be made.

The general pharmacological principle of using the lowest effective dose is particularly important and a patient's drug requirements must be periodically reassessed. Where possible, short-acting drugs should be administered as a single evening dose and the intervals between parenteral depôt preparations can often be gradually increased. Crane (1977) regards a total daily dose of 400 mg chlorpromazine as safe and effective but in patients over 55 the dose should not exceed 150 mg and in the very old an upper limit of 75 mg/d has been quoted.

It is probable, but as yet unproven, that the more prolonged the period of neuroleptic treatment the greater the likelihood that changes conducive to the emergence of tardive dyskinesias will occur. After a single acute psychotic episode it is usually possible to taper off neuroleptics within a few months without relapse. In chronic schizophrenics on therapy in hospital a reasonable approach is to reduce the dose by 10% every three to seven days until it has been discontinued or, alternatively, clear signs of worsening have occurred. If possible treatment should be witheld for at least 14 days. This strategy permits the detection of withdrawal dyskinesias which may signify a prodromal reversible variant of tardive dyskinesia and also enables the patient to have a 'drug holiday'. This strategy may also reduce the risk of receptor hypersensitivity and its use in preventing tardive dyskinesias is under study (American College of Neuropsychopharmacology, 1973). Psychiatric out-patients on chronic neuroleptics should probably be admitted annually to hospital to assess their continuing need for therapy.

Prompt recognition of the first signs of the disorder is another important aspect of management. Probably the earlier the syndrome is detected and the offending neuroleptic withdrawn the better the chances of full recovery (Crane,

1972b). Bradykinesia may mask the early signs of tardive dyskinesia (Degkwitz and Wenzel, 1967) and it is inadvisable to allow drug-induced Parkinsonism to persist for an extended period. Dosage reduction or a switch to another anti-psychotic drug with less powerful extrapyramidal side-effects is preferable to the use of an anticholinergic drug. Although it is generally agreed that anticholinergics aggravate established tardive dyskinesia, it is unclear at present whether prophylactic anticholinergics increase the risk of developing it. In fact drugs such as thioridazine and clozapine with strong inherent anticholinergic properties seem to be relatively less likely to induce tardive dyskinesias. Long-term prophylactic anticholinergic therapy is, however, probably unnecessary in most patients and their withdrawal in patients with emerging tardive dyskinesia may be helpful.

Immediate withdrawal of the offending neuroleptic is the ideal treatment for tardive dyskinesias. Temporary worsening may occur at first but there is then a trend towards gradual improvement over months or years. If on stopping medication the underlying psychosis worsens, there may be no alternative but to reinstitute drug treatment but efforts should always be made to keep the dosage as low as possible. Treatment with haloperidol or one of the relatively selective dopaminergic antagonists (D_2 antagonists) such as oxiperomide or sulpiride may be less hazardous and worth a trial. Increasing the dosage of the offending neuroleptic will usually temporarily suppress the symptoms (Kazamatzuri et al, 1972) but this is an irrational approach and in any case the dyskinesias will often again break through within a few months.

If discontinuation of the antipsychotic drug proves to be totally impossible or tardive dyskinesias become very pronounced after drug withdrawal, the use of pharmacological agents known to suppress hyperkinesias may have to be considered. However, in most instances, the abnormal movements are mild and insufficiently severe to warrant unproven therapies. If it is decided to embark on drug treatment a reasonable approach is to start with the most innocuous available therapy such as a benzodiazepine or lecithin, and, if these prove ineffective, to graduate sequentially to agents with potent effects on dopaminergic systems. A great many drugs have been tried in the treatment of tardive dyskinesia and the consensus view on the effects of some of those studied is shown in Table 12.3. However, the considerable methodological difficulties involved in assessing improvement and the variable diagnostic criteria and trial designs have led to disagreement with respect to the therapeutic worth of many of these drugs.

SOME ADVOCATED THERAPIES

CHOLINERGIC AGENTS

The occurrence of cholinergic hypofunction in tardive dyskinesia has led to attempts to treat the disorder by increasing brain choline levels. This approach also carries the attractive possibility of controlling symptoms without aggra-

Table 12.3. THE EFFECT OF DIFFERENT PHARMACOLOGICAL AGENTS ON TARDIVE DYSKINESIA

Drugs causing partial suppression	Drugs with uncertain or negligible effects	Drugs worsening dyskinesias
Catecholamine-synthesis inhibitor alpha methylpara tyrosine	Cholinergic agents physostigmine choline lecithin arecoline dimethylaminoethanol	Dopamine releasing agents amphetamines
Dopamine depleting agents reserpine tetrabenazene	GABA agents muscimol sodium valproate baclofen gamma acetylenic GABA	Dopamine receptor agonists L-dopa (high doses)
Dopamine receptor blocking drugs phenothiazines butyrophenones clozapine sulpiride oxiperomide	Serotonergic agents l-tryptophan	Anticholinergic agents benzhexol benztropine
Dopamine receptor agonists (sustained treatment) apomorphine L-dopa	Miscellaneous des-tyrosine-gamma-endorphin papaverine propranolol phenytoin	
Benzodiazepines phenobarbitone		

vating the underlying psychosis. The observation that physostigmine, a centrally acting reversible anticholinesterase, has a mild although somewhat inconsistent beneficial effect (Klawans and Rubovitz, 1974; Tarsy et al, 1974) led to the search for orally active, centrally active cholinergic agents. Oral choline has been administered with reputedly beneficial results (Klawans and Rubovitz, 1974; Growdon et al, 1977) but it is often poorly tolerated because of the fishy odour it causes. Lecithin is a more acceptable way to administer choline and may be beneficial occasionally (Growdon et al, 1978). Tacrine, a centrally acting anticholinesterase, has also been claimed to be beneficial in eight patients at a dose of 45–90 mg/d producing a mean 43% reduction in disability (Ingram and Newgreen, 1983). However, arecoline, a muscarinic agonist derived from the betel nut was ineffective in doses of up to 20 mg/d (Nutt et al, 1979). Dimethylaminoethanol (Deanol) which is converted to choline in the peripheral tissues of some animal species has also been extensively used, especially in the United States with mixed success (Granacher et al, 1975). Up to the present time the use of currently available cholinergic agents has proved generally disappointing.

DOPAMINE DEPLETING AGENTS

Reserpine causes pre-synaptic neuronal depletion of catecholamines by preventing their uptake into storage vesicles and thereby allowing degradation by monoamine oxidase. Despite the fact that chronic reserpine administration may induce supersensitivity changes in animals identical to those seen after phenothiazines it has rarely been reported to cause tardive dyskinesia. In several uncontrolled short duration studies reserpine 1–5 mg/d has in fact been reported to suppress tardive dyskinesias, although Parkinsonism frequently occurred (Villeneuve and Borszomenyi, 1970; Sato et al, 1971; Duvoisin, 1972). However, the low incidence of tardive dyskinesias in patients treated with reserpine may simply reflect the fact that relatively few people have been treated for long periods and the occurrence of disuse or denervation supersensitivity in animal models raises the possibility that the drug might eventually contribute to the pathophysiological process it is being used to treat. Tetrabenazene is a shorter-acting drug with similar dopamine depleting properties. In doses of 75–300 mg/d it has been shown to abolish tardive dyskinesia but depression, sedation and Parkinsonism are common complications (Brandrup, 1961; Godwin-Austen and Clark, 1971; Kazamatzuri et al, 1972a) and the effects of long-term administration are not known.

Alphamethylparatyrosine is an inhibitor of tyrosine hydroxylase, the rate-limiting enzyme for dopamine and noradrenaline synthesis, which in high doses is capable of reducing brain dopamine in animals. In a study on 24 psychiatric patients with tardive dyskinesia treatment with alphamethylparatyrosine 4 g for three days reduced hypermotility but did not change the amplitude of the movements (Gerlach and Thorsen, 1976). Improvement has also been reported in another study (Chase, 1972), and Fahn (1978) has claimed excellent results with the combined use of reserpine (4–6 mg/d) and alphamethylparatyrosine (250–750 mg/d).

Alphamethyldopa has poorly-understood and complicated actions on the synthesis, storage and post-synaptic actions of catecholamines. Two of three patients treated in doses of 750–1000 mg/d improved in one study (Villeneuve and Boszormenyi, 1970) but in a second controlled study no significant effect occurred (Kazamatsuri et al, 1972c).

DOPAMINE RECEPTOR BLOCKING DRUGS

Paradoxically drugs which block post-synaptic dopamine receptors attenuate tardive dyskinesia. If tardive dyskinesia develops during sustained neuroleptic therapy, an increase in the dose of the offending medicine often temporarily abolishes the dyskinesias. Pimozide has been shown to ameliorate tardive dyskinesias in a controlled study in 18 patients carried out over six weeks, but the abnormal movements recurred when the drug was discontinued (Claveria et al, 1975). Haloperidol (8–16 mg/d) and thiopropopazate (40–80 mg/d) have also been reported to improve neuroleptic-induced tardive orofacial dyskinesias over a four-week period (Kazamatsuri et al, 1972b). Improvement, however, is often short-lived and may only occur with the development of Parkinsonism or sedation. After a period of symptomatic relief tardive dyskinesias usually break through again often with increased vehemence.

There has been considerable interest recently in the use of neuroleptics with a reported low incidence of tardive dyskinesias. Clozapine and the newer dibenzodiazepines, the D_2 receptor antagonists, oxiperomide, sulpiride and tiapride, and chlorprothixene and oxypertine all effectively reduce tardive dyskinesias. It remains to be seen, however, whether their long-term use leads to the same problems of increasingly severe breakthrough dyskinesias as occur with more widely used antipsychotic drugs. For the present they probably represent the most effective available therapy for severe tardive dyskinesias, particularly in patients who still require antipsychotic medication.

DOPAMINERGIC AGONISTS

In view of the hypothesis that reduced dopaminergic activity and dopaminergic receptor hypersensitivity could be instrumental in inducing tardive dyskinesia it might be expected that large acute doses of dopaminergic agonists should aggravate the condition. This has been confirmed in a few studies although the effect is variable. For instance Hippius and Longemann (1970) increased the severity of tardive dyskinesia in only one-third of patients after an intravenous bolus of 100 mg L-dopa, and the administration of 1200 mg L-dopa in combination with 300 mg benserazide for 14 days in another study resulted in only a moderate exacerbation of dyskinesia (Gerlach et al, 1974).

Carroll et al (1977) found that 2–4 g/d of L-dopa actually reduced the severity of tardive dyskinesias over a 12-day period.

Apomorphine, a post-synaptic dopamine receptor agonist, might also be expected to exacerbate tardive dyskinesia. However, when administered to Parkinsonian patients, it may actually attenuate L-dopa-induced choreoathetosis (Duby et al, 1972) and in parenteral doses of 0.75–6 mg/d it has also been reported to reduce tardive dyskinesia (Carroll et al, 1977; Smith et al, 1977). The mechanism for this effect is unclear but may arise from selective pre-synaptic effects or the drug's partial agonist properties.

Both L-dopa and apomorphine can depress persistent dyskinesias in monkeys (Gunne and Barany, 1980) and the biochemical and behavioural signs of dopaminergic hypersensitivity are decreased by chronic L-dopa therapy in animals (Ezrin-Waters and Seeman, 1978; Friedhoff et al, 1980). Although early trials with high doses of L-dopa were disappointing (Klawans and McKendal, 1971; Gerlach et al, 1974) several recent studies using moderate doses of L-dopa and peripheral dopa decarboxylase inhibitor in patients with tardive dyskinesia alone or with coexistent drug-induced Parkinsonism have shown that after treatment for several weeks the tardive dyskinesias may improve to a degree not seen in controls (Alpert and Friedhoff, 1983; Shoulson, 1983). Others, however, have failed to confirm these findings (Bjørndal et al, 1980; Hardie et al, 1983). This approach to therapy is likely to be most effective in accelerating spontaneous resolution of tardive dyskinesias after neuroleptic withdrawal, but carries a slight risk of triggering a psychotic relapse.

OTHER DRUG TREATMENTS

Several agents that effect the inhibitory neurotransmitter gamma-aminobutyric acid (GABA) have been tried. A gabaminergic striato-nigral pathway projects on to the dopaminergic nigro-striatal bundle but the interplay of these two systems is still poorly understood. Muscimol, a GABA agonist, can reduce tardive dyskinesias in a modest way but sedation, confusion and accentuation of schizophrenic symptoms occur (Chase and Tamminga, 1979). The GABA-transaminase inhibitors, sodium valproate (Linnoila et al, 1976) and gamma-acetylenic GABA (Casey et al, 1980) have also been claimed to have anti-hyperkinetic effects and baclofen (p-chlorophenyl GABA) which has complex inhibitory effects on several central neurotransmitters may also produce benefit when added to antidopaminergic treatment (Gerlach et al, 1978). The indirect acting GABA agonist, gamma vinyl GABA, an irreversible inhibitor of GABA transaminase given in a dose of 3000 mg/d produced antidyskinetic effects in seven schizophrenics with tardive dyskinesia in which the offending neuroleptic had been withdrawn. Cerebrospinal fluid examination revealed a selective increase in GABA and homocarnosine and no psychotoxic or Parkinsonian side-effects were observed (Tamminga et al, 1983). Calcium hopantenate, another gabamimetic drug, has also been reported to be beneficial. These promising results raise the possibility that derangement of striatal and pallidal

GABA mechanisms may be an important primary aetiological factor in tardive dyskinesia but further clinical pharmacological studies are required.

Based on the notion that an imbalance between dopamine and 5-hydroxy-tryptamine might be involved in extrapyramidal disease, the natural serotonin precursor, 1-tryptophan has been tried in a small number of patients without substantial benefit (Prange et al, 1973; Jus et al, 1974).

A number of other drugs with poorly defined effects on the central nervous system have been reported to be beneficial, including lithium in modest dosage (Simpson et al, 1976), papaverine (Gardos and Cole, 1975), benzodiazepines (Bobruff et al, 1981), barbiturates (Sovner and Loadman, 1978), low dose propranolol (Bacher and Lewis, 1980) and the dopamine beta hydroxylase inhibitor fusaric acid (Viukari and Linnoila, 1977).

GENERAL MEASURES

The cosmetic impact of orofacial dyskinesias can be reduced by chewing gum or sucking sweets. The edentulous state can lead to mouthing movements *per se* and compound drug-induced dyskinesias; regular dental care, therefore, is an essential part of management. Biofeedback techniques may also prove valuable and Farrar (1976) has reported their use in spontaneous orofacial dyskinesia. Regular physical activity and relaxation techniques should also be encouraged as the abnormal movements are often at their worst during inactivity or stress.

SURGERY

Stereotactic surgery has occasionally been performed for severe disabling cases but the high frequency of axial involvement in tardive dyskinesia makes this an inappropriate approach to treatment for most patients. Nashold (1969) treated three patients with unilateral or bilateral ablative lesions to the region of the red nucleus and the pre-rubral field of Forel and there is also a further report of temporary surgical success on truncal movements (Druckman, et al, 1962).

2. PSYCHOMOTOR STIMULANT-INDUCED DYSKINESIAS

GENERAL INTRODUCTION

The various analogues and isomers of amphetamine, cocaine and pemoline are the principal drugs in this category that have found therapeutic application. The amphetamines are potent, indirect sympathomimetic drugs which when administered orally cause elevation in systolic and diastolic blood pressure, mild relaxation of bronchial muscle, and excitatory effects on the nervous system. These effects include stimulation of the medullary respiratory centre and facilitation of monosynaptic and polysynaptic transmission in the spinal cord. The psychic effects are dose-dependent and are affected by the personality and mood of the individual. Increased alertness, self-confidence and initiative, elation and euphoria, wakefulness, decreased fatigue with improved concentration and pressure of speech are among the most commonly reported effects.

Edeleano first synthesised amphetamine in 1887 but it was Alles in 1933 who first realised that it might be of use in clinical medicine, in the beginning as a nasal decongestant and then after self-experimentation as an antidepressant. Within a short time it was being widely administered as a psychic energiser and by the 1940s had been tried in conditions as diverse as obesity, urticaria, post-encephalitic Parkinsonism, caffeine mania, heart block and epilepsy. Since then indications for its use have steadily dwindled and it is now probably the drug of choice only for narcolepsy, and together with pemoline and methylphenidate, may be of benefit for the hyperkinetic behavioural disorders of childhood. Fenfluramine is prescribed by many physicians to suppress appetite in obese patients.

During the Spanish Civil War and World War Two amphetamines were given to pilots to maintain their alertness on long-range bombing missions and to army truck-drivers carrying out arduous nocturnal manoeuvres. Indeed they became a standard part of military survival kits and 72 million tablets were issued to the British forces. Objective testing confirmed that amphetamines increased the capacity for simple physical and mental tasks and could increase intelligence up to eight points on psychological test batteries.

Not unreasonably, therefore, they came to be regarded as a 'superman drug' essential for those who wanted 'to get places, do things and be somebody'. The essence of this sentiment was captured by Joseph Mankiewics, the Hollywood dramatist, who, as a volunteer subject in one of the early studies wrote:

> I felt like God . . . it was unbelievable . . . I wrote fifty pages of dialogue . . . I went into a story conference I was absolutely brilliant.

Needless to say widespread illicit use resulted from this attitude and the prevailing ignorance of the potential dangers. In the 1960s the drug became popular in Great Britain as a 'spree' drug for the fashion-conscious, dance-crazy mods who invented slang names for the many preparations such as Purple Hearts, black bombers and French blues. A weekend of thrills was generally followed by a miserable Monday with profound malaise, lethargy and exhaustion and thus, in some unstable individuals, led to a gradual escalation of drug intake. Dependency syndromes became a mounting social problem occurring particularly amongst adolescents with personality and identity problems and also in bored, understimulated housewives. Addiction was complicated by recurrent drug-induced psychoses, social disintegration and abuse of other drugs such as alcohol and barbiturates. Restrictions on the prescription of these drugs helped temporarily to curb their illegal use but there continues to be a flourishing black market in both cocaine and amphetamines.

Central nervous stimulants generally increase motor activity, and stereotyped movements (pundning) in chronic amphetamine and phenmetrazine addicts have been recognised for about 20 years. Choreo-athetosis, dystonia and tics have also been reported but are rare.

Large single doses of amphetamines produce stereotyped activity in mammalian and avian species consisting of the fixed repetition over long periods of time of purposeless motor acts. These are characteristic for each species and in rats, whose major means of exploring their environment is olfactory, they consist of sniffing, licking, gnawing and head bobbing, usually conducted hunched up in one corner of the cage (Randrup and Munkvad, 1967). In laboratory cats repetitive sniffing occurs whereas in less confined animals furtive side to side glancing movements occur. Non-human primates develop eye-hand examination, visual scanning and side to side tracking with self-picking and grooming behaviour. After chronic administration they also develop oral dyskinesias, dystonia and loss of normal social, sexual and maternal behaviour (Ellinwood and Kilbey, 1977).

Amphetamine, methylphenidate and cocaine all increase the release of catecholamines from synaptic terminals and also inhibit pre-synaptic re-uptake mechanisms. By one or other means, therefore, an increase in the quantities of noradrenaline and dopamine available for receptor stimulation occurs (Moore, 1977). After the injection of very high doses of d-amphetamine to rats, increased release and re-uptake inhibition of 5-hydroxy-tryptamine also occur which contribute to the bizarre circling and backward walking which is seen in some animals. (Curzon et al, 1979). 5-hydroxytryptamine release is a particularly important property of fenfluramine.

Compelling evidence now exists to implicate increased dopaminergic stimulation in the mediation of amphetamine-induced stereotypy in animals. This is drawn from work using the d- and l-isomers of amphetamine which have differential effects on noradrenaline and dopamine re-uptake, from selective lesioning of dopaminergic pathways, the use of dopamine B-hydroxylase inhibitors and, finally, from the micro-injection of amphetamine analogues and dopamine into the corpus striatum (Randrup and Munkvad, 1970; Snyder, 1972). It is now believed that stereotyped behaviour in rodents is controlled mainly by the dopaminergic nigrostriatal pathway whereas increased locomotor activity and rearing, which occurs with lower doses of amphetamine, involve the nucleus accumbens (Kelly et al, 1975) and possibly noradrenergic systems. The similarity of the stereotyped behavioural responses in animals to those occurring in amphetamine addicts is striking and suggests that increased dopamine release in the striatum might also be the mechanism responsible for pundning. The occasional occurrence of tics, chorea and dystonia at lower doses, however, may depend on some undetermined idiosyncratic response.

PUNDNING (KNICK-KNACKING)

Pundning, literally translated block-head, is a term used by Swedish amphetamine addicts to describe a purposeless fixed behaviour provoked by high doses of central nervous stimulants. The monograph by Bonhoff and Lewrenz, published in 1954, mentions a man who under the influence of amphetamine cleaned his car over and over again, and Bleuler described among cocaine users a 'preoccupation with various tasks that lead to nothing' (Bleuler, 1924). The first comprehensive accounts of this extraordinary condition, however, came from Scandinavia and California in the 1960s where stimulant abuse was rife (Kramer et al, 1967; Rylander, 1972).

As early as 1942 it was estimated that up to 3% of the Swedish population were taking amphetamines and, as a consequence of its strict restriction, many of the Swedish *habitués* had switched to phenmetrazine or methylphenidate by the early 1960s. Rylander studied 154 of these addicts in the Forensic Psychiatry Clinic in Stockholm and by skilful interrogation ascertained that doses as great as 1–2 g were being injected intravenously each day. The illegally obtained tablets would be crushed, added to water and the gruel-like mixture then crudely filtered through wads of cotton wool before injection. 101 individuals had experienced a drug-induced psychosis at some stage and 40 recollected periods of stereotyped motor behaviour. These 40 addicts were studied in some detail and asked to fill in a questionnaire. From this detailed enquiry and a similarly designed study by Schiorring (1977) conducted on 50 Swedish and Danish addicts a clear picture of the condition is now available. Schiorring's study is particularly valuable as he was able to observe six addicts during a 'run' (30 minutes after the intravenous injection of 200–350 mg phenmetrazine). Most of the informants had criminal records and more than half were considered to have an underlying sociopathic or schizoid personality disorder. 59% of Rylander's cases had been taking central nervous stimulants regularly for more than two years.

The constant ritualistic performance of a motor act is the hallmark of pundning and manipulation of technical equipment such as radio sets, clocks and car engines is the commonest activity in men. One man bought 12 radio sets and spent 24 hours assembling them and then immediately dismantling them. Tidying rooms and drawers, washing dishes, perpetual hair brushing, putting on make-up and manicuring were the commonest activities in women. Artistic pastimes, including drawing, painting and writing were also quite common. Distinctive walking patterns were also seen, such as pacing up and down the same part of the street, marching round in circles often lifting the legs high or occasionally walking backwards. Schiorring reports one gang of motorcyclists who after taking amphetamines drove 200 times round the same block of houses. Continuous searching in attics or houses, and extended monologues devoid of substantial content and peppered with perseverative phrases were other manifestations. Some addicts were in the habit of taking their cars out and driving nowhere in particular for hours on end. Scher (1966) describes the phenomenon as follows:

One of the most pecular phenomena which may occur in the course of the use of amphetamines especially methamphetamine is what is called 'being hung-up'. An individual who is 'hung-up' will literally get stuck in a repetitious act or thought for hours. He may sit in a tub and bathe all day long, clean up the house or a particular item, hold a note or phrase of music or engage in non-ejaculatory intercourse for extended periods.

The Scandinavian addicts' descriptions of pundning are equally instructive:

A rigid behaviour, a never ceasing repetition of certain actions like the otter in the zoo.

A girl I know can tidy up her handbag in a mechanical way for many hours (even a whole day). She takes the things out and puts them back. She has done this for 6–7 years now.

At the final examination I was really high on Preludin. I wrote my name a hundred times on the paper and thought that I had solved the problem.

One guy I know always worked with/fiddled with cars when high. Once I saw him lying under the car at 7 p.m. A lot of engine parts were spread on the ground around him. The next morning he was still there without having fixed the car.

Most addicts withdraw into themselves during pundning, becoming tacit and unresponsive and often giving the impression of absent-mindedness ('snowed under'). In fact all the six cases witnessed by Schiorring behaved psychotically, staring into space, with lack of eye contact, experiencing visual and tactile hallucinations and paranoid delusions. However, most regarded it as an enjoyable experience which not even the desire to micturate or defecate, nor even a sexual overture, would interrupt. Invitation to take more drugs or fear of imminent arrest were more likely to abort the abnormal behaviour. Most felt angry, irritable or anxious after enforced disruption of pundning. Interestingly the pundning act is consistently the same in each addict and tends to be something he or she enjoys doing; a swindler, for example, wrote out hundreds of counterfeit cheques oblivious of his impending arrest. Although it has been considered by many authors as an obsessional behaviour, Rylander has pointed out that it is only if the act is interrupted that any compulsive urge becomes apparent.

CHOREA (THE JERKING SYNDROME)

2.5 mg/d of d-amphetamine can occasionally provoke orofacial hyperkinesias and chorea of the limbs in susceptible children with minimal brain dysfunction (Mattson and Calverly, 1968; Case and McAndrew, 1974). Similar reactions have also occurred with methylphenidate (Palatucci, 1974; Weiner et al, 1978) and pemoline (Nausieda et al, 1981). In these susceptible individuals, repeated challenges with different central nervous stimulants always induce the same response, and discontinuation of the offending agent invariably leads to rapid resolution.

In chronic drug abusers, generalised choreo-athetosis is usually dose-dependent and typically is seen in the absence of any associated psychosis. Lundh and Tunving (1981) have reported four individuals who had injected themselves over years with gram doses of amphetamine and developed severe chorea of the trunk, limbs and face with hypotonia and ataxia. In one patient wild flinging movements of the limbs were seen while in another curious twisting of the trunk occurred earning him the nickname of 'the screw'. In some of these cases hyperkinesias persisted in mild form for up to three years after amphetamine discontinuation.

Buccolingual dyskinesias with bruxism have also been reported in an amphetamine addict following the ingestion of about 120 mg of fenfluramine (Brandon, 1969). Indeed, it has been suggested that continuous chewing movements, teeth grinding and incessant rubbing of the tongue against the lips are helpful signs in enabling chronic amphetamine users to be recognised. Face picking and stereotyped touching are other characteristic behaviours.

DYSTONIA

Torticollis has been described after low (Mattson and Calverly, 1968) and high doses of amphetamine (Lundh and Tunving, 1981). An acute dystonic reaction with retrocollis and tongue and throat spasms also occurred in a 43-year-old woman after fenfluramine (Sanamman, 1974).

TICS

Although relatively rare, there are a number of undoubted case reports of central nervous system stimulants provoking tics. Denckla et al (1976) studied 5000 children with minimal brain dysfunction seen over five years and noted that 2% of the 1254 neurologically referred children had pre-treatment tics compared with 5% of the psychiatrically referred cases. Forty-five (3%) of the 1520 children treated with methylphenidate had pre-treatment tics. In six of these aggravation of tics occurred during treatment and 14 further children developed tics for the first time. Eighteen of these 20 children were boys and most were considered to have obsessional personality traits. The age range was 7–14 years with a mean of 10 years and the mean daily dose of methylphenidate was 2.5 mg (10–60 mg). In three patients the tics appeared only when the dosage was increased and disappeared on dose reduction. Thirteen became symptom-free on stopping the drug. The onset or exacerbation of tic severity occurred in the first week in five patients, between one week and one month in two patients, one month to three months in four patients, after six months in two patients and one year in seven patients. Eye blinks, facial grimacing, head jerks and neck tics were the most frequent abnormal movements. Denckla and her colleagues concluded that tics related to methylphenidate administration were rare and might be due to an idiosyncratic response. Pollack et al (1977) described a 5-year-old boy with minimal brain dysfunction who, after

Table 12.4. CLINICAL FEATURES OF THE REPORTED CASES OF CNS STIMULANT-INDUCED GILLES DE LA TOURETTE SYNDROME

Author	Age of patient at onset (yrs)	Sex	Diagnosis	CNS stimulant	Duration of therapy	Dosage / day	Clinical features
Golden (1974)	9	M	Minimal brain dysfunction	Methylphenidate	8 weeks	20 mg*	Grimacing, grunts, cough barks, tics of face and arms
Golden (1977)	5	M	Minimal brain dysfunction	Methylphenidate	Immediate onset	Not specified	blinks, hoots, multifocal tics
	5	M	Deaf; minimal brain dysfunction	Methylphenidate	2nd challenge	Not specified	jerking tics, grunts
Pollack et al (1977)	5	M	Minimal brain dysfunction	Methylphenidate d-amphetamine	6 months 2nd challenge	10 mg 20 mg 60 mg*	Eye tics, facial grimaces Tics increased, limb tics, throat clearing, snorting
Bremness and Sverd (1979)	9	M		Minimal brain dysfunction	10 weeks		Barking, squeals, echolalia, facial tics, tics of head, shoulder
Mitchell and Matthews (1980)	10	M	Minimal brain dysfunction	Pemoline	8 weeks	37.5 mg*	Eye rolling, blinking, grunting, head neck jerk
Bachman (1981)	9	M	Minimal brain dysfunction	Pemoline	Few weeks	75 mg	Eye blinks, jaw jerks, arm jerks, hip turns, humming, yelping
Bonthala and West (1983)	52	M	Personality disorder	Pemoline	Overdosage	400 mg	Grunts, coprolalia, tongue protrusion, limb choreo-athetosis, neck twitches

* Complete resolution on drug discontinuation.

five months' methylphenidate treatment (10 mg/d), developed facial tics, eye blinks and grimacing and one year later, while receiving 20 mg/d of d-amphetamine, started to have additional vocal tics. This child had a first cousin with Gilles de la Tourette syndrome. A number of case reports of stimulant-induced Gilles de la Tourette syndrome can also be found in the literature (Table 12.4) and the fact that the tics disappeared in some on withdrawing the drug suggests a strong cause and effect relationship.

Central nervous stimulants may also rarely increase spontaneously occurring tics, an effect first reported by Singer (1963) and subsequently confirmed by others (Meyerhoff and Snyder, 1973; Fras and Karlavage, 1977; Cohen et al, 1978; Feinberg and Carroll, 1979; Sleator, 1980). Present evidence favours this as a dose-related phenomenon, more likely to occur with the d- than 1-isomer of amphetamine.

Golden (1977b) sent a questionnaire to members of the United States Tourette Syndrome Association to enquire about the use of central nervous system stimulants. He then sent a further detailed form to 32 of the 88 individuals who had received these drugs. There were 41 separate exposures nearly all to either methylphenidate or d-amphetamine and 25 individuals had taken the drug on 34 occasions after the diagnosis had been made, usually while receiving haloperidol. Symptoms worsened in 18 of these and in the seven cases in whom the drugs had been given for hyperactive behaviour before the onset of Gilles de la Tourette syndrome, three developed multiple vocal and bodily tics (Table 12.0). In the investigation by Denckla et al (1976) only 13.3% of the hyperkinetic children with pre-existing tics experienced worsening of symptoms with methylphenidate. Bachman (1981) has observed exacerbation in three of 14 patients who received stimulants and improvement occurred in one.

Shapiro and Shapiro (1981a) found that 21 of 134 patients with Gilles de la Tourette syndrome seen over a one-year period had received stimulants, in the majority after the diagnosis had been made. After a mean dose of 29 mg/d methylphenidate only four (19%) reported an increase in tics. They also drew attention to the fact that behavioural disorders indistinguishable from those seen in minimal brain dysfunction occur in at least 50% of patients with Gilles de la Tourette syndrome providing plenty of scope for diagnostic error. In fact these authors consider that the case for central nervous stimulants causing tics or aggravating those already present is unproven and recommend their use in combination with haloperidol to treat learning and concentration difficulties in patients with Gilles de la Tourette syndrome.

3. L-DOPA-INDUCED DYSKINESIAS

GENERAL INTRODUCTION

3:4 dihydroxyphenylalanine (dopa) is a naturally occurring amino-acid which is found in high concentrations in certain fungi and leguminous plants.

The broad bean (*Vicia faba*) and the Indian herbal medicine, cowhage (*Mucuna pruriens*), contain particularly large quantities and botanists have postulated that dopa's emetic properties are biologically advantageous in protecting these species from insect attack. Dopa was first synthesised in 1911 by Funk but it was not until 1960 when Hornykiewicz discovered a deficiency of dopamine in the corpus striatum of patients with Parkinson's disease that its potential medicinal properties were considered.

The biosynthetic pathway of catecholamines was first proposed by Blaschko in 1939, extrapolating from the properties of the recently discovered l-aromatic amino-acid decarboxylase. Tyrosine, the dietary amino-acid precursor is first hydroxylated by tyrosine hydroxylase and a pteridine co-factor, to form dopa. Although this is now considered to be the rate-limiting step and is controlled by catecholamine release, the constant for the Michaelis-Menton equation (Km) of the enzyme is such that it is normally more or less saturated in relation to its substrate. L-aromatic amino-acid decarboxylase then converts dopa to dopamine and in noradrenaline-rich areas of the brain such as the hypothala-

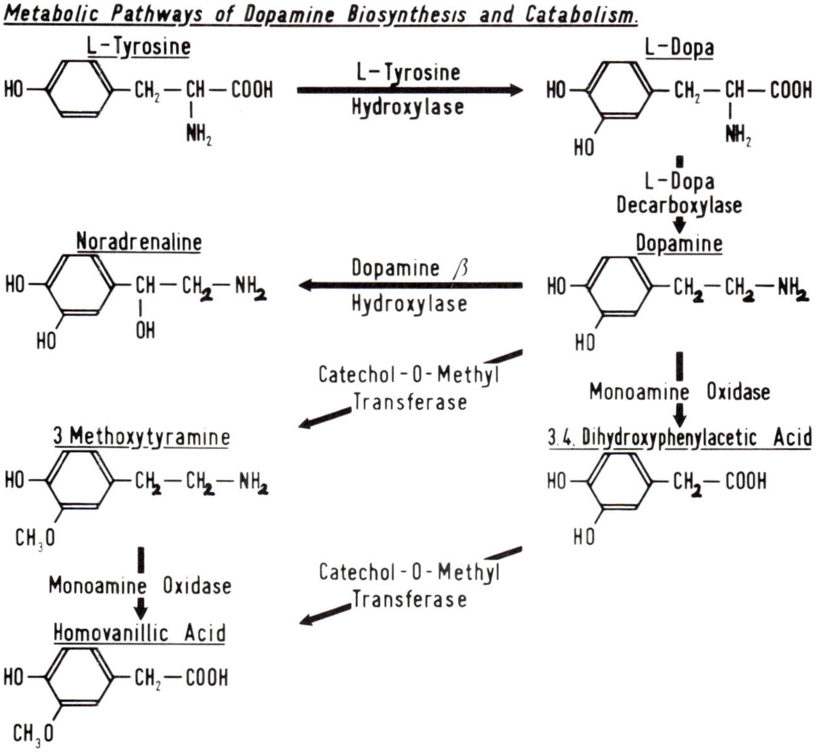

Figure 12.4. The metabolic pathways of dopamine biosynthesis and catabolism.

mus and locus coeruleus dopamine is converted to noradrenaline by dopamine-beta-hydroxylase. L-aromatic amino-acid decarboxylase is a ubiquitous enzyme in the brain and also converts 5-hydroxy-tryptophan to 5-hydroxy-tryptamine. 95% of the enzyme's activity may be inhibited without impairing dopamine synthesis. Catecholamines are mainly inactivated in the central nervous system by energy-dependent re-uptake mechanisms, although two relatively non-specific enzymes, monoamine oxidase and catechol-o-methyl transferase are also involved (Fig. 12.4).

The concept of Parkinson's disease as a dopamine deficiency state encouraged attempts to replenish the missing chemical. Dopamine itself is poorly absorbed from the gut and cannot cross the blood-brain barrier. As a result attention focused on the natural precursor dihydroxyphenylalanine. In 1960 Degkwitz showed that L-dopa could reverse reserpine-induced Parkinsonism and shortly after this Birkmayer in Vienna and Barbeau in Montreal confirmed its efficacy in the idiopathic disease. Only small quantities of the drug were available at this time and the really dramatic potential of this treatment had to await the studies of Cotzias in 1967. Working at the Brookhaven Laboratories in New York he administered large doses (3–16 g/d) of racemic dopa and reported 'a striking sustained clinical improvement in some patients. He had reasoned that the low melanin concentrations found in the substantia nigra of Parkinsonians might be responsible for the symptoms. He initially gave beta-melanocyte-stimulating hormone in the hope of repleting nigral neuromelanin but this actually aggravated the condition and produced skin pigmentation. This finding he interpreted as due to the shift of melanin precursors from brain to skin. By then administering large doses of the common precursor dopa, he hoped to saturate aromatic amino-acid decarboxylase and thereby replenish central dopamine and melanin.

In fact L-dopa probably works by replacing deficient dopamine at striatal receptor sites although this remains unproven. The reason such large quantities needed to be given was that 95% of orally administered L-dopa is metabolised peripherally by aromatic amino-acid decarboxylase in the gut wall and cerebral capillaries where it is converted to dopamine. The development of effective dopa decarboxylase inhibitors with a predominantly peripheral action has represented an extremely valuable refinement to treatment. The last decade has confirmed L-dopa as a valuable palliative agent in the management of Parkinsonism, relieving temporarily the cardinal features of the illness and improving quality of life. Sustained therapy, however, brought with it a number of challenging problems collectively called the long-term L-dopa syndrome. Paroxysmal, reversible, abnormal involuntary movements are the commonest drug-induced complication but capricious sudden swings in motor performance and visual pseudo-hallucinations may also mar the therapeutic response.

EPIDEMIOLOGY

Adventitious involuntary movements of a type not previously encountered in idiopathic Parkinson's disease are the major disabling and dose-limiting complication of long-term L-dopa treatment (Cotzias et al, 1969). It seems that a specific neuropathological substrate is an important predisposing factor for their occurrence in man as they have not as yet been reported in normal control subjects, acromegalics or patients with breast cancer (Barbeau, 1969; Markham, 1971) treated with dopaminergic agonists. Apart from a single case report occurring in a patient with motor neurone disease (Lieberman et al, 1972), they have in fact only been recorded in patients with neurological diseases known to damage the basal ganglia (Chase et al, 1973). L-dopa-induced dyskinesias commonly bear a close resemblance to chorea seen in Huntington's disease. In this context it is of interest that L-dopa may aggravate Huntington's chorea (Klawans, 1973) and that reversible chorea has been provoked by L-dopa in about half of the unaffected off-spring of sufferers with this disease (Klawans et al, 1972). However, other degenerative extrapyramidal syndromes affecting the corpus striatum such as striato-nigral degeneration, multiple cerebral infarcts with Parkinsonian features and the Steele-Richardson-Olszewski syndrome are in general refractory to both the anti-Parkinsonian and dyskinesia-promoting effects of L-dopa.

In marked contrast patients with post-encephalitic Parkinson's disease are exquisitely responsive to even small doses of the drug often exhibiting intolerable dyskinesias within the first two weeks of treatment. Previous stereotactic thalamotomy may temporarily protect against limb chorea but axial hyperkinesias and dystonia are just as common as in non-operated cases (Mones et al, 1971; Duvoisin, 1973). Present evidence does not exclude the possibility that, if much higher doses of L-dopa were given to normal individuals for very long periods of time dyskinesias might occur.

In Parkinson's disease their prevalence is directly related to the duration of treatment and with maximum tolerated doses of L-dopa in combination with a peripheral dopa decarboxylase inhibitor, at least 70% of cases have some abnormal involuntary movements within a year of starting therapy. Probably every patient would ultimately experience dyskinesias to some degree if the dose were pushed high enough and treatment continued for a sufficient length of time.

There is no absolute relationship between the onset of dyskinesias and dosage of L-dopa. A few susceptible individuals experience florid involuntary movements at subtherapeutic doses (100 mg L-dopa/d as combination therapy) whereas other patients tolerate with benefit 1750 mg/d for years without ever manifesting dyskinesias. Furthermore, relief of Parkinsonian disabilities usually peaks several months before the emergence of chorea. Once established, however, the dyskinesias are clearly dose-related and even small drops in dosage may abolish them completely.

A long pre-treatment duration of disease may predispose to L-dopa-induced dyskinesias (Cotzias et al, 1969; Klawans and Bergen, 1975) but this may to some extent be a function of disease severity and as Duvoisin (1976) has indicated could be explained by attempts to get a better result in the more disabled patient by pushing the dose higher. In fact, in the early years of high-dose therapy, the appearance of abnormal hyperkinetic movements was the end point used to titrate dosage to maximum levels.

Mones et al (1971) considered the elderly patient and those with long-standing disease to be most at risk. Klawans and Garvin (1969) found bucco-lingual dyskinesias to bear no relationship to pre-treatment disease severity whereas limb dyskinesias were more frequent in those with significant disability. On the other hand Markham (1971) and Chase et al (1973) found no correlation between the incidence of dyskinesias and either duration or severity of Parkinson's disease.

Controversy also exists with respect to the side of initial involvement in Parkinsonian patients with asymmetrical disease. Most authorities consider that in patients with predominantly unilateral disease, peak-dose choreo-athetosis usually starts on the more severely affected side and tends to remain more pronounced on the side with most Parkinsonian disability (Mones et al, 1973). Duvoisin (1976), however, believes that choreiform dyskinesias are greater on the side last affected chronologically in the evolution of the disease whereas the involuntary movements on the side with more severe Parkinsonism tend to be dystonic.

ANIMAL DATA

There is no shortage of putative paradigms for L-dopa-induced dyskinesias but it is not clear which, if any, of these is appropriate. L-dopa and the dopamine receptor agonists produce abnormal hyperactivity in rodents with stereotyped gnawing and rearing behaviour. Dyskinesias resembling those provoked in Parkinsonian patients also occur after the injection of large doses of L-dopa into monkeys. In one study the acute intraperitoneal injection of 100–400 mg/g of L-dopa together with 20–80 mg/g of peripheral dopa decarboxylase inhibitor produced, within one to two hours of the injection, twisting movements of the mouth, tongue, jaw and neck with choreas of the limbs. The movements abated within six hours but two of the monkeys collapsed and died. The peak plasma dopa levels recorded in the animals were four or five times the highest levels recorded during L-dopa treatment for Parkinson's disease (Mones, 1971, 1973). Sassin et al (1972) gave serially increasing doses of L-dopa (up to 400 mg/g) to eight macaque monkeys and observed chewing, lip smacking, tongue protrusion and increased grooming effects which could be reproduced by apomorphine. Paulson (1973) was unable to provoke dyskinesias in 10 healthy rhesus monkeys given 2 g L-dopa or more orally every day for six months. Nausea occurred initially but even at this huge dose, which is at least five times that used to treat Parkinsonians, dyskinesias were not seen. However, Paulson confirmed that acute parenteral administration of large doses could cause abnormal movements often with collapse, myoclonus, self-mutilation and death.

In rodents with unilateral lesions of the substantia nigra, torsion of the head and trunk occurs with circling activity following the administration of dopaminergic drugs (Ungerstedt, 1971). In male squirrel monkeys treated with intraventricular 6-hydroxy-dopamine, body swaying, lip smacking and dystonic posturing occur with doses of L-dopa which do not affect saline-treated controls (Ng et al, 1973).

Further support for this view comes from the recent observation that the meperidine analogue 1-methyl-4 phenyl-1,2,3,6 tetrahydropyridine (NMPTP) which appears to have selective neurotoxic effects on the zona compacta of the substantia nigra induces Parkinsonism in man and a rigid bradykinetic syndrome in monkeys. Dopaminergic agonists promptly reverse the Parkinsonian features in both NMPTP-treated animals and in the heroin addicts who developed Parkinsonism following NMPTP administration, and drug-induced dyskinesias rapidly appear (Burns et al, 1984; Langston and Ballard, 1984).

PATHOPHYSIOLOGY

Although the evidence is at present inconclusive, stimulation of striatal dopaminergic receptors by dopamine is probably important in causing L-dopa-induced dyskinesias. Drugs which block dopamine receptors such as pimozide attenuate the abnormal movements (Tarsy et al, 1975) whereas dopaminergic agonists such as piribedil and the synthetic ergolenes increase them. Production of minor metabolities with direct effects on dopamine receptors may also be involved (Sandler et al, 1973) and increased plasma O-methyldopa levels (Feuerstein et al, 1977) with a swing towards 4–0 methylated derivative production has been implicated (Lhermitte et al, 1977).

Cholinergic mechanisms may also be relevant and the centrally acting anticholinesterase physostigmine can reduce the dyskinesias (Tarsy et al, 1973) whereas anticholinergics can increase them (Horrocks et al, 1973). There are also a few reports of anticholinergic-induced dyskinesias in Parkinsonian patients not treated with L-dopa (Birket-Smith, 1974). Noradrenergic receptor stimulation is another possible contributory factor (Birket-Smith and Vang Anderson, 1973) which requires further exploration.

Degeneration of the nigrostriatal bundle in idiopathic Parkinson's disease probably leads to denervation hypersensitivity of the dopaminergic receptors on the striatal cholinergic interneurones. Although not the cause of the drug-induced movements, this compensatory response may well be a predisposing factor. Anden (1970) demonstrated that animals in whom he had destroyed the nigrostriatal pathway were responsive in behavioural test systems to quantities of dopamine which were ineffective in unlesioned controls. The clinical observation that dyskinesias tend to occur first on the more severely affected side would also be in keeping with the concept of denervation hypersensitivity as a dose-determining factor. Arguing from his contrary clinical observations and the data from animals that small lesions in the substantia nigra of non-human primates may prevent L-dopa-induced orofacial dyskinesias (Mones et al, 1973) and that large ventral tegmental lesions increase them (Battista et al, 1972), Duvoisin believes that the pathological substrate favouring the occurrence of

L-dopa-induced dyskinesia involves structures other than the substantia nigra and the corpus striatum.

Defective control mechanisms for the release of dopamine in the Parkinsonian brain leading to erratic delivery on to hypersensitive receptors may also be important and the simultaneous occurrence of Parkinsonian symptoms and hyperkinesias may be caused by an uneven pattern of receptor activation in different areas of the corpus striatum (Carlsson, 1970). Klawans has suggested that the increasing severity of dyskinesias with time and their progressive resistance to dosage reduction might be due to a direct effect of chronic L-dopa treatment on receptor sensitivity. After complete withdrawal of L-dopa, dyskinesias usually recur on recommencing treatment at a lower dose than that which initially provoked them. Similar preclinical observations derived from long-term studies with dopaminergic drugs such as amphetamine have led him to postulate a dopamine-induced dopaminergic supersensitivity as the cause (Klawans et al, 1977).

A further factor which must be taken into account in explaining peak-dose dyskinesias is that their appearance is not inextricably bound to the therapeutic properties of the drug. There is now physiological (McLennan and York, 1967), histological (Olson et al, 1972) and biochemical (Kebabian and Calne, 1979) support for the existence of at least two dopamine neuronal populations. A relatively selective stimulation of one subgroup of receptors might be important (Klawans, 1973b) and the relative degree of denervation supersensitivity of the different cell groups might determine the relationship between therapeutic success and severity of dyskinesias (Marsden, 1975). Of interest in this regard are the clinical observations that the dopamine receptor agonist bromocriptine can produce therapeutic effects comparable to those seen with L-dopa in previously untreated Parkinsonians with a much lower incidence of dyskinesias (Lees and Stern, 1981).

All the above remarks refer to peak-dose choreo-athetosis, and the other dopa-induced dyskinesia sequences are even less well understood. A long duration response to L-dopa lasting three to five days occurs in some young, mildly disabled patients. This causes a stable improvement throughout the day and, if therapy is stopped, several days elapse before Parkinsonian disabilities return to pre-treatment levels. Biphasic dyskinesias (Dystonia-Improvement-Dystonia) have been regarded as an integral feature of this response (Barbeau, 1975; Muenter et al, 1977). It has been suggested that post-synaptic depolarisation blockade might occur with rapidly rising or falling plasma dopa levels (Muenter et al, 1977). The commoner short duration response lasts only one to four hours and is associated with peak-dose dyskinesias at times of high plasma levels and oscillations in diurnal performance. Most patients with the long duration response are said to ultimately convert to the short-duration response as their disease progresses.

What determines which patients develop chorea and which dystonia following L-dopa is not clear although the studies of Parkes et al, (1976) on peak-dose phenomena suggest that the relative degree of damage in nigrostriatal and pallidal systems may be more important than imbalance of different dopamine receptor types. Early morning and end of dose dystonia is a further intriguing manifestation of chronic L-dopa therapy often occurring in the interludes between bouts of chorea. It is usually abolished by withdrawal of the drug but during treatment occurs at times when plasma dopa levels may be negligible and when Parkinsonian disabilities may be severe. Paradoxically it is relieved temporarily by each dose of L-dopa and may be improved the long-acting dopaminergic agonist bromocriptine (Lander et al, 1979). The gamma-aminobutyric acid analogue baclofen which has complex affects on several neurotransmitter systems may also help. Finally, a disturbance of dopamine 5-hydroxy-tryptamine (5HT) relationship may be involved in L-dopa-induced myoclonus as the 5HT antagonist methysergide can specifically relieve this complaint (Klawans et al, 1975).

CLINICAL DESCRIPTION

In most patients L-dopa-induced dyskinesias start imperceptibly with slight fidgetiness, restlessness or increased gesticulation and are first noticed by relatives or acquaintances. Rarely their onset is abrupt and explosively disabling. Each individual develops a characteristic pattern and distribution of dyskinesias which are in part determined by the pre-treatment clinical picture. Once the involuntary movements are well-established, patients can often predict the onset of each flurry by premonitory sensations of heat or paraesthesiae. A Jacksonian 'march' is occasionally apparent at the onset of each bout, and it is by no means exceptional to observe florid choreo-athetosis in one part of the body when severe Parkinsonism is still evident elsewhere.

DYSKINESIA TYPES

CHOREO-ATHETOSIS

This is the commonest form. The most severely affected patients have generalised violent movements of the whole body often with hypotonia and 'hung-up' stretch reflexes. The movements are in general tolerated surprisingly well but the interminable motion sometimes leads to depression in the patients' spouses. Orofacial dyskinesias are common particularly in patients over 60 years and include lip smacking, tongue rolling and twisting, gnawing, yawning, sniffing, pouting, sucking, grunting, chewing, nibbling, snarling, grimacing and eyebrow raising; speech may be nasal, jerky or drawling and interference with eating and breathing can result. Secondary hypertrophy of the tongue combined with lingual and oral dyskinesias may impede swallowing, and uncontrollable extrusion of the dentures may cause feeding difficulties. Tongue dryness and soreness with ulceration and scarring of the buccal cavity may lead to dental referral.

Cervical dyskinesias are nearly always a striking feature of the disturbance.

Head bobbing or twisting, with violent shoulder shrugging and neck extension, are characteristic and may lead to cervical radiculopathies as a consequence of severe cervical spondylosis. Recurrent furunculosis and skin abrasions are other occasional complications.

Flinging movements of the extended arm, continuous flapping abductions of the shoulder and writhing internal rotation movements may lead to a variety of musculo-skeletal injuries such as shoulder dislocation and fractures. Fragmentary mannerisms with fine 'piano playing' finger movements or sinuous wrist movements are also common and when severe may make handwriting jerky and illegible and lead to difficulty with feeding and drinking. Gross circumvolutions of the whole leg, sudden flexion-extension movements of the knee and constant shifting of weight-bearing are also seen when the patient is sitting whereas strong extension spasms may occur in the recumbent position (Fig. 12.5). Foot tapping with toe spreading and curling is also commonplace.

Swaying of the trunk, when standing or sitting, may lead to the mistaken conclusion that the individual is drunk especially when orofacial dyskinesias cause slurred speech. Sometimes the gait is wide-based with exaggerated lumbar lordosis and associated poor balance leading to falls. Other bizarre gaits

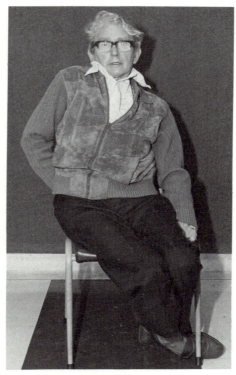

Figure 12.5. L-dopa-induced peak-dose chorea in a man with Parkinson's disease.

may be seen with prancing, tip-toe and crab-like movements. Hyperventilation, inspiratory gasps and intractable hiccoughs are occasional accompaniments.

DYSTONIA

This occurs either as an isolated phenomenon usually in the first year or two or develops later with a different diurnal sequence in patients already experiencing drug-induced chorea. Spasm of the foot is most frequently seen with a sustained equinovarus posture, clawing of the digits and dorsiflexion of the great toe. Torsion of the trunk, oromandibular dystonia, torticollis and dystonic finger cramps also occur.

MYOCLONUS

Rapid shock-like movements of the proximal limb musculature and occasionally the face are sometimes seen during the day but are particularly troublesome at night. Spouses report that patients jerk their legs throughout the night sometimes with kicking movements and shouting.

TICS

Clonic eye blinks, facial grimaces and rapid twitches together with shoulder shrugs are frequent, but vocalisations have not been reported in idiopathic Parkinson's disease. L-dopa exacerbates and frequently unmasks the tics of post-encephalitic Parkinson's disease.

DYSKINESIA SEQUENCES

(a) **Peak-dose dyskinesias** These usually consist of choreo-athetotic movements although in about 5% torsion of the trunk limbs and neck may occur. They usually begin 20–90 minutes after each L-dopa dose, usually at the time of maximum plasma dopa levels, and may last from 30 minutes to three hours, tending to be most severe midway through the interdose period. They bear a close inverse relationship to the relief of bradykinesia and are aggravated by emotion, fatigue, voluntary movement of other parts of the body and certain postures. They may not be present after every dose; some patients experience isolated morning dyskinesias but in other patients they tend to build up towards the evening. Occasionally the movements are severe and continuous for several months and then inexplicably disappear for long periods. Ingestion of L-dopa on an empty stomach leads to a more rapid and violent onset whereas a high protein meal may prevent them from occurring altogether. Increases in dose invariably aggravate the movements whereas dosage reduction leads to improvement.

Illustrative case history A 62-year-old man with a five-year of predominantly left-sided Parkinson's disease began L-dopa in 1969 and within two months improvement in bradykinesia and tremor occurred at a daily dose of 3.0 g. Rapid, jerking movements of the left hand, restlessness of the legs and lip smacking began after six months and became increasingly severe. Each episode began in the left toes 20–40 minutes after L-dopa and lasted from one to two and a half hours being most severe in the morning. Three months later similar movements started in the right arm, each attack being slower in onset and less severe than the left-sided disturbance. By 1973 the patient was obliged to reduce his daily dose to 2.0 g as a consequence of increasingly severe truncal dyskinesia. Closer spacing and reduction of individual doses failed to alter the sequence of the movements and by 1975 severe oscillations in motor performance were also present, the periods of chorea coinciding with residual periods of mobility.

(b) Early morning and end of dose dystonia Dystonic foot postures are a well-recognised, occasional feature of untreated Parkinson's disease (Purves Stewart, 1898) (Fig. 12.6). Chronic L-dopa therapy induces reversible focal dystonias in up to 50% of patients after 10 years. They occur most frequently in the early morning on rising, before the first daily dose of medication and may recur towards the end of each interdose period when Parkinsonian disabilities

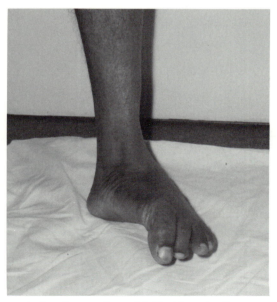

Figure 12.6. A dystonic foot in a patient with Parkinson's disease.

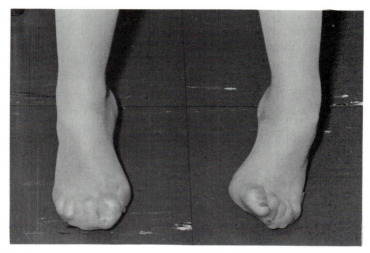

Figure 12.7. L-dopa-induced off period dystonic left foot in a patient with Parkinson's disease.

are returning (Fig. 12.7). Another common time for them to occur is just before retiring to bed in the evening. In contrast to peak-dose dyskinesias which usually appear in the first two years of treatment, end of dose dystonia is rarely a prominent symptom until treatment has been continued for at least five years. The disturbance is usually restricted to the foot but the whole leg, neck and jaw may occasionally be affected. In some cases the phenomenon is triggered by walking.

Illustrative case history A 61-year-old woman with a five-year history of mainly right-sided Parkinson's disease began to complain of severe generalised spasms four years after starting L-dopa (3.5 g/d). Examination in the early morning before the first dose revealed a sustained painful torsion of her right foot with dorsiflexion of the great toe and plantar flexion of the other digits with forced extension of her leg. Her jaw was forcibly deviated to the right preventing mouth opening, her neck was hyperextended and her right shoulder was elevated and internally rotated with flexion at the elbow. The foot posture prevented her putting her shoe on and was associated with a severe painful cramp of the calf. About half an hour after her morning dose of L-dopa, the dystonia was replaced by right-sided chorea. Severe torsion movements recurred in the early afternoon four hours after the morning L-dopa dose.

(c) **Diphasic dyskinesias (onset and end of dose dyskinesias)** In my own experience this is the least common sequence although others regard it as relatively frequent. It is most often seen in young predominantly bradykinetic patients who have derived a good response to L-dopa. It is characterised by two discrete episodes of dyskinesia within each interdose period, with a period of unimpeded mobility inbetween. Abnormal involuntary movements begin 15–30 minutes after a dose of L-dopa with an associated release from bradykinesia. The movements then subside after about 30 minutes leaving the patient mobile for one to two hours. Towards the end of the interdose period, a mounting sense of apprehension with profuse sweating precedes a second more violent burst of dyskinesias occasionally accompanied by fine tremor and lasting about half an hour. A final very short period of mobility without dyskinesia sometimes then follows before the return of bradykinesia. Smaller more frequent doses or an increase in dose convert the disturbance to peak-dose dyskinesia.

COURSE

At constant dosage L-dopa-induced peak-dose dyskinesias increase in severity with time (Fig. 12.8). Eventually they may become so incapacitating that the dose has to be steadily reduced in order to prevent embarrassment, self-injury and exhaustion. In the early years of therapy very small dosage reductions may rapidly abolish the movements, but after five or six years substantial decrements usually have to be made to afford relief. Exceptionally dyskinesias may continue for up to 24 hours after complete discontinuation of the drug and there is a single case report of persistent dystonic spasms eight

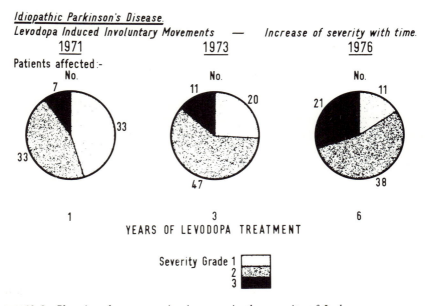

Figure 12.8. Showing the progressive increase in the severity of L-dopa-induced dyskinesias with time (personal data).

Table 12.5. DISTRIBUTION OF L-DOPA-INDUCED DYSKINESIAS AFTER ONE AND SIX YEARS' THERAPY (PERSONAL DATA)

Patients receiving L-dopa	1971–2	1976–7
No. with dyskinesias	75	65
Distribution %		
Cephalic	40	20
Cephalic and limbs	36	50
Cephalic, limbs and trunk	0	12
Cephalic and trunk	1	1
Limbs	18	13
Limbs and trunk	3	2
Trunk	2	2

months after complete withdrawal of L-dopa (Weiss et al, 1971). The abnormal movements also become increasingly generalised as treatment continues (Table 12.5) and late truncal and respiratory involvement may be seen.

TREATMENT

A modest reduction in L-dopa dosage is often temporarily effective in stemming the steady increase in dyskinesia severity. Eventually, however, dyskinesias re-emerge at a lower threshold and complete withdrawal of the drug may become necessary. Current practice is to use much smaller doses of L-dopa from the outset of treatment and this will probably reduce to some degree the incidence of severe peak-dose dyskinesias (Lees and Stern, 1982).

Based on the notion that overstimulation of dopamine receptors is involved in the pathogenesis of these abnormal movements, a number of neuroleptic drugs have been tried as treatment. Trifluoperazine (Yahr, 1970), haloperidol (Klawans and Weiner, 1974b) and pimozide (Tarsy et al, 1975) all effectively alleviate L-dopa-induced dyskinesias; unfortunately this occurs only at the expense of an increase in Parkinsonian disability and is no more effective than simply reducing the dose of L-dopa. A similar disappointing response occurs with the dopamine depleting drugs reserpine and tetrabenazene.

The realisation that several separate dopamine receptor populations exist in the corpus striatum and that the anti-Parkinsonian action and dyskinetic side-effects of L-dopa are not inextricably linked has stimulated the search for selective dopaminergic antagonists. In animals the peri-oral dyskinesias produced by direct intra-striatal injection of dopaminergic agonists have been dissociated from the increased locomotor activity produced by the systemic administration of such drugs. What is more, certain neuroleptics such as oxiperomide and the substituted benzamide tiapride reduce the dyskinesias more than the locomotor activity (Costall et al, 1977). At critical carefully titrated doses both these medications have been found to have selective anti-dyskinetic effects in Parkinson's disease. Oxiperomide (5–10 mg/d) reduced L-dopa and spontaneous hyperkinesias in one study without necessarily increasing Parkinsonism, although drowsiness was a limiting side-effect (Bédard et al, 1978). L'Hermitte et al (1977a) first reported the beneficial selective effects of tiapride (200 mg/d) in peak-dose dyskinesias and this observation was subsequently confirmed by Marsden and his group (mean dose 150 mg/d) (Price et al, 1978) although these latter authors were obliged to increase the dose of L-dopa to obtain selective effects. My own experience with tiapride in 16 Parkinsonian patients with the long-term L-dopa syndrome at doses ranging between 12.5 mg and 100 mg a day was disappointing; no selective antidyskinetic effects were demonstrated (Lees et al, 1979). If further studies do provide more convincing evidence that these dopamine receptor antagonists are of clinical value in some of the long-term complications of L-dopa therapy, this must be balanced against the potential hazards of irreversibly aggravating Parkinsonism or inducing tardive dyskinesia.

There is a report of the dopaminergic agonist apomorphine improving L-dopa-induced dyskinesias when administered parenterally (Duby et al, 1972) but this effect may have resulted from non-specific sedative effects. Orally administered dopaminergic agonists usually aggravate abnormal involuntary movements provoked by L-dopa.

A number of other drugs with widely differing effects on central neuro-transmitter systems have been tried without great success. Pyridoxine reduces L-dopa-induced dyskinesias but aggravates Parkinsonism whereas barbiturates, 1-tryptophan and 5-hydroxy-tryptophan (Yahr, 1970) have no effect. Physo-stigmine reduces dyskinesias but aggravates Parkinsonism and there is some evidence that stopping concurrently administered anticholinergics may also be beneficial (Klawans and Bergen, 1975). Deanol, despite enthusiastic early reports, is probably useless (Klawans et al, 1975). Sodium valproate which raises brain gamma-aminobutyric acid (GABA) levels produced a modest reduction in peak-dose dyskinesias without aggravating Parkinsonism (Price et al, 1978) whereas the GABA analogue baclofen had no beneficial effects on peak-dose dyskinesias and aggravated Parkinsonian disabilities (Lees et al, 1978). Drugs influencing noradrenergic systems have also been reported to be of value (Mena et al, 1971; Birket-Smith and Vang Andersen, 1973). Stereo-tactic surgery has also been suggested as a possible treatment but by the time dyskinesias become severe most patients carry a considerable operative risk.

Some patients with end of dose dystonia respond to baclofen (Lees, et al, 1978; Nausieda et al, 1980) and others do well with the addition of small amounts of bromocriptine (Lander et al, 1979). Myoclonus has been said to respond to methysergide (Klawans, et al, 1975).

References

Abe K, Oda N 1980 Incidence of tics in the offspring of childhood ticqueurs: a controlled follow-up study. Devel Med Child Neurol 22: 649–653

Aberle D F 1952 'Arctic hysteria' and latah in Mongolia. NY Acad Sci 14: 291–297

Abse D W 1966 In: Hysteria and related disorders. Wright, Bristol, pp 22–23

Abuzzahab F S, Anderson F O 1976 Gilles de la Tourette's syndrome: international registry. Mason, St Paul, Minnesota

Agras S, Marshall C 1965 The application of negative practice to spasmodic torticollis. Am J Psychiat 122: 579–582

Ajuriaguerra J, Garcia-Badaracco J, Trillat E, Soubiran G 1956 Traitement de la crampe des écrivains par relaxation. L'Encephalé 45: 141–171

Alajouanine T, Gastaut H 1958 La syncinésie-surtaut et l'epilepsie sursaut à declen-choment sensitif ou sensoriel inopiné les faits anatomo-cliniques. Rev Neurol 93: 29–41

Albrecht H 1949 Uber die Ticerscheinungen im Kindesalter. Nervenarzt 20: 314–320

Aldren Turner W, Critchley M 1925 Respiratory disorders in epidemic encephalitis. Brain 47: 72–104

Aldren Turner W, Critchley M 1928 The prognosis and the late results of postencephalitic respiratory disorders. J Neurol Psychopath 8: 191–208

Alles G A 1933 The comparative physiological actions of dL-β-phenylisopropylamines I pressor effect and toxicity. J Pharmacol Exp Ther 47: 339–354

Alpers B J, Drayer C S 1937 The organic background of some cases of spasmodic torticollis: report of a case with autopsy. Am J Med Sci 193: 378–384

Alpert M, Friedhoff A J, Diamond F 1983 Use of dopamine receptor agonists to reduce dopamine receptor number as treatment for tardive dyskinesia. In: Fahn S, Calne D B, Shoulson I (eds) Experimental therapeutics of movement disorders. Adv Neurol, vol 37. Raven Press, New York, pp 253–258

Altrocchi P H 1972 Spontaneous oral-facial dyskinesia. Arch Neurol 26: 506–512

Altrocchi P H, Forno L S 1983 Spontaneous oral-facial dyskinesia: neuropathology of a case. Neurology 33: 802–805

Ambani L H, Van Woert M H, Bowers M B 1973 Physostigmine effects on phenothiazine-induced extrapyramidal reactions. Arch Neurol 29: 444–446

American College of Neuropsychopharmacology — Food and Drug Administration Task Force 1973 Neurologic syndromes associated with antipsychotic drug use. New Engl J Med 289: 20–23

Aminoff M J 1972 Acanthocytosis and neurological disease. Brain 95: 749–760

Aminoff M J, Dedo H H, Izdebski K, 1978 Clinical aspects of spasmodic dysphonia. J Neurol, Neurosurg Psychiat 41: 361–365

Anden N-E 1970 Pharmacological and anatomical implications of induced abnormal movements with L-dopa. In: Barbeau A, McDowell F H (eds) L-dopa and Parkinsonism. Davis, Philadelphia, pp 173–198

Anden N-E 1972 Dopamine turnover in the corpus striatum and the limbic system after treatment with neuroleptic and anti-acetylcholine drugs. J Pharm Pharmacol 24: 905–906

Andermann F, Keene D L, Andermann E, Quesney L F 1980 Startle disease or hyper-ekplexia: further delineation of the syndrome. Brain 103: 985–997

Andrew J, Fowler C J, Harrison M J G 1983 Stereotaxic thalamotomy in 55 cases of dystonia. Brain 106: 981–1000

Ang L, Borison R, Dysken M, Davis J M 1982 Reduced excretion of MHPG in Tourette syndrome. In: Friedhoff A J, Chase T N (eds) Gilles de la Tourette syndrome. Adv Neurol, Vol 35. Raven Press, New York, pp 171–175

Angle C, McIntyre M 1968 Persistent dystonia in a brain-damaged child after ingestion of phenothiazine. J Pediat 73: 124–126

Angus J W S, Simpson G M 1970 Hysteria and drug-induced dystonia. Acta Psychiat Scand Suppl 212: 52–58

Ansari K, Webster D, Manning N 1972 Spasmodic torticollis and L-dopa. Neurology 22: 670–674

Antelman S M, Szechtman H, Chin P, Fisher A E 1975 Taillpinch-induced eating, gnawing and licking behaviour in rats: dependence on the nigrostriatal dopamine system. Brain Res 99(2): 319–337

Arnold G E 1959 Spastic dysphonia. Logos 2: 3–14

Aronson A E 1973 In: Psychogenic voice disorders: an interdisciplinary approach to detection, diagnosis and therapy. Saunders, Philadelphia

Aronson A E, Brown J R, Litin E M, Pearson J S 1968 Spastic dysphonia I voice neurologic and psychiatric aspects. J Speech Hear Dis 33: 203–218

Arseni C, Maretsis M 1971 The surgical treatment of spasmodic torticollis. Neurochirurgia 14: 177–180

Asam U 1979 Katamnestische Untersuchung von jugendlichen Patienten mit multiplen Tics unter spezieller Berücksichtigung des Gilles de la Tourette-Syndromes. Acta Paedopsychiat Basel 45: 51–63

Asam U 1982 A follow-up study of Tourette syndrome. In: Friedhoff A J, Chase T N (eds) Gilles de la Tourette syndrome. Adv Neurol, vol 35. Raven Press, New York, pp 285–286

Ascher E 1948 Psychodynamic considerations in Gilles de la Tourettes disease: with a report of five cases and discussion of the literature. Am J Psychiat 105: 267–276

Asnis G M, Leopold M A, Duvoisin R C, Schwartz A H 1977 A survey of tardive dyskinesia in psychiatric outpatients. Am J Psych 134: 1367–1370

Ayd F J 1960 Drug-induced extrapyramidal reactions: their clinical manifestations and treatment with akineton. Psychosomatics 1: 143–150

Ayd F J 1961 A survey of drug-induced extrapyramidal reactions. J Am Med Ass 175: 1054–1060

Ayd F J 1974 Neurological effects of abrupt withdrawal of neuroleptic medications in schizophrenic children. Int Drug Ther Newsletter 9: 25–28

Azrin N H, Nunn R G 1973 Habit reversal: a method of eliminating nervous habits and tics. Behav Res Ther 11: 619–628

Azrin N H, Nunn R G, Frantz S E 1980 Habit-reversal vs negative practice treatment of nervous tics. Behav Ther 11: 169–178

Babinski J 1900 Sur un cas d'hemispasme (contribution a l'étude de la pathogenie du torticollis spasmodique). Rev Neurol 8: 142–147

Bacher N M, Lewis H A 1980 Low-dose propranolol in tardive dyskinesia. Am J Psychiat 137: 495–497

Bachman D S 1981 Pemoline-induced Tourette's disorder: a case report. Am J Psychiat 138: 1116–1117

Baker E F W 1962 Gilles de la Tourette syndrome treated by bimedial frontal leucotomy. Canad Med Assoc J 86: 746–747

Ballinger B R 1970 The prevalence of nail-biting in normal and abnormal populations. Br J Psychiat 117: 445–446

Balthasar K 1957 Über das anatomische Substrat der generalisierten Tic-Krankheit (maladie des tics, Gilles de la Tourette Entwicklungshemmung des Corpus Striatum. Arch Psychiat Berlin 195: 531–549

Barbeau A 1969 L-dopa therapy in Parkinson's disease: a critical review of nine years experience. Canad Med Assoc J 101: 59–68

Barbeau A 1975 Diphasic dyskinesias during levodopa therapy. Lancet 1:756

Barbeau A 1980 Cholinergic treatment in the Tourette syndrome. New Engl J Med 302: 1310–1311

Baron M, Shapiro E, Shapiro A, Rainer J D 1980 Genetic analysis of Tourette syndrome suggesting major gene effect. Am J Hum Genet 32:138A

Barré J A 1952 La crampe des écrivains, maladie organique ses formes, ses causes. Rev Neurol 86:703

Barrett R E, Yahr M D, Duvoisin R C 1970 Torsion dystonia and spasmodic torticollis: results of treatment with L-dopa. Neurology 20 2: 107–113

Bartholini G 1976 Differential effect of neuroleptic drugs on dopamine turnover in the extrapyramidal and limbic system. J Pharm Pharmacol 28: 429–433

Battista A F 1982 Surgical approach to blepharospasm: nerve thermolysis. In: Marsden C D, Fahn S (eds) Movement disorders. Butterworth, London, pp 319–321

Battista A, Goldstein M, Ohmoto T 1972 The effects of 5-HTP (precursor of serotonin) on abnormal movements produced by L-dopa in monkeys with tegmental lesions and resting tremor. Trans Am Neurol Assoc 97:33

Battista A F, Goldstein M, Miyamoto T, Matsumoto Y 1976 Effort of centrally acting drugs on experimental torticollis in monkeys. In: Eldridge R, Fahn S (eds) Dystonia. Adv Neurol, vol 14. Raven Press, New York, pp 329–338

Beard G M 1880a Experiments with the 'jumpers of Maine'. Pop Sci Month 18: 170–178

Beard G 1880b Experiments with the 'jumpers' or 'jumping Frenchmen' of Maine. J Nerv Ment Dis 7: 487–490

Bédard P, Parkes J D, Marsden C D 1978 Effect of a new dopamine-blocking agent (oxiperomide) on drug-induced dyskinesias in Parkinson's disease and spontaneous dyskinesias. Br Med J 1: 954–6

Beech H R 1960 The symptomatic treatment of writer's cramp. In: Eysenck H J (ed) Behaviour therapy and the neurosés. Pergamon, Oxford, pp 349–372

Behan P, Geschwind N, Quadfasel F A 1981 Coprolalia in Sydenham's chorea. Abstracts of 1st International Gilles de la Tourette syndrome Symposium, New York and personal communication

Bell C 1833 In: The nervous system of the human body. Duff Green, Washington, p 221

Bell R C H, Smith R C 1978 Tardive dyskinesia: characterisation and prevalence in a statewide system. J Clin Psychiat 39: 39–47

Benedek W 1925 Zwangsmäßiges Schreien in Anfällen als postencephalitische Hyperkinese. Z Ges Neurol Psychiat 98: 17–26

Benson D F 1979 In: Aphasia, alexia and agraphia. Churchill Livingstone, Edinburgh, p 167

Bergen D, Tanner C M, Wilson R 1981 The electroencephalogram in Tourette syndrome. Ann Neurol 11: 382–385

Berkson G 1983 Repetitive stereotyped behaviours. Am J Ment Defic 88: 239–246

Berkson G, Davenport R K 1962 Stereotyped movements of mental defectives 1. initial survey. Am J Ment Defic 66: 849–852

Bertrand C M 1982 Peripheral versus central surgical approach for the treatment of spasmodic torticollis. In: Marsden C D, Fahn S (eds) Movement disorders. Butterworth, London, pp 315–318

Besson J O, Walker L G 1983 Hypnotherapy for writer's cramp. Lancet 1: 71–72

Betts J J, Nicholson J T, Critchley EMR 1970 Acanthocytosis with normolipoproteinaemia: biophysical aspects. Postgrad Med J 46: 702–707

Bickford R G 1957 New dimensions in electroencephalography. Neurology 7: 469–475
Billings A 1978 Self-monitoring in the treatment of tics: a single-subject analysis. J Behav Ther Exp Psychiat 9: 339–342
Binder R L, Levy R 1981 Extrapyramidal reactions in Asians. Am J Psychiat 138: 1243–1244
Bindman E, Tibbetts R W 1977 Writer's cramp: a rational approach to treatment. Br J Psychiat 131: 143–148
Bing R 1925 Über lokale Muskelspasmen und Tics nebst Bemerkungen zur Revision des Begriffes der 'Psychogenie'. Schweiz Med Wosch 55: 993–1000
Bing R 1936 Somatische Faktoren in der Gestaltung psychogener Symptome. Schweiz Med Wosch 17: 953–960
Bird A C, McDonald W I 1975 Essential blepharospasm. Trans Ophthalmol Soc UK 95: 250–253
Bird T D, Cederbaum S Volpey R W, Stahl W L 1978 Familial degeneration of the basal ganglia with acanthocytosis: a clinical, neuropathological and neurochemical study. Ann Neurol 3: 253–258
Birket-Smith E 1974 Abnormal involuntary movements induced by anticholinergic therapy. Acta Neurol Scand 50: 801–811
Birket-Smith E, Vang Andersen J 1973 Treatment of side-effects of L-dopa. Lancet 1:431
Bjørndal N, Casey D, Gerlach J 1980 In: Cattabeni F et al (eds) Long term effects of neuroleptics. Adv Biochem Psychopharm, vol 24. Raven Press, New York, pp 541–545
Blaschko, H 1939 The specific action of L-dopa decarboxylase. J Physiol 96: 50–51
Blaschko H 1957 Metabolism and storage of biogenic amines. Experientia 13: 9–13
Bleeker H E 1978 Gilles de la Tourette's syndrome with direct evidence of organicity. Psychiat Clin 11: 147–154
Bleuler E 1924 In: Textbook of psychiatry, trans A A Brill. Allen and Unwin, London
Bleuler E 1949 Dementia praecox. Int Univ Press, New York
Bliss J 1980 Sensory experiences of Gilles de la Tourettes syndrome. Arch Gen Psychiat 37: 1343–1347
Bloom F, Segal D, Ling N, Guillemin R 1976 Endorphins profound behavioural effects in rats suggest new aetiological factors in mental illness. Science 194: 630–632
Bobruff A, Gardos G, Tarsy D, Rapkin R M, Cole J O, Moore P 1981 Clonazepam and phenobarbital in tardive dyskinesia. Am J Psychiat 138: 189–193
Bockner S 1959 Gilles de la Tourette's disease. J Ment Sci 105: 1078–1081
Boenheim C 1930 Über den Tic im Kindesalter. Klin Wschr 9: 2005–2011
Boller F, Boller M, Denes G, Timberlake W H, Zieper I, Albert M 1973 Familial palilalia. Neurology 23: 1117–1125
Boncour G P 1910 Les tics chez l'écolier et leur interpretation. Prog Med 26: 495–496
Bond E D, Smith L H 1935 Post-encephalitic behaviour disorders. Am J Psychiat 92: 17–33
Bonhoff G, Lewrenz H 1954 Über Weckamine. Springer, Berlin
Bonnet K A 1982 Neurobiological dissection of Tourette syndrome a neurochemical focus on a human neuroanatomical model. In: Friedhoff A J, Chase T N (eds) Gilles de la Tourette syndrome. Adv Neurol, vol 35. Raven Press, New York, pp 77–82
Bonthala C M, West A 1983 Pemoline induced chorea and Gilles de la Tourette's syndrome. Br J Psychiat 143: 300–302
Borenstein P, Dabbah M, Bles G 1962 Contribution a L'étude des syndromes extrapyramidaux secondaires aux neuroleptiques. Ann Med Psych 120: 279–319
Borison R L, Ang L, Chang S, Dysken M, Comaty J E, Davis J M 1982 New pharmacological approaches in the treatment of Tourette syndrome. In: Friedhoff A J, Chase T N (eds) Gilles de la Tourette syndrome. Adv Neurol, vol 35. Raven Press, New York, pp 377–382
Bouteille E M 1810 In: Traité de la chorée ou danse de St Guy. Vincard, Paris, pp 329–362

Bowers M 1975 Thioridazine: central dopamine turnover and clinical effects of anti-psychotic drugs. Clin Pharmacol 17: 73–78

Brain W R 1934 The great convulsionary. Some reflections on genius and other essays. Pitman, London, p 69

Brandon S 1969 Unusual effect of fenfluramine. Br Med J 4: 557–558

Brandon S, McClelland H A, Protheroe C 1971 A study of facial dyskinesia in a mental hospital population. Br J Psych 118: 171–184

Brandrup E 1961 Tetrabenazene treatment in persisting dyskinesia caused by psychopharmaca. Am J Psychiat 118: 551–552

Braude W M, Barnes T R E, Gore S M 1983 Clinical characteristics of akathisia: a systematic investigation of acute psychiatric inpatient admissions. Br J Psychiat 143 139–150

Bremness A B, Sverd J 1979 Methylphenidate-induced Tourette syndrome case report. Am J Psych 136: 1334–5

Brenning R 1971 Motor manifestations in molimina crurum nocturna (including restless legs). J Am Geriat Soc 19: 700–708

Brierly H 1967 The treatment of hysterical spasmodic torticollis by behaviour therapy. Behav Res Ther 5: 139–142

Brissaud E 1895 Tics et spasmes cloniques de la face. In: Leçons sur les maladies nerveuses. 1er série, p 502

Brissaud E, Feindel E 1899 Sur le traitement du torticollis mental et des tics similaires. Journal de Neurologie 8

Bruck J 1831 In: Caspers Kritisches Repertorium, p 2

Brun R 1964 Psychoanalytische Behandlung und Heilung eines Schreibkrampfes verbunden mit Steifikgeit und Paraesthesien in den Armen. Acta Psychother et Psychosom Basel 12: 382–390

Bruun R D 1982a Clonidine treatment of Tourette syndrome. In: Friedhoff A J, Chase T N (eds) Gilles de la Tourette syndrome. Adv Neurol, vol 35. Raven Press, New York, pp 403–405

Bruun R D 1982b Dysphoric phenomena associated with haloperidol treatment of Tourette syndrome. In: Friedhoff A J, Chase T N (eds) Gilles de la Tourette syndrome. Adv Neurol, vol 35. Raven Press, New York, pp 433–436

Bunney B S, Aghajanian G K 1976 The effect of antipsychotic drugs on the firing of dopaminergic neurons: a reappraisal. In: Sedvall G, Uvnas B, Zotterman Y (eds) Antipsychotic drugs: pharmacodynamics and pharmacokinetics. Pergamon, pp 305–318

Bunney B S, Walters J R, Roth R H, Aghajanian G K 1973 Dopaminergic neurons: effect of anti-psychotic drugs and amphetamine on single cell activity. J Pharmacol Exp Ther 85: 560–571

Burke R E, Fahn S, Jankovic J, Marsden C D, Lang A E, Gollomp S et al 1982 Tardive dystonia: late-onset and persistent dystonia caused by antipsychotic drugs. Neurology 32: 1335–1341

Burns R S, Markey S P, Phillips J M, Chiueh C C 1984 The neurotoxicity of 1-methyl-4-phenyl-1,2,3,6-tetrahydropyridine in the monkey and man. Canad J Neurol Sci 11: 166–168

Burt D R, Creese I, Snyder S H 1977 Anti-schizophrenic drugs: chronic treatment elevates dopamine receptor binding in brain. Science 196: 326–328

Buser P, St Laurent J, Menini C 1966 Intervention du colliculus inférieur dans l' elaboration et le controle corticale spécifique des décharges cloniques au son chez le chat sous chloralose. Exp Brain Res 1: 102–126

Butler I J, Koslow S H, Seifert W E, Caprioli R M, Singer H S 1979 Biogenic amine metabolism in Tourette syndrome. Ann Neurol 6: 37–39

Caine E D, Polinsky R J 1981 Tardive dyskinesia in persons with Gilles de la Tourette's disease. Arch Neurol 38: 471–472

Caine E D, Polinsky R J, Ludlow C L, Ebert M H, Nee L E 1982 Heterogeneity and variability in Tourette syndrome. In: Friedhoff A J, Chase T N (eds) Gilles de la Tourette syndrome. Adv Neurol, vol 35. Raven Press, New York, pp 437–442

Cameron J 1947 In: The psychology of behaviour disorders. Houghton Mifflin, Boston, p 353

Canavan A G M, Powell G E 1981 The efficacy of several treatments of Gilles de la Tourette's syndrome as assessed in a single case. Behav Res Therapy 19: 549–556

Cantwell D 1972 Psychiatric illness in the families of hyperactive children. Arch Gen Psychiat 27: 414–417

Caparulo B K, Cohen D J, Rothman S L, Young J G, Katz J D, Shaywitz S E et al 1981 Computed tomographic brainscanning in children with developmental neuropsychiatric disorders. J Am Acad Child Psychiat 20: 338–357

Caprini G, Melotti V 1961 Un grave syndrome ticcosa guarita con haloperidol. Riv Sper Freniat 85: 191–196

Carlson K R 1977 Supersensitivity to apomorphine and stress two years after chronic methadone treatment. Neuropharmacology 16: 795–798

Carlson K R, Eibergen R D 1976 Susceptibility to amphetamine-elicited dyskinesias following chronic methadone treatment in monkeys. Ann NY Acad Sci 281: 336–349

Carlsson A 1970 Biochemical aspects of abnormal movements induced by L-dopa. In: Barbeau A, Mc Dowell F H (eds) L-dopa and Parkinsonism. Davis, Philadelphia, pp 205–213

Carlsson A, Lindqvist M 1963 Effect of chlorpromazine and haloperidol on formation of 3-methoxytyramine and normetanephrine in mouse brain. Acta Pharmacol Toxicol 20: 140–144

Carlsson A, Lindqvist M, Magnusson T 1957 3:4 dihydroxyphenylalanine, 5-hydroxytryptophan as reserpine antagonists. Nature 180:1200

Carlsson A, Kehr W, Lindqvist M, Magnusson T, Atack C V 1972 Regulation of monoamine metabolism in the central nervous system. Pharmacol Rev 24: 371–384

Carman J S 1972 Methylphenidate in akathisia. Lancet 2:1093

Carpenter M B 1956 A study of the red nucleus in the rhesus monkey, anatomical degenerations and physiological effects resulting from localised lesions of the red nucleus. J Comp Neurol 105: 195–249

Carrea R M E, Mettler F A 1954 Anatomy of primate brachium conjunctivum and associated structures. J Comp Neurol 101: 565–689

Carrea R M E, Mettler F A 1955 Function of the primate brachium conjunctivum and related structures. J Comp Neurol 102: 151–322

Carroll B J, Curtis G C, Kokmen E 1977 Paradoxical response to dopamine agonists in tardive dyskinesia. Am J Psychiat 134: 785–789

Carter C J, Pycock C J 1980 Behavioural and biochemical effects of dopamine and noradrenaline depletion within the medial prefrontal cortex of the rat. Brain Res 192(1): 163–176

Case Q, McAndrew J B 1974 Dexedrine dyskinesia: an unusual iatrogenic tic. Clin Pediat 13: 69–72

Casey D E 1980 Pharmacology of blepharospasm-oromandibular dystonia syndrome. Neurology 30: 690–695

Casey D, Denney D 1977 Pharmacological characterisation of tardive dyskinesia. Psychopharmacology 54: 1–8

Casey D, Rabins P 1978 Tardive dyskinesia as a life-threatening illness. Am J Psychiat 135: 486–488

Casey D, Gerlach J, Magelund G, Rosted Christensen T 1980 Gamma-acetylenic GABA (GAG) in tardive dyskinesia. Arch Gen Psychiat 37: 1376–1382

Cassirer R 1922 Halsmuskelkrampf und Torsionspasmus. Klin Wschr 1: 53–57

Catrou J 1890 Étude sur la maladie des tics convulsifs (jumping, latah, myriachit). Faculté de Médecine de Paris. Thèse pour le doctorat en médecine. Henri Jouve, Paris

Cavenar J O, Harris M A 1980 À folie à deux dystonic reaction. Am J Psychiat 137: 99–100

Cavenar J O, Brantley I J, Braasch E 1978 Blepharospasm: organic or functional? Psychosomatics 19: 623–628

Chapel J L 1966 Gilles de la Tourettes disease: the past and the present. Canad Psychiat Assoc J 11: 324–329

Chapel J L 1970 Latah, myriachit and jumpers revisited. NY State J Med 70(ii): 2201–2204

Chapman J, McGhie A 1964 Echopraxia in schizophrenia. Br J Psychiat 110: 365–374

Charcot J 1885 Intorno ad alcuni casi di tic convulsivo con coprolalia ed echolalia. Reported by Melotti G. La Riforma Medica, 184, 185, 186

Chase T N 1972 Drug-induced extrapyramidal disorders. Res Pub Assoc Res Nerv Ment Dis 50: 448–471

Chase T N 1976 Antipsychotic drugs, dopaminergic mechanisms and extrapyramidal function in man. In: Sedvall G, Uvnas B, Zotterman Y (eds) Antipsychotic drugs: pharmacodynamics and pharmacokinetics. Pergamon, pp 321–329

Chase T N, Tamminga C A 1979 GABA system participation in motor, cognitive and endocrine function in man. In: Krogsgaard-Larson P, Scheel-Kruger J, Kofod H (eds) GABA-neurotransmitters: pharmacochemical, biochemical and pharmacological aspects. Academic Press, New York, pp 283–295

Chase T N, Holden E M, Brody J A 1973 Levodopa-induced dyskinesias. Arch Neurol 29: 328–330

Chateau R, Fau R, Gros Lambert R, Perret J A 1966 À propos d'un cas de torticollis spasmodique au cours d'un traitement par neuroleptiques. Ann Med Psychol Paris 124: 110–111

Chen X 1981 Selective resection and denervation of cervical muscles in the treatment of spasmodic torticollis: results in 60 cases. Neurosurgery 2: 520–533

Chen Han Bai, Lu Fei Han-Quin 1983 Tourette syndrome: report of 19 cases. Chin Med J 96: 45–50

Chien C P, Cole J O 1973 Eighteen-months follow-up of tardive dyskinesia treated with various catecholamine-related agents. Psychopharmacol Bull 9: 37–40

Christensen A V, Møller-Nielsen I 1974 Influence of flupenthixol and flupenthixol decanoate on methylphenidate and apomorphine-induced compulsive gnawing in mice. Psychopharmacologia Berlin 34: 119–126

Christensen E, Møller J E, Faurbye A 1970 Neuropathological investigation of 28 brains from patients with dyskinesia. Acta Psychiat Scand 46: 14–23

Ciminero A R, Nelson R D, Lipinski D P 1977 Self-monitoring procedures. In: Ciminero A R, Calhoun K S, Adams H E (eds) Handbook of behavioral assessment. Wiley, New York

Clark L P, Atwood C E 1912 A study of the significance of habit movements in mental defectives. J Am Med Assoc 58: 838–843

Claude H, Baruk H, Lamache A 1927 Obsessions-impulsions consécutives Á l'encephalité epidémique. Encephalé 22: 716–720

Clauss J L, Balthasar K 1954 Zur Kenntnis der generalisierten Tic-Krankheit (maladie des tics, Gilles de la Tourette sche Krankheit). Arch Psychiat Berlin 191: 398–418

Claveria L E, Teychenne P F, Calne D B, Haskayne L, Petrie A, Pallis C A et al 1975 Tardive dyskinesia treated with pimozide. J Neurol Sci 24: 393–401

Cleveland S E 1959 Personality dynamics in torticollis. J Nerv Ment Dis 129: 150–161

Clifford H C 1898 Some notes and theories concerning latah. Studies in brown humanity. Grant Richards, London

Clow A, Jenner P, Marsden C D 1978 An experimental model of tardive dyskinesias. Life Sci 23: 421–424

Clow A, Jenner P, Marsden C D 1979a Changes in dopamine mediated behaviour during one year's neuroleptic administration. Eur J Pharmacol 57: 365–375

Clow A, Jenner P, Theodorou A, Marsden C D 1979b Striatal dopamine receptors become supersensitive while rats are given trifluoperazine for six months. Nature 278: 59–61

Cockburn J J 1971 Spasmodic torticollis: a psychogenic condition. J Psychosom Res 15: 471–477

Cohen D J, Shaywitz B A, Caparulo B, Young J G, Bowers M B 1978 Chronic multiple tics of Gilles de la Tourette's disease. Arch Gen Psychiat 35: 245–250

Cohen D J, Shaywitz B A, Young J G, Carbonare C M, Nathanson J A, Lieberman D et al 1979 Central biogenic amine metabolism in children with the syndrome of chronic multiple tics of Gilles de la Tourette: norepinephrine, serotonin and dopamine. J. Am. Acad. Child. Psychiat. 18: 320–341

Cohen D J, Detlor J, Young G, Shaywitz B A 1980 Clonidine Amelioratos Gilles de la Tourette syndrome. Arch Gen Psychiat 37: 1350–1357

Cole W H 1973 Essential blepharospasm. South Med J 66: 1407–1411

Collier J, Adie W J 1922 In: Price F W (ed) A textbook of practice of medicine. Hodder and Stoughton, London, pp 1462–1466

Comings D, Gursey B, Hecht T, Blume K 1982 HLA typing in Tourette syndrome. In: Friedhoff A J, Chase T N (eds) Gilles de la Tourette syndrome. Adv Neurol, vol 35. Raven Press, New York, pp 251–254

Cooper I S 1964 Effect of thalamic lesions upon torticollis. New Engl J Med 270: 967–972

Cooper I S 1977 Neurosurgical treatment of the dyskinesias. Clin Neurosurg 24: 367–390

Corbett, J A 1971 The nature of tics and Gilles de la Tourette's syndrome. J Psychosom Res 15: 403–409

Corbett J A 1976 The nature of tics and Gilles de la Tourettes syndrome. In: Abuzzahab F, Anderson F (eds) Gilles de la Tourette syndrome international registry. Mason, St Paul, Minnesota, pp 25–32

Corbett J A, Campbell H J 1980 In: Mittler P (ed) Frontier knowledge in mental retardation, vol 2. University Park Press, p 288

Corbett J A, Mathews A M, Connell P H, Shapiro D A 1969 Tics and Gilles de la Tourettes syndrome: a follow-up study and critical review. Br J Psychiat 115: 1229–1241

Costall B, Naylor R J, Olley J E 1972 On the involvement of the caudate-putamen globus Pallidus and substantia nigra with neuroleptic and cholinergic modification of locomotor activity. Neuropharmacology 11: 317–330

Costall B, Naylor R J, Cannon J C, Lee T 1977 Differentiation of the dopamine mechanisms mediating stereotyped behaviour and hyperactivity in the nucleus accumbens and caudate putamon. J Pharm, Pharmacol 29: 337–42

Cottraux J A, Juenet C, Collet L 1983 The treatment of writer's cramp with multimodal behaviour therapy and biofeedback: A study of 15 cases. Br J Psychiat 142: 180–183

Cotzias G C, Van Woert M H, Schiffer L M 1967 Aromatic amino acids and modification of Parkinsonism. New Engl J Med 276: 374–379

Cotzias G C, Papavasiliou P S, Gellene R 1969 Modification of Parkinsonism-chronic treatment with L-dopa. New Engl J Med 280: 337–345

Couch J R 1975 The relationship between spasmodic torticollis and essential tremor. Trans Am Neurol Assoc 100: 181–183

Couch J R 1976 General discussion of drug therapy in dystonia. In: Eldridge R, Fahn S (eds) Adv Neurol, vol 14. Raven Press, New York, p 419

Crane G E 1967 A review of clinical literature on haloperidol. Int J Neuropsychiat 3 Suppl 1: 110–123

Crane G E 1968a Dyskinesia and neuroleptics. Arch Gen Psych 19: 700–703

Crane G E 1968b Tardive dyskinesia in patients treated with major neuroleptics. Am J Psychiat 124 Suppl: 40–48

Crane G E 1971 Persistence of Neurological symptoms due to neuroleptic drugs. Am J Psychiat 127: 1407–1410

Crane G E 1972a Pseudoparkinsonism and tardive dyskinesia. Arch Neurol 27: 426–430

Crane G E 1972b Prevention and management of tardive dyskinesia. Am J Psychiat 129: 126–127

Crane G E 1973 Persistent dyskinesia. Br J Psychiat 122: 395–405

Crane G E 1977 The prevention of tardive dyskinesia. Am J Psychiat 134: 756–758

Crane G E, Naranjo E R 1971 Motor disorders induced by neuroleptics. Arch Gen Psych 24: 179–184

Creak M, Guttmann E 1935 Chorea, tics and compulsive utterances. J Ment Sci 81: 834–839

Crisp A H, Moldofsky H 1965 A psychosomatic study of writer's cramp. Br J Psychiat 111: 841–858

Critchley E M R 1982 Humoral influences on human speech: a discussion paper. J Roy Soc Med 75: 258–261

Critchley E M R, Clark D B, Wikler A 1968 Acanthocytosis and neurological disorder without abetalipoproteinaemia. Arch Neurol 18: 134–140

Critchley E M R, Betts J J, Nicholson J T, Weatherall D J 1970 Acanthocytosis, nor-molipoproteinaemia and multiple tics. Postgrad Med J 46: 698–701

Critchley M 1927 On palilalia. J Neurol Psychopath 8: 23–31

Critchley M 1931 The neurology of old age. Lancet 1: 1221–1230

Critchley M 1938 106th meeting of the British Medical Association: section of neurology and psychological medicine. Br Med J 2:241

Critchley M 1939 Spastic dysphonia (inspiratory speech). Brain 62: 96–103

Critchley M 1977 Occupational palsies in musical performers. In: Critchley M, Henson R A (eds) Music and the brain. Heinemann, London, pp 365–377

Crosley, C J 1979 Decreased serotonergic activity in Tourette syndrome. Ann Neurol 5: 596–597

Crossman A R, Sambrook M A 1978 Experimental torticollis in the monkey produced by unilateral 6-hydroxydopamine brain lesions. Brain Res 149: 498–502

Crown S 1953 An experimental enquiry into some aspects of the motor behaviour and personality of ticqueurs. J Ment Sci 99: 84–91

Cruchet R 1907 Traite des torticolis spasmodiques, spasmes, tics, rhythmes do cou, torticollis Masson, Paris

Culpin M 1931 In: Recent advances in the study of the psychoneuroses. Churchill, London, p 178

Cummings D E, Gursey B T, Avelino E, Kopp V, Hanin I 1982 Red blood cell choline in Tourette syndrome. In: Friedhoff A J, Chase T N (eds) Gilles de la Tourette syndrome. Adv Neurol, vol 35. Raven Press, New York, pp 255–258

Curling T B 1860 Torticollis following rheumatic fever. Lancet 1:348

Curzon G 1973 Involuntary movements other than Parkinsonism. Proc Roy Soc Med 66: 873–876

Curzon G, Fernando J C R, Lees A J 1979 Backward walking and circling: behavioural responses induced by drug treatments which cause simultaneous release of cate-cholamines and 5-hydroxytryptamine. Br J Pharmacol 66: 573–579

Dandy W E 1930 An operation for the treatment of spasmodic torticollis. Arch Surg 20: 1021–1032

David M, Hecaen H, Constans J 1952 Torticolis spasmodique consécutif a une lésion corticale traumatique discussion du resultat favorable obtenu après excision de la lesion corticale. Rev Neurol 86: 57–61

Davis J M 1975 Overview: maintenance therapy in psychiatry 1. Schizophrenia. Am J Psychiat 132: 1237–1245

Davis M 1980 Neurochemical modulation of sensory-motor reactivity: acoustic and tactile startle reflexes. Neurosci Biobehav Rev 4: 241–263

Davison K, Bagley C R 1969 Schizophrenia-like psychoses associated with organic disorders of the central nervous system: a review. In: Herrington R N (ed) Current problems in neuropsychiatry. Br J Psychiat, special publication no. 4. Headley, Ashford, Kent

Debray P, Messerschmitt P, Lonchap D, Herbault M 1972 L'utilization du pimozide en pédopsychiatrie. Nouv Presse Med 1: 2917–2918

Debray-Ritzen P, Dubois H 1980 Maladies des tics de l'enfant. Rev Neurol Paris 136: 15–18

Dedo H H 1976 Recurrent laryngeal nerve section for spastic dysphonia. Ann Otol Rhinol Laryngol 85: 451–459

Dedo H H, Izdebski K, Townsend J J 1977 Recurrent laryngeal nerve histopathology in spastic dysphonia: a preliminary study. Ann Otol Rhinol Laryngol 86: 806–812

Degkwitz R 1969 Extrapyramidal motor disorders following long-term treatment with neuroleptic drugs. In: Crane G, Gardner R (eds) Psychotropic drugs and dysfunction of the basal ganglia. Public Health Service Publications no 1938, Washington D C, pp 22–32

Degkwitz R, Wenzel W 1967 Persistent extrapyramidal side-effects after long-term application of neuroleptics. In: Brill H, Cole J O, Deniker P, Hippius H, Bradley P B (eds) Neuropsychopharmacology Int Cong Ser 129. Mouton, Amsterdam, pp 608–615

Degkwitz R, Frowein R, Kulenkampff C, Mohs U 1960 Über die Wirkungen des L-dopa beim Menschen und ihre Beeinflussung durch Reserpin, Chlorpromazin, Iproniazid und Vitamin B6. Klin Wosch 38: 120–123

Degkwitz R, Consbruch U, Haddenbrock S, Neusch B, Oehlert W, Unsold R 1976 Therapeutische Risiken bei der Langzeitbehandlung mit Neuroleptika und Lithium klinische, histologische und biochemische. Nervenarzt 47: 81–87

Déjérine J 1914 In: Sémiologie des affections du système nerveux. Masson, Paris, pp 499–504

De Jong H H 1945 In: Experimental catatonia. Williams and Wilkins, Baltimore, pp 3–84

Delay J, Deniker P 1969 Drug-induced extrapyramidal syndromes. In: Vinken P J, Bruyn G W (eds) Handbook of clinical neurology, vol 6. North Holland, Amsterdam, pp 248–266

Delay J, Deniker P, Green A, Mororet M, 1957 Le syndrome excito moteur provoqués par les medicaments neuroleptiques. Presse Med 65: 1771–1774

Delay J, Deniker P, Ropert R, Beek H, Barande R, Eurieult M 1959 Syndromes neurologiques experimentaux et therapeutique psychiatrique: effets neurologique d'un nouveau neuroleptique majeur le 7843 RP. Presse Med 67: 123–126

De Lissovoy V 1962 Head banging in early childhood. Child Dev 33: 43–56

Delwaide P J, Desseiles M 1977 Spontaneous buccolingual dyskinesia in the elderly. Acta Neurol Scand 756: 256–262

Demars J C A 1966 Neuro-muscular effects of long-term phenothiazine medication, electroconvulsive therapy and leucotomy. J Nerv Ment Dis 143: 73–79

Denckla M B, Bemporad J R, Mackay M C 1976 Tics following methylphenidate administration: a report of 20 cases. J Am Med Assoc 235: 1349–1351

Denham J, Carrick D J E L 1961 Therapeutic value of thioproperazine and the importance of the associated neurological disturbances. J Ment Sci 107: 326–345

Denny-Brown D 1962 The mid-brain and motor integration. Proc Roy Soc Med 55: 527–538

De Renzi E 1879 Sulla catafasia. Giorn Int Sci Med 1: 474–479

De Speville 1906 Deux cas de blépharospasme guéris par deux procédés differénts. Rec Ophthalmol 3 S 28: 232–235

DeVeaugh-Geiss J 1980 Tardive Tourette syndrome. Neurology 30: 562–563

Devinsky O 1983 Neuroanatomy of Gilles de la Tourettes syndrome: possible midbrain involvement. Arch Neurol 40: 508–514

Dewulf A, van Bogaert L 1941 Études anatomo-cliniques de syndromes hypercinetiques complexes III. Une observation anatomo-clinique de maladie des tics (Gilles de la Tourette). Monatschr Psychiat Neurol 104: 53–61

Diamond B, Reyes M, Borison 1982 A new animal model for Tourette syndrome. In: Friedhoff A J, Chase T N (eds) Gilles de la Tourette syndrome. Adv Neurol vol 35. Raven Press, New York, pp 221–226

Dieckmann G 1976 Stereotaxic treatment of extrapyramidal torticollis. Neurochirurgie 22: 568–571

Dincmen K 1966 Chronic psychotic choreo-athetosis. Dis Nerv Syst 27: 399–402

Drage W 1963 Mary Hall of Gadsden in Hertford. In: Hunter R, McAlpine I (eds) 300 years of psychiatry. OUP, London, pp 174–177

Drake W E 1968 Clinical and Pathological findings in a child with a developmental learning disability. J Learn Dis 1: 486–502

Druckman R, Seelinger D, Thulin B 1962 Chronic involuntary movements induced by phenothiazines. J Nerv Ment Dis 135: 69–76

Düby S E, Cotzias G C, Papavasiliou P S, Lawrence W H 1972 Injected apomorphine and orally administered levodopa in Parkinsonism. Arch Neurol 27: 474–480

Duchenne de Boulogne G B A 1872 In: De l'electrisation localisée. Bailliere, Paris

Duchenne da Boulogne G B A 1883 In: Selections from the clinical works of Dr Duchenne de Boulogne. New Sydenham Society, pp 399–409

Duffy F H, Denckla M B, Bartels P H, Sandini G, Kiessling L S 1980 Dyslexia: regional differences in brain electrical activity by topographical mapping. Ann Neurol 7: 412–420

Dugas M, Ferrand I, Fabiani M, Lejonc M 1975 L'enfant tiquer qui est-il? comment le soulager? quel est son devenir? Rev Practicien 25 47: 3669–3678

Dunlap K 1945 In: Habits their making and unmaking. Liveright, New York, p 195

Dunstan R, Jackson D M 1977 The demonstration of a change in responsiveness of mice to physostigmine and atropine after withdrawal from long-term haloperidol pretreatment. J Neural Transm 40: 181–189

Duvoisin R C 1972 Reserpine for tardive dyskinesia. New Engl J Med 286:611

Duvoisin R C 1973 Hyperkinetic reactions with L-dopa. In: Yahr M D (ed) Current concepts in the treatment of Parkinsonism. Raven Press, New York, pp 203–211

Duvoisin R C 1976 Levodopa-induced involuntary movements. In: Birkmayer W, Hornykiewicz O (eds) Advances in Parkinsonism. Roche, Basel, pp 574–581

Duvoisin R C 1983 Meige syndrome: relief on high-dose anticholinergic therapy. Clin Neuropharm 6: 63–66

Earl C J C 1934 The primitive catatonic psychosis of idiocy. Br J Med Psychol 14: 230–253

Eisenberg L, Ascher E, Kanner L 1959 A clinical study of Gilles de la Tourettes disease in children. Am J Psychiat 115: 715–723

Ekbom K A 1960 Restless legs syndrome. Neurology 10: 868–873

Ekbom K, Lindholm H, Ljungberg L 1972 New dystonic syndrome associated with butyrophenone therapy. J Neurol 20 2: 94–103

Eldridge R 1970 The torsion dystonias: literature review and genetic and clinical studies. Neurology 202: 1–78

Eldridge R, Gottlieb R 1976 The primary hereditary dystonias: genetic classification of 768 families and revised estimate of gene frequency, autosomal recessive form and selected bibliography. In: Eldridge R, Fahn S (eds) Dystonia. Adv Neurol, vol 14. Raven Press, New York, pp 457–474

Eldridge R, Sweet R, Lake R, Ziegler M, Shapiro A K 1977 Gilles de la Tourettes syndrome: clinical genetic, psychologic and biochemical aspects in 21 selected cases. Neurology 27: 115–124

Ellinwood E H, Kilbey M M 1977 Chronic stimulant intoxication models of psychosis. In: Hanin, Usdin E (eds) Animal models in psychiatry and neurology. Pergamon, Oxford, pp 61–74

Engel P 1970 Could this be a new syndrome? Report of seven cases with characteristic mental and physical degeneracy. Dev Med Child Neurol 12: 282–289

Eriksson B, Persson T 1969 Gilles de la Tourette's syndrome: two cases with an organic brain injury. Br J Psychiat 115: 351–353

Esquirol J E D 1845 Mental maladies: a treatise on insanity. Trans E K Hunt. Lea and Blanchard, Philadelphia, p 469

Ettigi P, Nair N P V, Lal S, Cervantes P, Guyd A 1976 Effect of apomorphine on growth hormone and prolactin secretion in schizophrenic patients with or without oral dyskinesia withdrawn from chronic neuroleptic therapy. J Neurol Neurosurg Psychiat 39: 870–876

Ezrin-Waters C, Seeman P 1978 L-dopa reversal of hyperdopaminergic behaviour. Life Sci 22: 1027–1032

Fabinyi G, Dutton J 1980 The surgical treatment of spasmodic torticollis. Aust NZ J Surg 50: 155–157

Fabricius A B Aquapendente 1687 In: Opera omnia anatomica et physiologica. Leipzig, Bonn, 1922, p 135

Fahn S 1978 Treatment of tardive dyskinesia with combined reserpine and alphamethyltyrosine. Trans Am Neurol Assoc 103: 100–102

Fahn S 1982 A case of post-traumatic tic syndrome. In: Friedhoff A J, Chase T N (eds) Gilles de la Tourette syndrome. Adv Neurol, vol 35. Raven Press, New York, pp 349–350

Fairweather D S 1947 Psychiatric aspects of the post-encephalitic syndrome. J Ment Sci 93: 201–254

Fann W E 1966 Use of methylphenidate to counteract acute dystonic effects of phenothiazines. Am J Psych 122: 1293–1294

Fariello R G, Schwartzman R J, Beall S S 1983 Hyperekplexia exacerbated by occlusion of posterior thalamic arteries. Arch Neurol 40: 244–246

Farrar W B 1976 Using electromyographic biofeedback in treating orofacial dyskinesia. J Prosthet Dent 35: 384–387

Faurbye A, Rasch P J, Peterson P B, Brandborg G, Pakkenberg H 1964 Neurological symptoms in pharmacotherapy of psychoses. Acta Psychiat Scand 40: 10–27

Feinberg M, Carroll B J 1979 Effects of dopamine agonists and antagonists in Tourettes disease. Arch Gen Psychiat 36: 979–985

Fenichel O 1945 In: The psychoanalytic theory of neurosis. Norton Press, New York, pp 317–321

Féré C 1906 Note sur quelques cas de trichotillomanie chez des aliénés. Nouv Icon Salpetriere 19: 168–170

Ferenczi S 1921 Psycho-analytical observations on tic. Int J Psychoanal 2: 1–30

Ferguson D 1971 An Australian study of telegraphist's cramp. Br J Indust Med 28: 280–285

Fernando S J M 1967 Gilles de la Tourette's syndrome: a report on 4 cases and a review of published case reports. Br J Psychiat 113: 607–617

Fernando S J M 1976 Six cases of Gilles de la Tourette's syndrome. Br J Psychiat 128: 436–441

Feser Prof 1875 Apomorphinum Hydrochloratum Ein Heilmittel gegen die Saug Lecksucht der Rinder, Schafe und Schweine. Z Praktische Veterinärwissenschaft 111–113

Feuerstein C, Serre F, Gavend M, Pellat J, Perret J, Tanche M 1977 Plasma o-methyldopa in levodopa-induced dyskinesias. Acta Neurol Scand 56: 509–524

Finney J M T, Hughson W 1925 Spasmodic torticollis. Ann Surg 81: 255–269

Finney J W, Christophersen E R, Ziegler D K 1981 Deanol and Tourette syndrome. Lancet 2:989

Fischer-Williams M 1969 The neurological aspects of mental subnormality. J Ment Subnorm 15: 21–36 and 16: 63–70

Fish F J 1976 In: Hamilton M (ed) Fish's schizoprenia. Wright, Bristol, pp 56–66

Fisher C M 1963 Reflex blepharospasm. Neurology 13: 77–78

Fishman R A 1965 Neurological aspects of magnasium metabolism. Arch Neurol 12: 562–569

Fitzgerald M X, Fitzgerald O 1969 Reaction to trifluoperazine abuse. Lancet 1:1100

Foerster O 1933 Mobile spasm of the neck muscles and its pathological basis. J Comp Neurol 58: 725–735

Fog R, Pakkenberg H 1980 Theoretical and clinical aspects of the Tourette syndrome (chronic multiple tic). J Neural Transm Suppl 16: 211–215

Fog R, Pakkenberg H 1981 Neuroleptic-induced tardive Tourette's syndrome and neuro-toxicity. In: Usdin E, Dahl S, Gram L, Linejaerde O (eds) Clinical pharmacology in psychiatry. Macmillan London, pp 385–387

Fog R, Pakkenberg H, Juul P, Bock E, Jørgensen O S, Andersen J 1976 High-dose treatment of rats with perphenazine enanthate. Psychopharmacology 50: 305–307

Foley J 1975 In: Kirman B, Bicknell J (eds) Neurological examination in mental handicap. Churchill Livingstone, Edinburgh, pp 321–335

Foley J 1983 The athetoid syndrome: a review of a personal series. J Neurol Neurosurg Psychiat 46: 289–298

Foltz E L, Knopp L M, Ward A A 1959 Experimental spasmodic torticollis. J Neurosurg 16: 55–72

Forrest D V, Fahn S 1979 Tardive dysphrenia and subjective akathisia. J Clin Psychiat 40:206

Forrest F M 1974 Evolutionary origin of extrapyramidal disorders in drug-treated mental patients. Its significance and the role of neuro-melanin. In: Forrest I S, Carr C J, Usdin E (eds) The phenothiazines and structurally related drugs. Raven Press, New York, pp 255–268

Forrest F M, Forrest, I S, Roizin L 1963 Clinical biochemical and post-mortem studies on a patient treated with chlorpromazine. Agressologie 4: 259–265

Foster J 1977 Putting on the agony. World Med June 29th: 26–27

Frank S M 1978 Psycholinguistic findings in Gilles de la Tourette syndrome. J Commun Disord 11: 349–363

Fras I, Karlavage J 1977 The use of methylphenidate and imipramine in Gilles de la Tourette's disease in children. Am J Psychiat 134: 195–197

Freeman T, Gathercole C E 1966 Perseveration: The clinical symptoms in chronic schizophrenia and organic dementia. Br J Psychiat 112: 27–32

Frey E 1914 Beitrage zur Klinik und pathologischen Anatomie der Alzheimerschen Krankheit. Z Neurol Psychiat 27: 397–434

Freyhan F A 1957 Psychomotility and Parkinsonism in treatment with neuroeptic drugs. Arch Neurol Psychiat 78: 465–472

Freyhan F A 1959 Extrapyramidal symptoms and other side-effects. In: Brill H (ed) Trifluperazine-clinical and pharmacological aspects. Kimpton, London, pp 195–205

Friedhoff A J, Rosengarten H, Bonnet K 1978 Receptor cell sensitivity modification as a model for the pathogenesis and treatment of tardive dyskinesia. Psychopharmacol Bull 14: 77–79

Friedhoff A J, Rosengarten H, Bonnet K 1980 Receptor cell sensitivity modification (RSM) as a model for pathogenesis and treatment of tardive dyskinesia. In: Fann W E, Smith R D, Davis J M, Domino E F (eds) Tardive dyskinesia research and treatment. Medical and Scientific Books, New York, 11: 139–143

Friedman S 1980 Self-control in the treatment of Gilles de la Tourettes syndrome: case-study with 18 month follow-up. J Con Clin Psychiat 48: 400–402

Friedreich N 1881 Ueber Koordinierte Erinnerungskrämpfe. Virchows Archiv für Pathologische Anatomie und Physiologie und für Klinische Medizin 86: 430–434

Friend J 1701 De spasmi rarioris historia. In: Philosophical transactions, pp 799–804

Gagrat D, Hamilton J, Belmaker R H 1978 Intravenous diazepam in the treatment of neuroleptic-induced dystonia and akathisia. Am J Psychiat 135: 1232–1233

Gailitis J, Knowles R R, Longobardi A 1960 Alarming Neuromuscular reactions due to prochlorperazine. Ann Int Med 52: 538–543

Galaburda A M, Kemper T L 1979 Cytoarchitectonic abnormalities in developmental dyslexia: a case study. Ann Neurol 6: 94–100

Garcia-Alba E, Franch O, Munoz D, Ricoy J R 1981 Brueghel's syndrome: report of a case with postmortem studies. J Neurol Neurosurg Psychiat 44: 437–440

Gardos G, Cole J O 1975 Papaverine for tardive dyskinesia? New Engl J Med 292:1355

Gardos G, Cole J O 1980 Public health issues in tardive dyskinesia. Am J Psychiat 137: 776–781

Gardos G, Orzack M H, Finn G, Cole J O 1974 High and low dose thiothixene treatment in chronic schizophrenia. Dis Nerv Syst 35: 53–58

Gardos G, Cole J O, Tarsy D 1978 Withdrawal syndromes associated with antipsychotic drugs. Am J Psychiat 135: 1321–1324

Garver D L, Davis J M, Dekirmenjian H, Ericksen S, Gosenfeld L, Haraszti J 1976a Dystonic reactions following neuroleptics: time course and proposed mechanisms. Psychopharmacology 47: 199–201

Garver D L, Davis J M, Dekirmenjian H, Jones F D, Casper R, Haraszti, J 1976b Pharmacokinetics of red blood cell phenothiazine and clinical effects: acute dystonic reactions. Arch Gen Psychiat 33: 862–866

Garver D L, Dekirmenjian H, Davis J M, Casper R, Ericksen S 1977 Neuroleptic drug levels and therapeutic response: preliminary observations with red blood cell bound butaperazine. Am J Psychiat 134: 304–307

Gastaut H, Tasinari C A 1966 Triggering mechanisms in epilepsy. Epilepsia 7: 85–138

Gastaut H, Villeneuve A 1967 The startle disease or hyperekplexia: pathological surprise reaction. J Neurol Sci 5: 523–542

Gaussel M 1904 Spasme bilateral des muscles du cou et de la face. Nouv Icon Salpetriere 17: 337–342

Gelenberg A J 1976a The catatonic syndrome. Lancet 1: 1339–1341

Gelenberg A J 1976b Computerised tomography in patients with tardive dyskinesia. Am J Psychiat 133: 578–579

Gerlach J 1975 Long-term effect of perphenazine on the substantia nigra in rats. Psychopharmacology 45: 51–54

Gerlach J 1977 Relationship between tardive dyskinesia, L-dopa induced hyperkinesia and Parkinsonism. Psychopharmacology 51: 259–263

Gerlach J 1979 Tardive dyskinesia. Dan Med Bull 26: 209–45

Gerlach J, Simmelsgaard H 1978 Tardive dyskinesia during and following treatment with haloperidol, haloperidol & biperiden, thioridazine and clozapine. Psychopharmacology 59: 105–112

Gerlach J, Thorsen K 1976 The movement pattern of oral tardive dyskinesia in relation to anti-cholinergic and antidopaminergic treatment. Int Pharmacopsychiat 11: 1–7

Gerlach J, Reisby N, Randrup A 1974 Dopaminergic hypesensitivity and cholinergic hypofunction in the pathophysiology of tardive dyskinesias. Psychopharmacology 34: 21–35

Gerlach J, Rye J, Kristjansen P 1978 Effect of baclofen on tardive dyskinesia. Psychopharmacology 56: 145–151

Gessa R, Tagliamonte A, Gessa G L 1972 Blockade by apomorphine of haloperidol-induced dyskinesia in schizophrenic patients. Lancet 2: 981–982

Gilbert G J 1972 The medical treatment of spasmodic torticollis. Arch Neurol 27: 503–506

Gilbert G J 1977 Familial spasmodic torticollis. Neurology 27: 11–13

Gilles de la Tourette G 1884 Jumping, latah, myriachit. Arch Neurol 8: 68–84

Gilles de la Tourette G 1885 Étude sur une affection nerveuse caracterisée par de l'incoordination motrice accompagnée d'écholalie et de coprolalie. Arch Neurol 9: 19–42, 158–200

Gilles de la Tourette G 1899 La maladie des tics convulsifs. Sem Med 19: 153–156

Gleckman R, Maddoff M A, Edsall G 1969 Tetanus or phenothiazine reaction? A differential diagnostic problem. New Eng J Med 280:1244

Godwin-Austen R B, Clark T 1971 Persistent phenothiazine dyskinesia treated with tetrabenazine. Br Med J 4: 25–26

Golden G S 1974 Gilles de la Tourette's syndrome following methylphenidate administration. Dev Med Child Neurol 16: 76–78

Golden G S 1977a Tourette syndrome: the paediatric perspective. Am J Dis Child 131: 531–534

Golden G S 1977b The effect of central nervous system stimulants on Tourette syndrome. Ann Neurol 2: 69–70

Golden G S, Greenhill L 1981 Tourette syndrome in mentally retarded children. Ment Retard 19: 17–19

Goldman D 1961 Parkinsonism and related phenomena from administration of drugs: their production and control under clinical conditions and possible relation to therapeutic effect. In: Bordeleau J (ed) Extrapyramidal system and neuroleptics. Editions Psychiatriques, Montreal, 453–464

Gollomp S, Illson J, Burke R, Fahn S 1981 Meige syndrome: a review of 31 cases. Neurology 31(2):A78

Gollomp S, Fahn S, Burke R E, Reches A, Ilson J 1983 Therapeutic trials in Meige syndrome. In: Fahn S, Calne D B, Shoulson I (eds) Experimental therapeutics of movement disorders. Adv Neurol, vol 37. Raven Press, New York pp 207–214

Gowers W R 1877 Writer's cramp. Med Times Gaz Lond 11: 536–538

Gowers W R 1893 A manual of diseases of the nervous system (Reprinted 1970). Hafner, Darien, Connecticut

Granacher R P, Baldessarini R J, Cole J O 1975 The pharmacologic evaluation of tardive dyskinesia. New Engl J Med 292: 926–927

Greenblatt D L, Dominick J R, Stotsky B A, Dimascio A 1968 Phenothiazine-induced dyskinesia in nursing home patients. J Am Ger Soc 16: 27–34

Greenfield J G, Wolfsohn J M 1922 The pathology of Sydenham's chorea. Lancet 2: 603–606

Gresty M A, Ell J J 1981 Spasmus nutans or congenital nystagmus? Classification according to objective criteria. Br J Ophthalmol 65: 510–511

Gresty M A, Halmagyi G M 1979 Abnormal head movements. J. Neurol Neurosurg Psychiat 42: 705–714

Grinker R R, Walker A E 1933 The pathology of spasmodic torticollis with a note on respiratory failure from anaesthesia in chronic encephalitis. J Nerv Ment Dis 78: 630–637

Gross H, Kaltenbäch E 1968 Neuropathological findings in persistent dyskinesia after neuroleptic long-term therapy. In: Cerletti A, Bové F J (eds) The present status of psychotropic drugs. Excerpta Medica, Amsterdam, pp 474–76

Growdon J H, Hirsch M J, Wurtman R J, Wiener W 1977 Oral choline administration to patients with tardive dyskinesia. New Engl J Med 297: 524–527

Growdon J H, Gelenberg A J, Doller J 1978 Lecithin can suppress tardive dyskinesia. New Engl J Med 298:1029

Grünthal V E, Walther-Buel H 1960 Über Schädigung der Oliva inferior durch Chlorperphenazine (Trilafon). Psychiat Neurol Basel 140: 249–257

Guggenheim M A 1979 Familial Tourette syndrome. Ann Neurol 5:104

Guillain G, Bize R 1933 Sur un cas de sclérose en plaques avec torticolis spasmodique. Rev Neurol 40(ii): 133–138

Guinon G 1886 Sur la maladie des tics convulsifs. Rev Med 6: 50–80

Guinon G 1887 Tics convulsifs et hysterie. Rev Med 7: 509–519

Gunne L M, Barany S 1976 Haloperidol-induced tardive dyskinesia in monkeys. Psychopharmacology 150: 237–40

Gunne L M, Barany S 1980 A primate model for tardive dyskinesia. In: Fann W E, Smith R C, Davis J M (eds) Tardive dyskinesia research and treatment. Spectrum, New York

Gupta J M, Lovejoy F H 1967 Acute phenothiazine toxicity in childhood: A five-year survey. Pediatrics 39: 771–774

Haase H J, Janssen P A 1965 The action of neuroleptic drugs. North Holland, Amsterdam

Hall M 1852 On muscular tic. Lancet 2:510

Hammer M 1965 A case of coprolalia in an adolescent boy. Psychother Theory Res Pract 2: 169–176

Hammond W A 1884 Miryachit: newly described disease of nervous system and its analogues. NY Med J 39: 191–192

Hammond G M 1892 Convulsive tic: its nature and treatment. Med Record 41: 236–239

Hardie R J, Lees A J, Stern G M 1983 Sustained levodopa therapy in tardive dyskinesia. J Neurol Neurosurg Psychiat 46:685

Hardison J E 1980 Are the jumping frenchmen of Maine goosey? J Am Med Assoc 70:244

Harenko A 1967 Retrocollis as an irreversible late complication of neuroleptic medications. Acta Neurol Scand 43 Suppl 31: 145–146

Harnack G 1958 In: Nervöse Verhaltensstörungen beim Schulkind. Thieme, Stuttgart

Haskovec M L 1901 L'akathisie. Rev Neurol 9: 1107–1109

Haskovec M L 1903 Nouvelles remarques sur l'akathisie. Nouv Icon Salpetriere 16: 287–296

Hassler R 1953 Extrapyramidal-motorische Syndrome und Erkrankungen. In: Handbuch der inneren Medizin Bd 13 Neurologie. Springer, Berlin, pp 676–904

Hassler R, Dieckmann G 1970 Traitement stereotaxique des tics et cris inarticules ou coprolalique considérés comme phénoméne d'obsession motrice au cours de la maladie Gilles de la Tourette. Rev Neurol 123: 89–100

Hassler R, Riechert T 1958 Über die Symptomatik und operative Behandlung der extrapyramidalen Bewegungsstörungen. Med Klin 53: 817–824

Heaver L 1959 Spastic dysphonia II. Logos 2: 15–24

Heinrich K, Wegener I, Bender H J 1968 Späte extrapyramidale Hyperkinesen bei neuroleptischer Langzeittherapie. Pharmakopsychiat Neuropsychopharmakol 1: 169–195

Henderson J W 1956 Essential Blepharospasm. Trans Am Ophthal Soc 54: 453–520

Hernesniemi J, Laitenen L 1977 Résultats tardifs de la chirurgie dans le torticollis spasmodique. Neurochirurgie 23: 123–131

Hershon H I, Kennedy P F, McGuire R J 1972 Persistence of extra-pyramidal disorders and psychiatric relapse after withdrawal of long-term phenothiazine therapy. Br J Psychiat 120: 41–50

Herz E, Glaser G H 1949 Spasmodic torticollis II. Clinical evaluation. Arch Neurol Psychiat 61: 227–239

Hess W R 1949 Funktionen des Zwischenhirns im Rahmen der extrapyramidalen Motorik. Bull Schweiz Akad D Med Wissensch 5: 221–225

Hippius H, Longemann G 1970 Zur Wirkung des Dioxyphenylalanin auf extrapyramidal motorische Hyperkinesen nach langfristiger neuroleptischer Therapie. Arzneimittelforsch 20: 894–895

Hochberg F H, Leffert R D, Heller M D 1983 Hand difficulties among musicians. J Am Med Assoc 249: 1869–1872

Hoffmann H, 1845 Der Struwwelpeter: oder lustige Geschichten und drollige Bilder. Inse Leipzig

Horrocks P M, Vicary D J, Rees J E, Parkes J D, Marsden C D 1973 Anticholinergic withdrawal and benzhexol treatment in Parkinson's disease. J Neurol Neurosurg Psychiat 36: 936–941

Huessy H 1967 Study of the prevalence and therapy of the choreatiform syndrome or hyperkinesis in rural Vermont. Acta Paedopsychiat 34: 130–135

Humphrey E, Warner L 1934 In: Working dogs. John Hopkins Press

Hunter R, Earl C J, Janz D 1964a A syndrome of abnormal movements and dementia in leucotomized patients treated with phenothiazines. J Neurol Neurosurg Psychiat 27: 219–223

Hunter R, Earl C J, Thornicroft S 1964b An apparently irreversible syndrome of abnormal movements following phenothiazine medication. Proc Roy Soc Med 57: 758–762

Hunter R, Blackwood W, Smith M C, Cumings J N 1968 Neuropathological findings in three cases of persistent dyskinesia following phenothiazine medication. J Neurol Sci 7263–7273

Hutzell, R R, Platzek D, Logue P E 1974 Control of symptoms of Gilles de la Tourette's syndrome by self-monitoring. J Behav Ther Exp Psychiat 5: 71–76

Hyttel J 1977a Levels of HVA and dopac in mouse corpus striatum in the supersensitivity phase after neuroleptic treatment. J Neurochem 28: 227–228

Hyttel J 1977b Changes in dopamine synthesis rate in the supersensitivity phase after treatment with a single dose of neuroleptics. Psychopharmacology 51: 205–207

Incagnoli T, Kane R 1982 Neuropsychological functioning in Tourette syndrome. In: Friedhoff A J, Chase T N (eds) Gilles de la Tourette syndrome. Adv Neurol, vol 35. Raven Press, New York, pp 305–310

Ingram N A W, Newgreen D B 1983 The use of tacrine for tardive dyskinesia. Am J Psychiat 140: 1629–1631

Ireland W W 1877 In: On idiocy and imbecility. Churchill, London, p 274

Irvine A R, Daroff R B, Sanders M D, Hoyt W F 1968 Familial reflex blepharospasm. Am J Ophthalmol 65: 889–890

Ismeuth A 1979 Gilles de la Tourette's syndrome. J Ment Def Res 23: 25–27

Itard J M G 1825 Mémoire sur quelques fonctions involontaires des appareils de la locomotion de la préhension et de la voix. Arch Gen Med 8: 385–407

Iverson S, Alpert J 1982 Functional organisation of the dopamine system in normal and abnormal behaviour. In: Friedhoff A J, Chase T N (eds) Gilles de la Tourette syndrome. Adv Neurol, vol 35. Raven Press, New York, pp 69–76

Jackson J H 1884 Case XXXII. Loss of speech and hemiplegia on the right side — recovery of power to swear — no valvular disease. Clinical Lectures and Reports to the London Hospital 1: 452–455

Jacobson G, Baldessarini R J, Manschreck T 1974 Tardive and withdrawal dyskinesia associated with haloperidol. Am J Psychiat 131: 910–913

Jaeger G F 1737 Inaugural dissertation. Roebelianis, Tubingen, 1953

James I, Cook P 1983 Bromocriptine for Horn Player's palsy. Lancet 1:1450

Janet P 1925 In: Psychological Healing, vol 2. Allen and Unwin, London, pp 710–783

Jankovic J, Ford J 1983 Blepharospasm and orofacial-cervical dystonia: clinical and pharmacological findings in 100 patients. Ann Neurol 13: 402–411

Jayne D, Lees A J, Stern G M 1984 Remission in spasmodic torticollis. J Neurol Neurosurg Psychiat 47: 1236–1237

Jelliffe S E 1910 Migraine, Neuralgia, professional spasms occupational neuroses. In: Osler W, McRae T (eds) A system of medicine, vol 7. OUP, London, pp 786–795

Jelliffe S E 1927 The mental pictures in schizophrenia and in epidemic encephalitis. Am J Psychiat 6: 413–465

Jelliffe S E 1929 Psychological components in post-encephalitic oculogyric crises. Arch Neurol Psych 21: 491–541

Jellinger K 1977 Neuropathologic findings after neuroleptic long-term therapy. In: Roizin L, Shiraka M, Grcevic N (eds) Neurotoxicology. Raven Press, New York, pp 25–42

Jenkins R L, Ashby H B 1983 Gilles de la Tourette's syndrome in identical twins. Arch Neurol 40: 249–251

Jeste D V, Potkin S G, Sinha S, Feder S, Wyatt R J 1979 Tardive dyskinesia: reversible and persistent. Arch Gen Psychiat 36: 585–590

John E R, Karmel B Z, Corning W E et al 1977 Neurometrics. Science 196: 1393–1410

Jones I H 1965 Observations on schizophrenic stereotypies. Comp Psych 6: 323–335

Jones M, Hunter R 1969 Abnormal movements in patients with chronic psychiatric illness. In: Crane G, Gardner R (eds) Psychotropic drugs and dysfunctions of the basal ganglia. Public Health Service Publication 1938, US Government Printing Office, Washington, pp 53–65

Joschko M, Rourke B 1982 Neuropsychological dimensions of Tourette syndrome: test-retest stability and implications for intervention. In: Friedhoff A J, Chase T N (eds) Gilles de la Tourette syndrome. Adv Neurol, vol 35. Raven Press, New York, pp 297–304

Jung R, Hassler R 1960 In: Handbook of physiology (section on Neurophysiology), vol 2. The extrapyramidal motor system. Williams and Wilkins, Baltimore

Jurgens U, Ploog D 1970 Cerebral representation of vocalisation in the squirrel monkey. Exp Brain Res 10: 532–554

Jus K, Villeneuve A, Jus A 1972 Tardive dyskinesia and the rabbit syndrome during wakefulness and sleep. Am J Psychiat 129:765

Jus K, Jus A, Gautier J, Villeneuve A, Pires P, Pineau R et al 1974 Studies on the action of certain pharmacological agents on tardive dyskinesia and on the rabbit syndrome. Int J Clin Pharmacol 9: 138–145

Kaiser H E 1954 Zentbl Allg Path Anat 91:196

Kameyama M, Yamanouchi H, Suda E 1975 Oral dyskinesia in the aged. Acta Geron Jap 59: 5–15

Kane J M, Weinhold P, Kinon B, Wegner J, Leader M 1982a A prospective study of tardive dyskinesia development: preliminary results.J Clin Psychopharmacol 2(5): 345–349

Kane J M, Weinhold P, Kinon B, Wegner J, Leader M 1982b Prevalence of abnormal involuntary movements (spontaneous dyskinesias) in the normal elderly. Psychopharmacology 77: 105–108

Kanner L 1948 In: Child Psychiatry. Blackwell, Oxford, pp 411–418

Karson C N, Jeste D V, Le Witt P A, Wyatt R J 1983 A comparison of two iatrogenic dyskinesias. Am J Psychiat 140: 1504–1506

Kaufman M E, Levitt H 1965 A study of three stereotyped behaviours in institutionalised mental defectives. Am J Ment Defic 69: 467–473

Kazamatsuri H, Chien C P, Cole J O 1972a Treatment of tardive dyskinesia I. clinical efficacy of a dopamine-depleting agent tetrabenazene. Arch Gen Psychiat 27: 95–99

Kazamatsuri H, Chien C, Cole, J O 1972b Treatment of tardive dyskinesias II. short-term efficacy of dopamine-blocking agents, haloperidol and thiopropazate. Arch Gen Psychiat 27: 100–103

Kazamatzuri H, Chien C P, Cole J O 1972c Treatment of tardive dyskinesia III. clinical efficacy of a dopamine competing agent, methyldopa. Arch Gen Psychiat 27: 824–827

Kebabian J W, Calne D B 1979 Multiple receptors for dopamine. Nature 277: 93–96

Keegan D L, Rajput A H 1973 Drug-induced dystonia tarda: treatment with L-dopa. Dis Nerv Syst 34: 167–169

Kehr W, Carlsson A, Lindqvist M, Magnusson T, Atack C 1972 Evidence for a receptor-mediated feedback control of striatal tyrosine hydroxylase activity. J Pharm Pharmacol 24: 744–747

Kellmer Pringle M L, Butler N R, Davie R 1967 1st report of national child development study. In: 11 000 seven-year-olds. National Bureau for Co-operation in Child Care, London, p 185

Kelly P H, Seviour P W, Iversen S D 1975 Amphetamine and apomorphine responses in the rat following 6 OHDA lesions of the nucleus accumbens septi and corpus striatum. Brain Res 94: 507–522

Kendler K 1976 A medical student's experience with akathisia. Am J Psychiat 133: 454–455

Kennedy P F, Hershon H I, McGuire R J 1971 Extrapyramidal disorders after prolonged phenothiazine therapy. Br J Psychiat 118: 509–518

Kidd K K, Pauls D L 1982 Genetic hypotheses for Tourette syndrome. In: Friedhoff A J, Chase T N (eds) Gilles de la Tourette syndrome. Adv Neurol, vol 35. Raven Press, New York, pp 243–250

Kidd K K, Prusoff B A, Cohen D J 1980 Familial pattern of Gilles de la Tourette syndrome. Arch Gen Psychiat 37: 1336–1339

Kito S, Itoga E, Hiroshige Y, Matsumoto N, Miwa S 1980 A pedigree of amyotrophic chorea with acanthocytosis. Arch Neurol 937: 514–517

Kjellin K G, Stibler H 1974 Protein pattern of cerebrospinal fluid in spasmodic torticollis. J Neurol Neurosurg Psychiat 37: 1128–1132

Klawans H L 1973a The pharmacology of tardive dyskinesia. Am J psychiat 130: 82–86

Klawans H L 1973b In: The pharmacology of extrapyramidal disorders. Neurol Monographs, vol 2. Karger, Basel, pp 1–136

Klawans H L, Barr A 1982 Prevalence of spontaneous lingual-facial buccal dyskinesias in the elderly. Neurology 32: 558–559

Klawans H L, Bergen D 1975 Side-effects of levodopa. In: Stern G M (ed) The clinical uses of levodopa. Medical and Technical Publishing, Lancaster, pp 73–107

Klawans H L, Garvin J S 1969 Treatment of Parkinsonism with L-dopa. Dis Nerv Syst 30: 737–746

Klawans H L, McKendal R 1971 Observations on the effects of L-dopa on tardive linguo-facial-buccal dyskinesia. J Neurol Sci 14: 189–192

Klawans H L, Rubovitz R 1974 Effect of cholinergic and anticholinergic agents on tardive dyskinesia. J Neurol Neurosurg Psychiat 27: 941–947

Klawans H L. Weiner W J 1974a The effect of d-amphetamine on choreiform movement disorders. Neurology 24: 312–318

Klawans H L, Weiner W J 1974b Attempted use of haloperidol in the treatment of L-dopa induced dyskinesias. J Neurol Neurosurg Psychiat 37: 427–430

Klawans H L, Paulson G W, Ringel S P, Barbeau A 1972 Use of L-dopa in the detection of presymptomatic Huntington's chorea. New Engl J Med 286: 1332–1334

Klawans H L. Bergen D, Bruyn G W, Paulson G W 1974 Neuroleptic-induced tardive dyskinesias in non-psychotic patients. Arch Neurol 30: 338–339

Klawans H L, Goetz C, Bergen D 1975a Levodopa-induced myoclonus. Arch Neurol 32: 331–334

Klawans H L, Topel J L, Bergen D 1975b Deanol in the treatment of levo-dopa induced dyskinesias. Neurology 25: 290–294

Klawans H L, Goetz C, Nausieda P A, Weiner W J 1977 Levodopa-induced receptor hypersensitivity. Ann Neurol 2: 125–132

Klawans H L, Falk D K, Nausieda P A, Weiner W J 1978 Gilles de la Tourette syndrome after long-term chlorpromazine therapy. Neurology 28: 1064–1068

Kleist K 1960 Schizophrenic symptoms and cerebral pathology. J Ment Sci 106: 246–255

Knopp W, Fisher R, Beck J, Teitelbaum A 1966 Clinical implications of the relation between taste sensitivity and the appearance of extrapyramidal side-effects. Dis Nerv Syst 27: 729–735

Koella W P 1955 Motor effects from electrical stimulation of basal cerebellum in unrestrained cat. J Neurophysiol 18: 559–573

Koester G 1899 Über die Maladie des Tics impulsifs (mimische Krampfneurose) Dt Nerven heilk 15: 147–159

Koizumi J, Shiraishi H 1973a Synaptic changes in the rabbit pallidum following long-term haloperidol administration. Folia Psychiat Neurol Japan 27: 51–57

Koizumi J, Shiraishi H 1973b Synaptic alterations in the hypothalamus of the rabbit following long-term chlorpromazine administration. Folia Psychiat Neurol Japan 27: 59–67

Kolbe H, Clow A, Jenner P, Marsden C D 1981 Neuroleptic-induced acute dystonic reactions may be due to enhanced dopamine release on to supersensitive postsynaptic receptors. Neurology 31: 434–439

Korczyn A, Goldberg G J 1972 Intravenous diazepam in drug-induced dystonic reactions. Br J Psychiat 121: 75–77

Korein J, Brudny J 1976 Integrated emg feedback in the management of spasmodic torticollis and focal dystonia: a prospective study of 80 patients. In: Yahr M D (ed) The basal ganglia. Raven Perss, New York, pp 385–424

Kraepelin E 1919 Dementia praecox and paraphrenia. Robertson G M (ed), Barclay R M (trans). E α S Livingstone, Edinburgh

Kramer F, Pollnow H 1932 Über eine hyperkinetische Erkrankuncg Kindesalter. Mschr Psychiat Neurol 82: 654–690

Kramer J C, Fischman V S, Littlefield D C 1967 Amphetamine abuse: pattern and effects of high doses taken intravenously. J Am Med Assoc 201: 305–309

Krauss S 1934 Persönlichkeitsveränderungen nach Chorea minor Schweiz Arch Psychiat Neurol 34: 94–142

Kravitz H, Boe hm J J 1971 Rhythmic habit patterns in infancy their sequence, age of onset and frequency. Child Devel 42: 399–413

Kravitz H, Rosenthal V, Teplitz Z, Murphy J B, Lesser R E 1960 A study of headbanging in infants and children. Dis Nerv Syst 21: 203–208

Krumholz A, Singer H S, Niedermeyer E, Burnite R, Harris K 1983 Electrophysiological studies in Tourette's syndrome. Ann Neurol 14: 638–641

Kruse W 1960 Persistent muscular restlessness after phenothiazine treatment: report of 3 cases. Am J Psychiat 117: 152–153

Kulenkampff C, Tarnow G 1956 Ein eigentümliches Syndrom im oralen Bereich bei Megaphenapplikation. Nervenarzt 27: 178–180

Kunkle E C 1967 The 'jumpers' of Maine: a reappraisal. Arch Int Med 119: 355–358

Kurczynski T W 1983 Hyperekplexia. Arch Neurol 40: 246–248

Labhardt F 1953 Technik, Nebenerscheinungen und komplikationen der Largactiltherapie. Schweiz Arch Neurol Psych 73 (1–2): 309–338

Lakke J P W 1981 Classification of extrapyramidal disorders: proposal for an international classification and glossary of terms. J Neurol Sci 51: 311–327

Lal S 1979 Pathophysiology and pharmacotherapy of spasmodic torticollis: a review. Canad J Neurol Sci 6: 427–435

Lal S, Hoyte K, Kiely M E, Soulkes T L, Baxter D W, Missala K et al 1979 Neuropharmacological investigation and treatment of spasmodic torticollis. In: Poirier L J, Soulkes T L, Bédard P J (eds) Adv Neurol vol 23. Raven Press, New York, pp 335–352

Lancet Editorial 1982 Writer's cramp. p 969

Lander C M, Lees A, Stern G 1979 Oscillations in performance in levodopa-treated Parkinsonians: treatment with bromocriptine and l-deprenyl. Clin Exp Neurol Proc Aust Assoc Neurol 16: 197–203

Landis C, Hunt W A 1939 The startle pattern. Farrar Strauss-Adaby, New York

Lang A E, Marsden C D 1982 Alphamethylparatyrosine and tetrabenazene in movement disorders. Clin Neuropharmacol 5: 375–387

Lang A E, Marsden C D 1983 Spasmodic dysphonia in Gilles de la Tourettes disease. Arch Neurol 40: 51–52

Lang A E, Sheehy M P, Marsden C D, 1982 Anticholinergics in adult-onset focal dystonia. Canad J Neurol Sci 9: 313–319

Lang A E, Sheehy M P, Marsden C D 1983 Acute anticholinergic action in focal dystonia. in: Fahn S, Calne D B, Shoulson I (eds) Adv Neurol, vol 37. Raven Press, New York, pp 193–200

Langston J W, Ballard P 1984 Parkinsonism Induced by 1-methyl-4-phenyl 1,2,3,6 tetrahydrophyridine (MPTP): implications for treatment and the pathogenesis of Parkinson's disease. Canad J Neurol Sci 11 Suppl 1: 160–165

Langworthy O R 1952 Emotional issues related to certain cases of blepharospasm and facial tics. Arch Neurol 68: 620–628

Lapouse R, Monk M 1964 Behaviour deviations in a representative sample of children:

variation by sex, age, race, social class and family size. Am J Orthopsychiat 34: 436–446

Lavy S, Melamed E, Penchas S 1978 Tardive dyskinesias associated with metoclopramide. Br Med J 1: 77–78

Lees A J, Stern G M 1981 Sustained bromocriptine therapy in previously untreated patients with Parkinson's disease. J Neurol Neurosurg Psychiat 44: 1020–1023

Lees A J, Stern G M 1982 Sustained low dose L-dopa therapy in Parkinson's disease: a 3-year follow-up. In: Fahn S, Calne D B, Shoulson I (eds) Experimental therapeutics of movement disorders. Adv Neurol, vol 37. Raven Press, New York, pp 9–16

Lees A J, Shaw K M, Stern G M 1976 Bromocriptine and spasmodic torticollis. Br Med J 1:1343

Lees A J, Shaw K M, Stern G M 1977 Off-period dystonia and on period choreoathetosis in levodopa treated patients with Parkinsons disease. Lancet 2:1034

Lees A J, Shaw K M, Stern G M 1978 Baclofen in Parkinson's disease. J Neurol Neurosurg Psychiat 41: 707–708

Lees A J, Lander C M, Stern G M 1979 Tiapride in levodopa-induced involuntary movements. J Neurol Neurosurg Psychiat 42: 380–383

Lees A J, Robertson M, Trimble M R, Murray N M F 1984 A clinical study of Gilles de la Tourette syndrome in the United Kingdom. J Neurol Neurosurg Psychiat 47: 1–8

Lehmann H B 1955 Therapeutic results with chlorpromazine (largactil) in psychiatric conditions. Canad Med Assoc J 72: 91–99

Levine I M, Estes J W, Looney J M 1968 Hereditary neurological disease with acanthocytosis. Arch Neurol 19: 403–409

Levy B S, Ascher E 1968 Phenothiazines in the treatment of Gilles de la Tourette's disease. J Nerv Ment Dis 146: 36–40

Levy D M 1944 On the problem of movement restraint (tics, stereotyped movements, hyperactivity). Am J Orthopsychiat 14: 644–671

Levy G 1922 Contribution à l'étude des manifestations tardives de l'encéphalite épidemique (formes prolongées et reprises tardives): syndrome excitomoteur-syndrome Parkinsonien forme respiratoire, forme insomnique et hypomaniac de l'enfant. Thèse, Paris

Lewin P M 1938 Restlessness in children. Arch Neurol Psych Chicago 39: 764–770

Lewin W, Whitty C W M 1960 Effects of antorior cingulate stimulation in conscious human subjects. J Neurophysiol 23: 445–447

L'hermitte F, Signoret J-L, Agid Y 1977a Étude des effets d'une molécule originale, le tiapride dans le traitement des mouvements anormaux d'origine extrapyramidale. Sem Hôp Paris 53 (39B): 9–15

L'hermitte F, Rosa A, Comoy E 1977b Mouvements anormaux des Parkinsoniens traité par la L-dopa et anomalies du metabolisme de la dopamine. Rev Neurol 133: 3–11

Lichtigfeld F J 1964 Opisthotonus in drug-induced dystonic syndrome. Br J Psychiat 110: 734–735

Lieberman A N, Goodgold A L, Goldstein M 1972 Treatment failures with levodopa in Parkinsonism. Neurology 22: 1205–1210

Liebman, J Neale R 1980 Neuroleptic-induced acute dyskinesias in squirrel monkeys: correlation with propensity to cause extrapyramidal side-effects. Psychopharmacology 68: 25–29

Lieh Mak F, Chung S Y, Lee P, Chen S 1982 Tourette syndrome in the Chinese: a follow-up of 15 cases. In: Friedhoff A J, Chase T N (eds) Gilles de la Tourette syndrome. Adv Neurol, vol 35. Raven Press, New York pp 277–283

Lindner H, Stevens H 1967 Hypnotherapy and psychodynamics in the syndrome of Gilles de la Tourette. Int J Clin Exp Hypnosis 15: 151–155

Linnoila M, Viukari M, Hietala O 1976 Effect of sodium valproate on tardive dyskinesia. Br J Psychiat 129: 114–119

Liversedge L A 1961 Writer's cramp and the conditioned reflex. In: Garland H (ed) Scientific aspects of neurology. E α S Livingstone, Edinburgh, pp 168–176

Lloyd K G, Hornykiewicz O, Davidson L, Shannak K, Farley I, Goldstein M et al 1981 Biochemical evidence of dysfunction of brain neurotransmitters in the Lesch-Nyhan syndrome. New Engl J Med 305: 1106–1111

Long C F 1929 Rumination in man. Am J Med Sci 178: 814–822

Lourie R S 1949 Role of rhythmic patterns in childhood. Am J Psychiat 105: 653–660

Lucas A R 1976 Follow-up of tic syndrome. In: Abuzzahab F S, Anderson F O (eds) Gilles de la Tourette syndrome. Vol 1, International Registry. Mason, Minnosota, pp 13–18

Lucas A R, Kauffman P E, Morris E M 1967 Gilles de la Tourette's disease: a clinical study of 15 cases. J Am Acad Child Psychiat 6: 700–722

Lucas A R, Beard C M, Rajput A H, Kurland L T 1982 Tourette syndrome in Rochester Minnesota, 1968–1979. In: Friedhoff A J, Chase T N (eds) Gilles de la Tourette syndrome. Adv Neurol, vol 35. Raven Press, New York pp 267–269

Ludlow C L, Polinsky R J, Caine E D, Bassich C J, Ebert M H 1982 Language and speech abnormalities in Tourette syndrome. In: Friedhoff A J, Chase T N (eds) Gilles de la Tourette syndrome. Adv Neurol, vol 35. Raven Press, New York, pp 351–362

Lundh H, Tunving K 1981 An extrapyramidal choreiform syndrome caused by amphetamine addiction. J Neurol Neurosurg Psychiat 44: 728–730

MacDonald I J 1963 A case of Gilles de la Tourette syndrome with some aetiological observations. Br J Psychiat 109: 206–210

Macé de Lépinay 1909 Études sur les crampes professionnelles. Nouv Icon Salpêtriere 22: 65–79, 189–225

MacFarlane J W, Honzik M P, Allen L 1954 In: Behaviour problems in normal children. University of California Publications in Child Development

Mackiewicz J, Gershon S 1964 An experimental study of the neuropathological and toxicological effects of chlorpromazine and reserpine. J Neuropsychiat 5: 159–169

Magoun H W, Atlas D, Ingersoll E H, Ranson S W 1937 Associated facial vocal and respiratory components of emotional expression: an experimental study. J Neurol Psychopathol 17: 241–255

Mahler M S, Rangell L 1943 A psychosomatic study of maladie des tics (Gilles de la Tourette's disease). Psychiat Quart 17: 579–603

Mahler M S, Luke J A, Daltroff W 1945 Clinical and follow-up study of the tic syndrome in children. Am J Orthopsychiat 15: 631–647

Marie P, Levy G 1920 Le syndrome excito-moteur de l'encéphalité epidemique. Rev Neurol 36: 513–525

Marie P, Lévy G 1922 Le syndrome excitomoteur de l'encéphalité épidemique prolongée. Rev Neurol 38: 1233–1247

Markand O N, Garg B P, Weaver D D 1984 Familial startle disease (hyperexplexia): electrophysiologic studies. Arch Neurol 41: 71–74

Markham C H 1971 The choreo-athetoid movement disorder induced by levodopa. Clin Pharm Ther 12: 340–343

Marmor M F 1982 Wilson strokes and zebras. New Engl J Med 307: 528–535

Marsden C D 1975 The neuropharmacology of abnormal involuntary movement disorders. In: Williams D W (ed) Modern trends in neurology, no 6. Butterworth, London, pp 141–166

Marsden C D 1976a The problem of adult-onset idiopathic torsion dystonia and other isolated dyskinesias in adult life (including blepharospasm, oromandibular dystonia, dystonic writer's cramp and torticollis or axial dystonia). In: Eldridge R, Fahn S (eds) Adv Neurol, vol 14. Raven Press, New York, pp 259–276

Marsden C D 1976b Blepharospasm-oromandibular dystonia syndrome (Brue ghel's syndrome): a variant of adult-onset torsion dystonia? J Neurol Neurosurg Psychiat 39: 1204–1209

Marsden C D, Harrison M J G 1974 Idiopathic torsion dystonia (dystonia musculorum deformans): a review of 42 patients. Brain 97: 793–810

Marsden C D, Jenner P 1980 The pathophysiology of extrapyramidal side-effects of neuroleptic drugs. Psychol Med 10: 55–72

Marsden C D, Sheehy M P 1982 Spastic dysphonia, Meige disease and torsion dystonia. Neurology 32: 1202–1203

Marsh H O 1965 Diazepam in incapacitated cerebral-palsied children. J Am Med Assoc 191: 797–800

Martin J P 1967 The basal ganglia and posture. Pitman Medical, London, p 101

Martindale C 1977 Syntactic and semantic correlates of verbal tics in Gilles de la Tourette's syndrome: a quantitative study. Brain Lang 4: 231–247

Martres M P, Costentin J, Baudry M, Marcais H, Protais P, Schwartz J C 1977 Long-term changes in the sensitivity of pre and post-synaptic dopamine receptors in mouse striatum evidenced by behavioural and biochemical studies. Brain Res 136: 319–337

Matthews W B, Beasley P, Parry-Jones W, Garland G 1978 Spasmodic torticollis: a combined clinical study. J Neurol Neurosurg Psychiat 41: 485–492

Matthysse S 1973 Implications of feedback control in catecholamine neuronal systems. In: Usdin E, Snyder S (eds) Frontiers in catecholamine research. Pergamon, New York, pp 1139–1142

Mattson R H, Calverley J R 1968 Dexamphetamine sulphate-induced dyskinesias. J Am Med Assoc 204: 400–402

McCall C N, Skolnik M L, Brewer D W 1971 A preliminary report of some atypical movement patterns in the tongue palate hypopharynx and larynx of patients with spasmodic dysphonia. J Speech Hear Dis 36: 466–470

McHenry L C 1967 Samuel Johnson's tics and gesticulations. J Hist Med 22: 152–168

McLennan H, York D H 1967 The action of dopamine on neurons of the caudate nucleus. J Physiol 189: 393–402

Meares R 1971a An association of spasmodic torticollis and writer's cramp. Br J Psychiat 119: 441–442

Meares R 1971b Features which distinguish groups of spasmodic torticollis. J Psychosom Res 15: 1–11

Meares R 1971c Natural history of spasmodic torticollis and effect of surgery. Lancet 2: 149–151

Meares R 1973 Spasmodic torticollis. Br J Hosp Med 235–241

Meige H 1910 Les convulsions de la face, une forme clinique de convulsion faciale bilaterale et mediane. Rev Neurol 21: 437–443

Meige H 1914 Dysphasie singultueuse avec reactions motrices tetaniformes et gestes stereotypes. Rev Neurol 27: 310–315

Meige H, Feindel E 1902 Les tics et leur traitement. Masson, Paris

Meige H, Feindel E 1907 In: Wilson S A K (trans) Tics and their treatment. Appleton, London

Meldrum B S, Anlezark G M, Marsden C D 1977 Acute dystonia as an idiosyncratic response to neuroleptics in baboons. Brain 100: 313–326

Mena I, Court J, Cotzias G C 1971 Levodopa involuntary movements and fusaric acid. J Am Med Assoc 218: 1829–1830

Mendelson W, Johnson N, Stewart M 1971 Hyperactive children as teenagers: a follow-up study. J Nerv Ment Dis 153: 273–279

Menkes M, Rowe J, Menkes J 1967 A twenty-five year follow-up study on the hyperkinesic child with minimal brain dysfunction. Paediatrics 39: 393–399

Merskey H 1974 A case of multiple tics with vocalisation (partial syndrome of Gilles de la Tourette) and XYY karyotype. Br J Psychiat 125: 593–594

Merson R M, Ginsberg A P 1979 Spasmodic dysphonia: abductor type: a clinical report of acoustic, aerodynamic and perceptual characteristics. Laryngoscope 89: 127–139

Mettler F A, Crandell A 1959 Neurologic disorders in psychiatric institutions. J Nerv Ment Dis 128: 148–159

Meyerhoff J L, Snyder S H 1973 Catecholamines in Gilles de la Tourette's disease. In: Barbeau A, Chase T, Paulson G (eds) Adv Neurol. Raven Press, New York, pp 123–134

Michael R P 1957 Treatment of a case of compulsive swearing. Br Med J 1: 1506–1508

Micheli F, Pardal N M F, Leiguarda R C 1982 Beneficial effects of lisuride in Meige disease. Neurology 32: 432–434

Mikkelsen E J, Detlor J, Cohen D J 1981 School avoidance and social phobia triggered by haloperidol in patients with Tourette's disorder. Am J Psychiat 138: 1572–1576

Milman D H 1976 Gilles de la Tourette's syndrome: report of four cases with extended follow-up. In: Abuzzahab F S, Anderson F O (eds) Gilles de la Tourette's syndrome. Vol 1, International Registry. Mason, Minnesota, pp 143–150

Mitchell E, Matthews K L 1980 Gilles de la Tourette's disorder associated with pemoline. Am J Psychiat 137: 1618–1619

Moldofsky H J 1971 Occupational cramp. Psychosom Res 15: 439–444

Moldofsky H, Tullis C, Lamon R 1974 Multiple tic syndrome (Gilles de la Tourette's syndrome: clinical, biological and psychosocial variables and their influence with haloperidol. J Nerv Ment Dis 15: 282–292

Mones R J 1971 Levodopa-induced dyskinesia in the normal rhesus monkey. Mt Sinai J Med NY 39: 197–201

Mones R J 1973 Experimental dyskinesias in normal rhesus monkeys. In: Barbeau A, Chase T N, Paulson G W (eds) Huntington's chorea 1872–1972. Adv Neurol, vol 1. Raven Press, New York, pp 665–669

Mones R J, Elizan T S, Siegel G J 1971 Analysis of L-dopa induced dyskinesias in 51 patients with Parkinsonism. J Neurol Neurosurg Psychiat 34: 668–673

Mones R J, Pasik P, Pasik T, Wilk S 1973 The modification of L-dopa-induced dyskinesias in the monkey by unilateral nigral lesions. Trans Am Neurol Assoc 98: 234–237

Montgomery M A, Clayton P J, Friedhoff A J 1982 Psychiatric illness in Tourette syndrome patients and first-degree relatives. In: Friedhoff A J, Chase T N (eds) Gilles de la Tourette syndrome. Adv Neurol, vol 35. Raven Press, New York, pp 335–339

Moore K E 1977 The actions of amphetamines on neurotransmitters: a brief review. Biol Psychiat 12: 451–462

Morphew J A, Sim M 1969 Gilles de la Tourette's syndrome: a clinical and psychopathological study. Br J Med Psychol 42: 293–301

Morrison J R 1973 Catatonia: retarded and excited types. Arch Gen Psychiat 28: 39–41

Morrison J, Stewart M 1971 A family study of the hyperactive child syndrome. Biol Psychiat 3: 189–195

Mowat A P 1973 Dystonic reactions to drugs. Dev Med Child Neurol 15: 654–655

Mueller J, Aminoff M J 1982 Tourette-like syndrome after long-term neuroleptic drug treatment. Br J Psychiat 141: 191–193

Muenter M D, Sharpless N S, Tyce G M, Darley F L 1977 Patterns of dystonia ('I-D-I' and 'D-I-D') in response to L-dopa therapy for Parkinson's disease. Mayo Clin Proc 52: 163–174

Murphy E L 1955 Observations on craft palsies. Trans Ass Industr Med Offrs 5: 113–120

Murray T J 1979 Dr Samuel Jonnson's movement disorders. Br Med J 1: 1610–1614

Murugaiah K, Theodorou A, Mann S, Clow A, Jenner P, Marsden C D 1982 Chronic continuous administration of neuroleptic drugs alter cerebral dopamine receptors and increases spontaneous dopaminergic action in the striatum. Nature 296: 570–572

Nadvornick P, Sramka M, Lisy L, Svicka I 1972 Experiences with dentatotomy. Confin Neurol 34: 320–324

Nashold B S 1969 The effect of central tegmental lesions on tardive dyskinesia. In: Crane C E, Gardner R J (eds)Psychotropic drugs and dysfunctions of the basal ganglia. US Public Health Service Publication No 1938, Washington pp 111–116

Nashold B S, Wilson W P, Boone E 1979 Depth recordings and stimulation of the human brain: a twenty year experience. In: Rasmussen T, Marino R (eds) Functional neurosurgery. Raven Press, New York, pp 181–195

National Institute of Mental Health Psychopharmacology Service Centre Collaborative Study Group 1964 Phenothiazine treatment in acute schizophrenia. Arch Gen Psych 10: 246–261

Nausieda P A, Weiner W J, Klawans H L 1980 Dystonic foot response of Parkinsonism. Arch Neurol 37: 132–136

Nausieda P A, Koller W C, Weiner W J, Klawans H L 1981 Pemoline-induced chorea. Neurology 31: 356–360

Nee, L E, Caine E D, Polinsky R J, Eldridge R, Ebert M H 1980 Gilles de la Tourette syndrome: clinical and family study of 50 cases. Ann Neurol 7: 41–49

Ng L K Y, Gelhard R E, Chase T N, Maclean P D 1973 Drug-induced dyskinesia in monkeys: a pharmacologic model employing 6-hydroxydopamine. In: Barbeau A, Chase T N, Paulson G W (eds) Adv Neurol, vol 1. Raven Press, New York, pp 651–655

Nielsen E B, Lyon M 1978 Evidence for cell loss in corpus striatum after long-term treatment with a neuroleptic drug (flupenthixol) in rats. Psychopharmacology 59: 85–89

Noir J 1893 Étude sur les tics. Thèse, Bureaux du Progrès Médical, p 170

Nomura Y, Segawa M 1982 Tourette syndrome in oriental children: clinical and pathophysiological considerations. In: Friedhoff A J, Chase T N (eds) Gilles de la Tourette syndrome. Raven Press, New York, pp 277–280

Nutt J G, Hammerstad J P 1981 Blepharospasm and oromandibular dystonia (Meige's syndrome) in sisters. Ann Neurol 9: 189–191

Nutt J G, Tamminga C A, Eisler T, Chase T N 1979 Clinical experience with a cholinergic agonist in hyperkinetic movement disorders. In: Barbeau A, Growdon J H, Wurtman R J (eds) Nutrition and the brain. Raven Press, New York, pp 317–324

Nutt J G, Hammerstad J P, Carter J H, de Garmo P 1983 Meige syndrome: Treatment with trihexyphenidyl. In: Fahn S, Calne D B, Shoulson I (eds) Experimental therapeutics of movement disorders. Adv Neurol, vol 37. Raven Press, New York, pp 201–208

Nuwer M R 1982 Coprolalia as an organic symptom. In: Friedhoff A J, Chase T N (eds) Gilles de la Tourette syndrome. Adv Neurol, vol 35. Raven Press, New York, pp 363–368

Nyback H, Sedvall G, Kopin I J 1967 Accelerated synthesis of dopamine C^{14} from tyrosine C^{14} in rat brain after chlorpromazine. Life Sci 6: 2307–2312

Nyhan W L 1973 The Lesch-Nyhan syndrome. Ann Rev Med 24: 41–60

Oberndorf C P 1916 Simple tic mechanism. J Am Med Assoc 16: 99–100

Obeso J A, Rothwell J C, Marsden C D 1981 Simple tics in Gilles de la Tourette's syndrome are not prefaced by a normal premovement EEG potential. J. Neurol Neurosurg Psychiat 44: 735–738

O'Brien H A 1883 Latah. J Straits Branch Roy Asiat Soc Singapore 11: 143–153

Ogita K, Yagi G, Itoh H 1975 Comparative analysis of persistent dyskinesia of long-term usage with neuroleptics in France and Japan. Folia Psychiat Neurol Japan 29: 315–320

O'Keefe R, Sharman D F, Vogt M 1970 Effect of drugs used in psychoses on cerebral dopamine metabolism. Br J Pharmacol 38: 287–304

Olson L, Seiger A, Fuxe K 1972 Heterogeneity of striatal and limbic dopamine innervation. Brain Res 44: 283–288

Oppenheim H 1887 Eine seltene motilitätsneurose. Berl Klin Wschr 24:309

Osler W 1892 Principles and practice of medicine. Young Pentland, Edinburgh pp. 963–965

Osler W 1894 In: On chorea and choreiform affections. Blakiston, Philadelphia

Ossipowa (1930) Über die konstitutionellen Eigenschaften bei Chorea minor. Z ges Neurol Psych 125: 69–82

Østerberg G 1937 On spasmus nutans. Acta Ophthal 15: 457–467

Ounsted C 1955 Hyperkinetic syndrome in epileptic children. Lancet 2: 303–311

Owens D G C, Johnstone E C, Frith C D 1982 Spontaneous involuntary disorders of movement. Arch Gen Psychiat 39: 452–461

Owens D G C, Johnstone E C, Crow T J, Frith C D, Jagoe R 1984 A cт scan study of involuntary movement disorder in schizophrenia. Abstracts from 14th CINP Congress, Florence, p 119

Pai M N 1947 Nature and treatment of writer's cramp. J Ment Sci 93: 68–81

Pakkenberg H, Fog R 1974 Spontaneous oral dyskinesia: results of treatment with tetrabenazene, pimozide or both. Arch Neurol 31: 352–353

Palatucci D M 1974 Single case study: iatrogenic dyskinesia, a unique reaction to parenteral methylphenidate. J Nerv Ment Dis 159: 73–76

Parkes J D, Bédard P, Marsden C D 1976 Chorea and torsion in Parkinsonism. Lancet 2:155

Pasamanick B, Kawi A 1956 A study of the association of prenatal and paranatal factors in the development of tics in children. J Pediat 48: 596–601

Paterson M T 1945 Spasmodic torticollis: results of psychotherapy in 21 cases. Lancet 2: 556–559

Patrick H T 1905 Convulsive tic. J Am Med Assoc 44: 437–442

Patterson R M, Little S C 1943 Spasmodic torticollis. J Nerv Ment Dis 98: 571–599

Pauls D L, Cohen D J, Heimbuch R, Detlor J, Kidd K K 1981 Familial pattern and transmission of Gilles de la Tourette syndrome and multiple tics. Arch Gen Psychiat 38: 1091–1093

Paulson G W 1972a Meige's syndrome: dyskinesia of the eyelids and facial muscles. Geriatrics 27: 69–73

Paulson G W 1972b Dyskinesias in rhesus monkeys. Trans Am Neurol Soc 97: 109–110

Paulson G W 1973 Dyskinesias in monkeys. In: Barbeau A, Chase T N, Paulson G W (eds) Huntington's chorea 1872–1972. Adv Neurol, vol 1. Raven Press, New York, pp 647–650

Penfield W, Jasper H 1954 In: Epilepsy and the functional anatomy of the human brain. Little Brown, Boston

Perez L M 1961 Treatment of extrapyramidal reactions. New Engl J Med 264: 1269–1270

Pernikoff M 1964 Treatment of acute and chronic muscle spasm with diazepam. Clin Med 71: 699–705

Pfohl B, Winokur G 1982 The evolution of symptoms in institutionalised hebephrenic/catatonic schizophrenics. Br J Psychiat 141: 567–572

Pick A 1921 Die neurologische Forschungsrichtung in der Psychopathologie und andere Aufsätze. Abhandl Neurol Berl 13: 1–247

Pind K, Faurbye A 1970 Concentration of homovanillic acid and 5-hydroxyindoleacetic acid in the cerebrospinal fluid after treatment with probenecid in patients with drug-induced tardive dyskinesia. Acta Psychiat Scand 46: 323–326

Piotrowski Z A 1945 The Rorschach records of children with a tic syndrome. Nerv Child 4: 342–352

Podivinsky F 1968 Torticollis. In: Vinken P J, Bruyn G W (eds) Handbook of clinical neurology, vol 6. North Holland, Amsterdam, pp 567–603

Polinsky R J, Ebert M H, Caine E D, Ludlow C, Bassich C J 1980 Cholinergic treatment in the Tourette syndrome. New Engl J Med 302:1310

Polizos P, Engelhardt D M, Hoffman S P 1973 C.N.S. consequences of psychotropic drug withdrawal in schizophrenic children. Psychopharmacol Bull 9: 34–35

Pollack M A, Cohen N L, Friedhoff A J 1977 Gilles de la Tourette syndrome: familial occurrence and precipitation by methylphenidate therapy. Arch Neurol 34: 630–632

Poore G V 1873 Writer's cramp: its pathology and treatment. Practitioner 10: 341–350

Poore G V 1878 An analysis of seventy-five cases of writer's cramp and impaired writing power. Med Chir Trans Lond 61: 111–145

Poore G V 1897 Nervous affections of the hand and other clinical studies. Smith Elder, London, pp. 26–34

Post R M, Goodwin F K 1975 Time-dependent effects of phenothiazines on dopamine turnover in psychiatric patients. Science 190: 488–489

Poursines Y, Alliez J, Toga M 1959 Syndrome Parkinsonien consecutif à la prise prolongée de chlorpromazine avec ictus mortel intercurrent. Rev Neurol 100: 745–751

Prange A J, Wilson I C, Morris C E, Hall C D 1973 Preliminary experience with tryptophan and lithium in the treatment of tardive dyskinesia. Psychopharmacol Bull 9: 36–37

Prechtl H F R, Stemmer C J 1962 The choreiform syndrome in children. Dev Med Child Neurol 4: 119–127

Price P A, Parkes J D, Marsden C D 1978a Sodium valproate in the treatment of levodopa-induced dyskinesia. J Neurol Neurosurg Psychiat 41: 702–706

Price P, Parkes J D, Marsden C D 1978b Tiapride in Parkinson's disease. Lancet 2:1106

Prince M 1906 Case of multiform tic including automatic speech and purposive movements. J Nerv Ment Dis 33: 29–34

Priori R, Schettini E 1958 Un syndrome moteur particulier au cours d'un traitement par reserpine. Riv Di Neurol 28: 512–518

Pryce I G, Edwards H 1966 Persistent oral dyskinesia in female mental hospital patients. Br J Psychiat 112: 983–987

Pulst S M, Walshe T M, Romero J A 1983 Carbon monoxide poisoning with features of Gilles de la Tourette syndrome. Arch Neurol 40: 443–444

Purves Stewart 1898 Paralysis agitans with an account of a new symptom. Lancet 2: 1258–1260

Quitkin F, Rifkin A, Gochfeld L, Klein D F 1977 Tardive dyskinesia: are first signs reversible? Am J Psychiat 134: 84–87

Rabinovitch R 1965 An exaggerated startle reflex resembling a kicking horse. Canad Med Assoc J 93:130

Rafi A A 1962 Learning theory and the treatment of tics. J Psychosom Res 6: 71–76

Railton T C 1886 Notes on a case of involuntary muscle movements accompanied by coprolalia. Med Chron Manchester 4: 24–29

Ramazzini B 1713 In: Cave W (trans) O morbus artificum diatriba. Wright, Chicago, 1940

Randrup A, Munkvad I 1967 Stereotyped activities produced by amphetamine in several animal species and man. Psychopharmacologia 11: 300–310

Randrup A, Munkvad I 1970 Biochemical, anatomical and psychological invetigations of stereotyped behaviour induced by amphetamines. In: Costa E, Garattini S (eds) Amphetamines and related compounds. Raven Press, New York, pp 695–713

Rapoport J 1959 Maladie des tics in children. Am J Psychiat 116: 177–178

Rapoport J L, Nee L, Mitchell S, Polinsky R, Ebert M 1982 Hyperkinetic syndrome and Tourette syndrome. In: Friedhoff A J, Chase T N (eds) Gilles de la Tourette syndrome. Adv Neurol, vol 35. Raven Press, New York, pp 423–426

Raskin D E 1972 Akathisia: a side-effect to be remembered. Am J Psychiat 129: 345–347

Raymond F, Janet P 1902 Le syndrome psychasthénique de 'l'akathisie'. Nouv Icon Salpêtrière 15: 241–246

Reckless J 1972 Hysterical blepharospasm treated by psychotherapy and conditioning procedures in a group setting. Psychosomatics 13: 263–264

Reiter P J 1926 Extrapyramidal motor disturbances in dementia praecox. Acta Psychiat Neurol Scand 1: 287–309

Richardson E P 1982 Neuropathological studies of Tourette syndrome. In: Friedhoff A J, Chase T N (eds) Gilles de la Tourette syndrome. Raven Press, New York, pp 83–88

Rifkin A, Quitkin F, Carrillo C, Klein D F, Oaks G 1971 Very high dosage fluphenazine for non-chronic treatment-refractory patients. Arch Gen Psychiat 25: 398–403

Robe E, Brumlik J, Moore P A 1960 Study of spastic dysphonia: neurologic and electroencephalographic abnormalities. Laryngoscope 70: 219–245

Rochon-Duvigneaud M, Weill A 1907 Blepharospasme. Rev Neurol 18: 1296–1297

Roizin L, True C, Knight M 1959 Structural effects of tranquillisers. Res Publ Assoc Res Nerv Ment Dis 37: 285–324

Rosenberger P B, Hier D B 1980 Cerebral asymmetry and verbal intellectual deficits. Ann Neurol 8: 300–304

Ross M S, Moldofsky H 1978 A comparison of pimozide and haloperidol in the treatment of Gilles de la Tourette's syndrome. Am J Psychiat 135: 585–587

Roth D C 1850 Histoire de la masculation irrésistible ou de la chorée anormale. Germer-Baillière, Paris

Rouquier A 1951 Crampe des écrivains, Parkinsonisme syndrome anxieux guérison par topectomie prefrontale bilatérale. Bull Soc Méd Hôp Paris 67: 65–67

Rubovitz R, Klawans H 1972 Implications of amphetamine-induced stereotyped behaviour as a model for tardive dyskinesias. Arch Gen Psychiat 27: 502–507

Rudler F, Chomel C 1903 Le tic de l'ours chez le cheval et les tics d'imitation chez l'homme. Rev. Neurol 11: 541–550

Rudler F, Chomel C 1904 Des stigmates physiques physiologiques et psychiques de la dégénérescence chez l'animal en particulier chez le cheval. Nouv Icon Salpêtrière 17: 471–489

Rutter M, Graham P, Birch H G 1966 Interrelations between the choreiform syndrome, reading disability and psychiatric disorder in children of 8–11 years. Dev Med Child Neurol 8: 149–159

Rutter M, Tizard J, Yule W, Graham P, Whitmore K 1976 Isle of Wight studies 1964–1974. Psychol Med 6: 313–332

Rylander G 1972 Psychoses and the punding and choreiform syndromes in addiction to central stimulant drugs. Psychiat Neurol Neurochir Amst 75: 203–212

Sacks O 1973 Awakenings. Duckworth, London

Sacks O 1981 Witty ticcy ray. London Review of Books, 19 March–1 April, pp 3–4

Sacks O 1982a Awakenings re-visited. In: Sarner M (ed) Advanced medicine, vol 18. Pitman Medical, London, pp 326–340

Sacks O 1982b Acquired Tourettism in adult life. In: Friedhoff A J, Chase T N (eds) Gilles de la Tourette syndrome. Adv Neurol, vol 35. Raven Press, New York, pp 89–92

Saenz-Lope E, Herranz-Tanarro F J, Masdeu J C, Chacon-Pena J R 1984 Hyperexplexia: a syndrome of pathological startle responses. Ann Neurol 15: 36–41

Safer J 1971 Unpublished observations. In: Arieti S (ed) American handbook of psychiatry, vol 2. Quoted by Wender P H and Eisenberg L. Basic Books, New York, 1974, p 138

Sainsbury P 1954 A method of measuring spontaneous movements by time-sampling motion pictures. J Ment Sci 100: 742–748

Sakai T, Mawatari S, Iwashita H, Goto I, Kuroiwa Y 1981 Choreoacanthocytosis: clues to clinical diagnosis. Arch Neurol 38: 335–338

Sakuta M, Takemura T, Kamekura K 1980 An autopsy case of chorea-acanthocytosis. Rinsho Shinkeigaku 20: 1059–1061

Sanamman M L 1974 Dyskinesia after fenfluramine. New Engl J Med 291:422

Sand P L, Carlson C 1973 Failure to establish control over tics in the Gilles de la Tourette syndrome with behaviour therapy techniques. Br J Psychiat 122: 665–670

Sandler M, Bonham-Carter S, Hunter K R, Stern G M 1973 Tetrahydroisoquinoline alkaloids in vivo metabolites of L-dopa. Nature 241: 439–443

Sandras C M S 1851 In: Traité pratique des maladies nerveuses. Germer-Baillière, Paris, pp 531–534

Sarkari N B, Mahendru R K, Singh S S, Rishi R P 1976 An epidemiological and neuropsychiatric study of writer's cramp. J Assoc Phys India 24: 587–591

Sarwer-Foner G J 1960 Recognition and management of drug-induced extrapyramidal reactions and 'paradoxical' behavioral reactions in psychiatry. Canad Med Assoc J 83: 312–318

Sassin J F 1975 Drug-induced dyskinesias in monkeys. In: Meldrum B S, Marsden C D (eds) Adv Neurol, vol. 10. Raven Press, New York, pp 47–54

Sassin J F, Taub S, Weitzman E D 1972 Hyperkinesia and changes in behaviour produced in normal monkeys by L-dopa. Neurology 22: 1122–1125

Sato S, Daly R, Peters H 1971 Reserpine therapy of phenothiazine-induced dyskinesia. Dis Nerv Syst 32: 680–685

Scatton B 1977 Differential regional development of tolerance to increase in dopamine turnover upon repeated neuroleptic administration. Eur J Pharmacol 46: 363–369

Scatton B, Garret C, Julou L 1975 Acute and sub-acute effects of neuroleptics on dopamine synthesis and release in the rat striatum. Naunyn-Schmiedeberg's Arch Pharmacol 289: 419–434

Schaaf M, Payne C A 1966 Dystonic reactions to prochlorperazine in hypoparathyroidism. New Engl J Med 275: 991–995

Schaeffer H, Bize R 1934 Torticolis spasmodique avec syndrome cérébello-pyramide d'origine spécifique. Rev Neurol 41(ii): 579–583

Scheel-Kruger J 1970 Central effects of anti-cholinergic drugs measured by the apomorphine gnawing test in mice. Acta Pharmacol Toxicol 28: 1–16

Scher J 1966 Patterns and profiles of addiction and drug abuse. Arch Gen Psychiat 15: 539–551

Schiørring E 1977 Changes in individual and social behaviour induced by amphetamine and related compounds in monkeys and man. In: Ellinwood Jr E H, Kilbey M M (eds) Cocaine and other stimulants. Adv Behav Biol, vol 21. Plenum Press, New York, pp 481–522

Schnitzler J 1875 Aphonia spastica. Wien Med Presse 16: 429–432, 477–479

Schöneker M 1957 Ein eigentümliches Syndrome im oralen Bereich bei Megaphenapplikation. Nervenarzt 28:35

Schwab R S, Fabing H D, Prichard J S 1951 Psychiatric symptoms and syndromes in Parkinson's disease. Am J Psychiat 107: 901–907

Seignot M J N 1961 Un cas de maladie des tics de Gilles de la Tourette guéri par le R-1625. Ann Med Psychol 119: 578–579

Selling L 1929 The role of infection in the aetiology of tics. Arch Neurol Psychiat 22: 1163–1171

Sethy V H 1976 Effects of chronic treatment with neuroleptics on striatal acetylcholine concentration. J Neurochem 27: 325–326

Shapiro A K, Shapiro E 1981a Do stimulants provoke, cause or exacerbate tics and Tourette syndrome? Compr Psychiat 22: 265–273

Shapiro A K, Shapiro E K 1981b Tic disorders. J Am Med Assoc 245: 1583–1585

Shapiro A K, Shapiro E 1982 Clinical efficacy of haloperidol, pimozide, penfluridol and clonidine in the treatment of Tourette syndrome. In: Friedhoff A J, Chase T N (eds) Gilles de la Tourette syndrome. Adv Neurol, vol 35. Raven Press, New York, pp 383–386

Shapiro A K, Shapiro E, Wayne H L, Clarkin J 1972 The psychopathology of Gilles de la Tourette's syndrome. Am J Psychiat 129: 427–434

Shapiro A K, Shapiro E S, Bruun R D, Sweet R, Wayne H, Solomon G 1976 Gilles de la Tourette's syndrome: summary of clinical experience with 250 patients and suggested nomenclature for tic syndromes. In: Eldridge R, Fahn S (eds) Dystonia. Adv Neurol, vol 14. Raven Press, New York, pp 277–281

Shapiro A K, Shapiro E S, Bruun R D, Sweet R D 1978 Gilles de la Tourette syndrome. Raven Press, New York

Shapiro A K, Shapiro E, Eisenkraft G J 1983 Treatment of Gilles de la Tourette's syndrome with clonidine and neuroleptics. Arch Gen Psychiat 40: 1235–1242

Shapiro A K, Baron M, Shapiro E, Levitt M 1984 Enzyme activity in Tourette's syndrome. Arch Neurol 41: 282–285

Sharman D F 1978 Brain dopamine metabolism and behavioral problems of farm animals. In: Roberts P J et al (eds) Adv in Biochem Psychopharmacol, vol 19. Raven Press, New York, pp 249–254

Sharpe R 1974 Behavior therapy in a case of blepharospasm. Br J Psychiat 124: 603–604

Shaw K M, Hunter K R, Stern G M 1972 Medical treatment of spasmodic torticollis. Lancet 1:1399

Sheehy M P, Marsden C D 1980 Trauma and pain in spasmodic torticollis. Lancet 1: 777–778

Sheehy M P, Marsden C D 1982 Writer's cramp: A focal dystonia. Brain 105: 461–480

Shelley E, Reister A 1972 Syndrome of minimal brain damage in young adults. Dis Nerv Syst 33: 335–338

Shibasaki H, Sakai T, Nishimura H, Sato Y, Goto I, Kuroiwa Y 1982 Involuntary movements in chorea: acanthocytosis: a comparison with Huntington's chorea. Ann Neurol 12: 311–314

Shoulson I 1983 Carbidopa/levodopa therapy of coexistent drug-induced Parkinsonism and tardive dyskinesia. In: Fahn S, Calne D B, Shoulson I (eds) Experimental therapeutics of movement disorders. Adv Neurol, vol 37. Raven Press, New York, pp 259–266

Sicard J A 1923 Akathisia and Tasikinesia. Presse Méd 31: 265–266

Sicard J A, Haguenaud J 1925 Paraspasm facial bilateral. Rev Neurol 32: 228–232

Siegfried J, Crowell R, Perret E 1969 Cure of tremulous writer's cramp by stereotaxic thalamotomy: case report. J Neurosurg 30: 182–185

Sigwald J, Piot C 1953 Les dyskinésies de la langue, étude clinique de 17 cas de mouvements anormaux de la langue et des muscles peribuccaux de nature post-encephalitique. Sem Hôp 29: 373–380

Sigwald J, Grossiord A, Duriel P, Dumont G 1947 Le traitement de la maladie de Parkinson et des manifestations extra pyramidales par le diéthylaminoéthyl-n-thiodiphénylamine (2987 RP) résultats d'une année d'application. Rev Neurol 79: 683–687

Sigwald J, Bouttier D, Raymondeaud C I, Piot C R 1959a Quatre cas de dyskinésie facio-bucco-linguo-masticatrice a evolution prolongée secondaire a un traitement par les neuroleptiques. Rev Neurol 100: 751–755

Sigwald J, Bouttier D, Courvoisier S 1959b Les accidents neurologiques des médications neuroleptiques. Rev Neurol 100: 553–595

Simmons V P 1982 Writer's cramp. Lancet 2:1220

Simons R C 1980 The resolution of the latah paradox. J Nerv Ment Dis 168: 195–206

Simpson G M 1973 Tardive dyskinesia. Br J Psychiat 122:618

Simpson G M, Shrivastava R K 1978 Abnormal gaits in tardive dyskinesia. Am J Psych 135:865

Simpson G M, Branchey M H, Lee J H 1976 Lithium in tardive dyskinesia. Pharmakopsychiat Neuropsychopharmakol 9: 76–80

Singer H S, Tune L E, Butler I J, Zaczek R, Coyle J T 1982 Clinical symptomatology, CSF neurotransmitter metabolites, and serum haloperidol levels in Tourette syndrome. In: Friedhoff A J, Chase T N (eds) Gilles de la Tourette syndrome. Adv Neurol, vol 35. Raven Press, New York, pp 177–183

Singer K 1963 Gilles de la Tourette's disease. Am J Psych 120: 80–81

Singer K 1976 Gilles de la Tourette's syndrome: a report on three cases in the Chinese. In: Abuzzahab F, Anderson F (eds) Gilles de la Tourette syndrome, vol 1. Int Registry, Mason St Paul, Minnesota, pp 19–24

Skirboll L R, Bunney B S 1979 Effects of chronic haloperidol treatment of spontaneous activity in the caudate nucleus. In: Usdin E, Kopin I J, Barchas J (eds) Catecholamines: basic and clinical frontiers. Pergamon, New York, pp 634–636

Sleator E K 1980 Deleterious effects of drugs used for hyperactivity on patients with Gilles de la Tourette syndrome. Clin Paediat Phil 19: 453–454

Smith J M, Baldessarini R 1980 Changes in prevalence, severity and recovery in tardive dyskinesia with age. Arch Gen Psychiat 37: 1368–1375

Smith J M, Oswald W J, Kucharski L T, Waterman L J 1978 Tardive dyskinesia: age and sex differences in hospitalised schizophrenics. Psychopharmacology 58: 207–211

Smith M, Culpin M, Farmer J 1927 A study of telegraphist's cramp. Med Res Coun Indust Fatigue Res Bd Lond Report No 43, 1943

Smith R C, Tamminga C A, Haraszti J, Pandey G N, Davis J M 1977 Effect of dopamine agonists in tardive dyskinesia. Am J Psychiat 134: 763–768

Snyder S H 1972 Catecholamines in the brain as mediators of amphetamine psychosis. Arch Gen Psychiat 27: 169–179

Solcher H 1957 Über einen Fall von überstandener fataler Kohlenoxydvergiftung. J Hirnforsch 3: 49–55

Solly S 1864 Clinical lectures on scrivener's palsy or the paralysis of writers. Lancet 2: 709–711

Sorensen B F, Hamby W B 1965 Spasmodic torticollis results in 71 surgically treated patients. J Am Med Assoc 194: 706–708

Souques A 1908 Palilalie. Rev Neurol 16: 340–349

Sovner R, Dimascio A 1977 The effect of benztropine mesylate in the rabbit syndrome and tardive dyskinesia. Am J Psychiat 134: 1301–1302

Sovner R, Loadman A 1978 More on barbiturate and tardive dyskinesia. Am J Psychiat 135:382

Sprengler J 1489 In: Summers M (trans) Malleus maleficarum. Pushkin, London, 1948

Stahl S M 1980 Tardive Tourette syndrome in an autistic patient after long-term neuroleptic administration. Am J Psychiat 137: 1267–1269

Stahl S M, Berger P A 1980a Physostigmine in Gilles de la Tourette's syndrome. New Engl J Med 302:298

Stahl S M, Berger P A 1980b Cholinergic treatment in the Tourette syndrome. New Engl J Med 302:1311

Steck H 1954 Le syndrome extrapyramidal et diēncēphalique au cours des traitements au largactil et au serpasil. Ann Med Psychol 112: 737–743

Stejskal L, Tomanek Z 1981 Postural laterality in torticollis and torsion dystonia. J Neurol Neurosurg Psychiat 44: 1029–1034

Stengel E 1947 A clinical and psychological study of echo reactions. J Ment Sci 93: 598–612

Stern F 1936 Epidemische encephalitis. In: Bumke O, Foerster O (eds) Handbuch der Neurologie. Springer, Gottingen-Heidelberg, Bd XIII, pp 307–500

Stern T A, Anderson W H 1979 Benztropine prophylaxis of dystonic reactions. Psychopharmacology 61: 261–262

Stevens H 1964 The syndrome of Gilles de la Tourette and its treatment. Med Ann DC 33: 277–279

Stevens H 1965 Jumping Frenchmen of Maine. Arch Neurol 12: 311–314

Stevens H 1971 Gilles de la Tourette and his syndrome by serendipity. Am J Psychiat 128: 489–492

Stevens J R 1978 Disturbances of ocular movements and blinking in schizophrenia. J Neurol Neurosurg Psychiat 41: 1024–1030

Stewart M, Pitts F, Craig A, Dieruf W 1966 The hyperactive child syndrome. Am J Orthopsychiat 36: 861–867

Still G F 1909 In: Common diseases and disorders of childhood. OUP, pp 653–663

Straus E 1927a Untersuchungen über die postchoreatischen Motilitätsstörungen insbesondere über die Beziehungen der Chorea minor zum tic. Monatschr Psychiat Neurol 66: 261, 294–299

Straus E 1927b Über die organische Natur der Tics und der Koprolalie. Zbl Ges Neurol 47: 698–699

Strombom U 1977 Antagonism by haloperidol of locomotor depression induced by small doses of apomorphine. J Neural Transm 40: 191–194

Suhren O, Bruyn G W, Tuynman J A 1966 Hyperexplexia: a hereditary startle syndrome. J Neurol Sci 3: 577–605

Surwillo W W, Shafii M, Barrett C L 1978 Gilles de la Tourette syndrome: a 20 month study of the effects of stressful life events and haloperidol on symptom frequency. J Nerv Ment Dis 169: 812–816

Sutcher H D, Underwood R B, Beatty R A, Sugar O 1971 Orofacial dyskinesia: a dental dimension. J Am Med Assoc 216: 1459–1463

Sutherland R J, Kolb B, Schoel W M, Whishaw I Q, Davies D 1982 Neuropsychological assessment of children and adults with Tourette syndrome: a comparison with learning difficulties and schizophrenia. In: Friedhoff A J, Chase T N (eds) Gilles de la Tourettes syndrome. Adv Neural, vol 35. Raven Press, New York, pp 311–322

Sutula T, Hobbs W R 1983 Senile-onset vocal and motor tics. Arch Neurol 40: 825–826

Svien H J, Cody D T R 1969 Treatment of spasmodic torticollis by suppression of labyrinthine activity report of a case. Mayo Clin Proc 44: 825–827

Swash M, Roberts A H, Zakko H, Heathfield K W G 1972 Treatment of involuntary movement disorders with tetrabenazene. J Neurol Neurosurg Psychiat 35: 186–191

Sweet R D, Solomon G E, Wayne H, Shapiro E, Shapiro A K 1973 Neurological features of Gilles de la Tourette syndrome. J Neurol Neurosurg Psychiat 36: 1–9

Sweet R D, Bruun R D, Shapiro A K, Shapiro E 1976 The pharmacology of Gilles de la Tourette's syndrome (chronic multiple tic). In: Klawans H L (ed) Clin Neuropharm Raven Press, New York, pp 81–105

Swett C 1975 Drug-induced dystonia. Am J Psychiat 132: 532–534

Tailarach J, Bancaud J, Geier S, Bordas-Ferrer M, Bonis A, Szilka G et al 1973 The cingulate gyrus and human behaviour. Electroencephalogr Clin Neurophysiol 34: 45–52

Talbot J F, Gregor Z, Bird A C 1982 The surgical management of essential blepharospasm. In: Marsden C D, Fahn S (eds) In: Movement disorders. Butterworth, London, pp 322–329

Talkow J 1870 Klonische Krämpfe der augenlider: Neurotomie der Supraorbitalnerven. Klin Monatschr Augeheilk 8: 129–145

Tamminga C, Smith R, Pandey G, Frohmann L A, Davis J M A neuroendocrine study of supersentivity in tardive dyskinesia. Arch Gen Psychiat 34: 1199–1203

Tamminga C A, Thaker G K, Ferraro T N, Hare T A 1983 GABA agonist treatment improves tardive dyskinesia. Lancet 2: 97–98

Tanner, C M, Glantz R H, Klawans H L 1982a Meige disease: acute and chronic cholinergic effects. Neurology 32: 783–785

Tanner C M, Goetz C G, Klawans H L 1982b Cholinergic mechanisms in Tourette syndrome. Neurology 32: 1315–1317

Tarlov E 1969 The postural effect of lesions of the vestibular nuclei: A note on species differences among primates. J Neurosurg 31: 187–195

Tarlov E 1970 On the problem of the pathology of spasmodic torticollis in man. J Neurol Neurosurg Psychiat 33: 457–463

Tarsy D, Baldessarini R J 1974 Behavioural supersensitivity to apomorphine following chronic treatment with drugs which interfere with the synaptic function of catecholamines. Neuropharmacology 13: 927–940

Tarsy D, Sax D S, Leopold N, Feldman R G 1973 The effect of physostigmine on Huntington's chorea and L-dopa dyskinesia. In: Barbeau A, Chase T N, Paulson G W (eds) Huntington's chorea, 1872–1972. Adv Neural, vol 1. Raven Press, New York, pp 777–788

Tarsy D, Leopold N, Sax D S 1974 Physostigmine in choreiform movement disorders. Neurology 24: 28–33

Tarsy D, Parkes J D, Marsden C D 1975 Metoclopramide and pimozide in Parkinson's disease and levodopa induced dyskinesias. J Neurol Neurosurg Psychiat 38: 331–338

Tasker R R 1976 The treatment of spasmodic torticollis by peripheral denevation: the

McKensie operation. In: Morley T P (ed) Current controversies in neurosurgery. Saunders, Philadelphia, pp 443–447

Task Force on late neurological effects of antipsychotic drugs 1980 tardive dyskinesia: summary of a task force report of the American Psychiatric Association. Am J Psychiat 137: 1163–72

Tassin J P Stinus L, Simon M, Blanc G, Thierry A M, le Moal M et al 1978 Relationship between the locomotor hyperactivity induced by A10 lesions and the destruction of the fronto-cortical dopaminergic innervation in the rat. Brain Res 141: 267–281

Thomas, E J, Abrams K S, Johnson J B 1971 Self-monitoring and reciprocal inhibition in the modification of multiple tics of Gilles de la Tourette's syndrome. J Behav Ther Exp Psychiat 2: 159–171

Thompson H T, Sinclair J 1912 Telegraphist's cramp. Lancet 1: 889–890, 941–944, 1008–1010

Thompson J H 1896 A wry-necked family. Lancet 2: 24

Thorley G 1984 Hyperkinetic syndrome of childhood: clinical characteristics. Br J Psychiat 144: 16–24

Thorne F C 1944 Startle Neurosis. Am J Psychiat 101: 105–109

Thornton W E, Thornton B P 1973 Tardive dyskinesia. J Am Med Assoc 226: 674

Tibbetts R W 1971 Spasmodic Torticollis. J Psychosom Res 15: 461–469

Tierney I R, Fraser W I, McGuire R J, Walton H J 1981 Stereotyped behaviours: prevalence, function and management in mental deficiency hospitals. Health Bull 39: 320–326

Tiller J W 1978 Brief family therapy for childhood tic syndrome. Fam Process 17: 217–223

Tolosa E S 1981 Clinical features of Meige's disease (Idiopathic orofacial dystonia): A report of 17 cases. Arch Neurol 38: 147–151

Tolosa E S, Lai Chi-Wan 1979 Meige disease: striatal dopaminergic preponderance. Neurology 29: 1126–1130

Torup E 1962 A follow-up study of children with tics. Acta Paediat 51: 261–268

Traube L 1871 Spastische Form der nervüsen Heiserkeit. In: Gesammelte Beiträge zur Pathologie und Physiologie, vol 2. Hirschwald, Berlin p 677

Trillet M, Joyeux O, Masson R 1977 Tiapride et mouvements anormaux. Sem Hôp Paris 53: 21–27

Trimble M R, Perez M M, Pratt RTC 1980 Some uses of prolactin in psychiatry. In: Adv Biol Psychiat, vol 5. Karger, Basel, pp 46–57

Trousseau A 1973 Clinique médical de l'hôtel Dieu de Paris 2:267

Tuke D H 1892 A dictionary of psychological medicine, vol 1. Churchill, London

Turpin G 1983 Behavioural management of tic disorders: a critical review. In: Adv Behav Res Ther, vol.5. Pergamon, Oxford, pp 203–245

Uhrbrand L, Faurbye A 1960 Reversible and irreversible dyskinesia after treatment with perphenazine, chlorpromazine, reserpine and electroconvulsive therapy. Psychopharmacologia 1: 408–18

Ungerstedt U 1971 Postsynaptic supersensitivity after 6-hydroxydopamine induced degeneration of the nigro-striatal dopamine systems in the rat brain. Acta Physiol Scand 82 suppl 367: 69–94

Ungher J, Ciurea E, Volanschi D 1962 EEG analysis of motor neurosis in children (infantile tics). Electroencaphalogr clin neurophysiol 14:147

Van Bogaert L 1934 Ocular paroxysms and palilalia. J Nerv Ment Dis 80: 48–61

Van Bogaert L 1941 Études anatomo-cliniques de syndromes hypercinétiques complexes II un torticollis heréditaire et familial avec tremblement. Monatschr Psychiat Neurol 103: 321–342

Vance In: quoted by Gowers W R 1893 Diseases of the nervous system, vol 2. Churchill London, p 658

Van Putten T 1975 The many faces of akathisia. Compr Psychiatry 16: 43–47

Van Woert M H, Jutkowitz R, Rosenbaum D, Bowers M B 1976 Gilles de la Tourette's syndrome: biochemical approaches. In: Yahr M D (ed) The Basal Ganglia. Raven Press, New York, pp 459–466

Van Woert M H, Yip L C, Balis M E 1977 Purine phosphoribosyltransférase in Gilles de la Tourette syndrome. New Eng J Med 296: 210–212

Van Woert M H, Rosenbaum D, Enna S J 1982 Overview of pharmacological approaches to therapy for Tourette syndrome. In: Friedhoff A J, Chase T N (eds) Gilles de la Tourette syndrome. Adv Neurol, vol 35. Raven Press, New York, pp 369–375

Villeneuve A 1972 The Rabbit syndrome: a peculiar extrapyramidal reaction. Canad Psychiat Assoc J 17 suppl: 69–72

Villeneuve A, Boszormenyi Z 1970 Treatment of drug-induced dyskinesias. Lancet 1: 353–354

Viukari M, Linnoila M 1977 Effect of fusaric acid on tardive dyskinesia and mental state in psychogeriatric patients. Acta Psychiat Scand 56: 57–61

Volow M R, Cavenar J O, Grosch W N, Shipley R H, Myers M 1980 The diagnostic dilemma of blepharospasm. Am J Psychiat 137: 620–621

Von Economo C 1931 In: Newman K O (trans) Encephalitis lethargica, its sequelae and treatment. OUP, London

Walsh L S 1974 Spasmodic torticollis. J Neurol Neurosurg Psych 37: 1285–1286

Waltz J M 1982 Surgical approach to dystonia. In: Marsden C D, Fahn S (eds) Movement disorders. Butterworth, London, pp 300–307

Waserman J, Lal S, Gauthier S 1983 Gilles de la Tourettes syndrome in monozygotic twins. J Neurol Neurosurg Psychiat 46: 75–77

Wassman E R, Eldridge R, Abuzzahab F S, Nee L 1978 Gilles de la Tourette syndrome: clinical and genetic studies in a mid-western city. Neurology 28: 304–307

Weiner W J, Nausieda P A 1982 Meige's syndrome during long-term dopaminergic therapy in Parkinson's disease. Arch Neurol 39: 451–452

Weiner W J, Nausieda P A, Klawans H L 1978 Methylphenidate-induced chorea: case report and pharmacological implications. Neurology 28: 1041–1044

Weiner W J, Nausieda P A, Glantz R H 1981 Meige syndrome (blepharospasm-oromandibular dystonia) after long-term neuroleptic therapy. Neurology 31: 1555–1556

Weingarten K 1968 Tics. In: Vinken P J, Bruyn G W (eds) Handbook of clinical neurology. Diseases of the basal ganglia, vol 6. North Holland, Amsterdam, pp 782–808

Weiss B, Santelli S, Lusink G 1977 Movement disorders induced in monkeys by chronic haloperidol treatment. Psychopharmacology 53: 289–293

Weiss J L, Ng L K Y, Chase T N 1971 Long-lasting dyskinesia induced by levodopa. Lancet 1: 1016–17

Wepfer J J 1727 Observationes medico-practicae de affectibus capitis internis et externis. Scaphusii Ziegleri J A

Werry J, Minde K, Guzman A, Weiss G, Dogan K, Hoy E 1972 Studies on the hyperactive child VII. Neurological status compared with neurotic and normal children. Amer J Orthopsychiat 42: 441–450

West H H 1977 Treatment of spasmodic torticollis with amantidine: a double-blind study. Neurology 27: 198–199

Whiles W H 1940 Treatment of spasmodic torticollis by psychotherapy. Br Med J 1: 969–971

Whitty C W M, Duffield J E, Tow P M, Cairns H 1952 Anterior cingulectomy in the treatment of mental disease. Lancet 1: 475–481

Wieser S 1958 Studie zum Schreiverhalten beim Säugling und beim Kleinkind. Wien Med Wschr 50: 1105–1108

Wilder J 1946 Pancreo-pituitary hypoglycaemia. Confin Neurol 7: 96–112

Wilder J, Silbermann J 1927 Beitrage zum Tic-problem. In: Abhandlungen aus der Neurologie, Psychiatrie, Psychologie, und ihren Grenzgebieten. Karger, Berlin

Willerman L 1973 Activity level and hyperactivity in twins. Child Dev 44: 288–293

Wilson R S, Garron D C, Klawans H L 1978 Significance of genetic factors in Gilles de la Tourette syndrome: a review. Behav Gen 8: 503–510

Wilson R S, Garron D C, Tanner C M, Klawans H L 1982 Behaviour disturbance in children with Tourette syndrome. In: Friedhoff A J, Chase T N (eds) Gilles de la Tourette syndrome. Adv Neurol, vol 35. Raven Press New York, pp 329–334

Wilson S A K 1927 The tics and allied conditions. J Neurol Psychopath 8: 93–109

Wimmer A 1929 Le spasme de torsion. Rev Neurol 1: 904–915

Winkelman N W 1961 The inter-relationship between the physiological and psychological etiologies of akathisia. Rev Canad Biol 20: 659–664

Winnicott D W 1931 Fidgetiness. In: Clinical notes on disorders of childhood. Heinemann, London, p 654

Wohlfart G, Ingvar D H, Hellberg A-M 1961 Compulsory shouting (Benedeks klazomania) associated with oculogyric spasms in chronic epidemic encephalitis. Acta Psychiat Scand 36: 369–377

Wolf S M 1973 Reserpine: cause and treatment of oral-facial dyskinesia. Bull Los Angeles Neurol Soc 38: 80–84

Wolff H, Hurwitz I 1966 The choreiform syndrome. Dev Med Child Neurol 48: 160–165

Yahr M D 1970 Clinical aspects of abnormal movements induced by L-dopa. In: Barbeau A, McDowell F H (eds) L-dopa and Parkinsonism. Davis, Philadelphia, pp 101–108

Yankovsky 1885 Miryatschenye, miryachit, meryajet. Vratch 6:602

Yap P M 1952 The latah reaction: its pathodynamics and nosological position. J Ment Sci 98: 515–564

Yarden P E, Discipio W J 1971 Abnormal movements and prognosis in schizophrenia. Am J Psychiat 128: 317–323

Yates A 1958 The application of learning theory to the treatment of tics. J Abnorm Soc Psychol 56: 175–182

Zarcone V, Thorpe B, Dement W 1972 Sleep parameters in two patients with Gilles de la Tourette's syndrome. Sleep Res 1: 155–157

Zausmer D M 1954 Treatment of tics in childhood. Arch Dis Child 29: 537–542

Zeman W, Kaebling R, Pasaminick B 1960 Idiopathic dystonia musculorum deformans II the formes frustes. Neurology 10: 1068–1075

Index

acanthocytosis and neurological disease, *see* neuro-acanthocytosis
aerophagy, 107–108
akathisia, 185–191
  clinical description, 187–189
  course, 189
  differential diagnosis, 189–190
  epidemiology, 185–186
  pathophysiology, 186–187
  treatment, 190–191
ambitendencies, 124
anticholinergics
  in acute neuroleptic-induced dyskinesias, 184
  in akathisia, 190–191
  in Meige syndrome, 152–153
  in spasmodic torticollis, 138
arithomania, 11
attention deficit disorder, 97; *see* hyperactivity syndrome
automatic obedience
  in latah, 85–86
  in schizophrenia, 122

Barking girls of Blackthorn, 22
biting nail, *see* nail-biting
blepharospasm, *see* Meige syndrome
blind
  disorders of movement associated with the, 109–116
blocking, 124
body rocking, 114–115
Brissaud's muscular drill, 20
broad bean, 221
Brueghel's syndrome, *see* Meige syndrome

cataplexy, 96
catatonia, 117
cholinergic drugs

in Gilles de la Tourette syndrome 49
in tardive dyskinesias, 208–209
chorea
  acanthocytosis and, *see* neuro-acanthocytosis
  definition, 5
  Dubini's electric, 1
  electrophysiology, 4
  habit, *see* tic idiopathic
  Huntington's, *see* Huntington's disease
  1-dopa-induced, 227–228, 229–230
  pseudo, *see* tic idiopathic
  psychomotor stimulant-induced, 217–218
  Sydenham's *see* Sydenham's chorea
  variable of Brissaud, 1; *see* Gilles de la Tourette syndrome
choreo-acanthocytosis, *see* neuro-acanthocytosis
Condé, Prince. 23
coprolalia
  in Gilles de la Tourette syndrome, 33–34, 37–39
  in schizophrenia, 123
copropraxia, 39
cortex anterior cingulate, 32–33
cowhage, 221
cramp, writers, *see* dystonia, writers

Dampierre, Marquise de, 23
dart players' dystonia, 169–170
dopa, 220–222
dopamine, 8, 172–173, 175
  220–222
  abnormalities in acute neuroleptic-induced dyskinesias, 180
  abnormalities in akathisia, 187
  abnormalities in animals, 11
  abnormalities in l-dopa-induced dyskinesias, 225–227

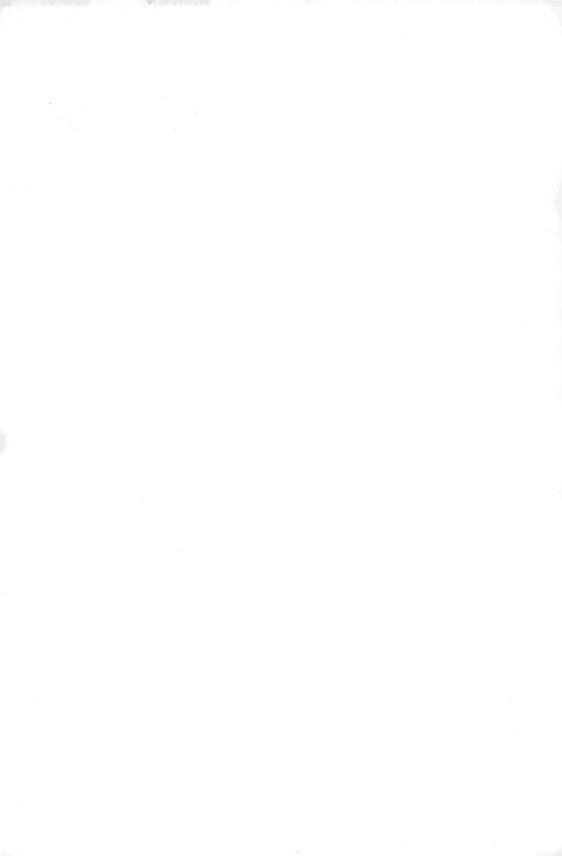